# Hybrid Data Processing by Combining Machine Learning, Expert, Safety and Security

# Hybrid Data Processing by Combining Machine Learning, Expert, Safety and Security

Guest Editors

**Zhiming Cai**
**Wencai Du**
**Zhihai Wang**
**Zuobin Ying**

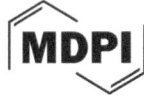

Basel • Beijing • Wuhan • Barcelona • Belgrade • Novi Sad • Cluj • Manchester

*Guest Editors*

Zhiming Cai
Faculty of Digital Science and
Technology
Macau Millennium College
Macau
China

Wencai Du
Institute for Data Engineering
and Sciences
University of Saint Joseph
Macau
China

Zhihai Wang
School of Computer &
Information Technology
Beijing Jiaotong University
Beijing
China

Zuobin Ying
Faculty of Data Science
City University of Macau
Macau
China

*Editorial Office*
MDPI AG
Grosspeteranlage 5
4052 Basel, Switzerland

This is a reprint of the Special Issue, published open access by the journal *Mathematics* (ISSN 2227-7390), freely accessible at: https://www.mdpi.com/si/mathematics/2H222N4970.

For citation purposes, cite each article independently as indicated on the article page online and as indicated below:

Lastname, A.A.; Lastname, B.B. Article Title. *Journal Name* **Year**, *Volume Number*, Page Range.

ISBN 978-3-7258-3545-4 (Hbk)
ISBN 978-3-7258-3546-1 (PDF)
https://doi.org/10.3390/books978-3-7258-3546-1

© 2025 by the authors. Articles in this book are Open Access and distributed under the Creative Commons Attribution (CC BY) license. The book as a whole is distributed by MDPI under the terms and conditions of the Creative Commons Attribution-NonCommercial-NoDerivs (CC BY-NC-ND) license (https://creativecommons.org/licenses/by-nc-nd/4.0/).

# Contents

**About the Editors** . . . . . . . . . . . . . . . . . . . . . . . . . . . . . . . . . . . . . . . . . . . . . . . . . . . . . . . . . . . . . . . . vii

**Yichuan Wang, Junxia Ding, Tong Zhang, Yeqiu Xiao and Xinhong Hei**
From Replay to Regeneration: Recovery of UDP Flood Network Attack Scenario Based on SDN
Reprinted from: *Mathematics* 2023, *11*, 1897, https://doi.org/10.3390/math11081897 . . . . . . . 1

**Zefeng Zhao, Haohao Cai, Huawei Ma, Shujie Zou and Chiawei Chu**
Optimal Multi-Attribute Auctions Based on Multi-Scale Loss Network
Reprinted from: *Mathematics* 2023, *11*, 3240, https://doi.org/10.3390/math11143240 . . . . . . . 23

**Xuefei Huang, Ka-Hou Chan, Wei Ke and Hao Sheng**
Parallel Dense Video Caption Generation with Multi-Modal Features
Reprinted from: *Mathematics* 2023, *11*, 3685, https://doi.org/10.3390/math11173685 . . . . . . . 34

**Linkai Zhu, Shanwen Hu, Xiaolian Zhu, Changpu Meng and Maoyi Huang**
Enhancing the Security and Privacy in the IoT Supply Chain Using Blockchain and Federated Learning with Trusted Execution Environment
Reprinted from: *Mathematics* 2023, *11*, 3759, https://doi.org/10.3390/math11173759 . . . . . . . 50

**Shujie Zou, Chiawei Chu, Ning Shen and Jia Ren**
Healthcare Cost Prediction Based on Hybrid Machine Learning Algorithms
Reprinted from: *Mathematics* 2023, *11*, 4778, https://doi.org/10.3390/math11234778 . . . . . . . 69

**Shujie Zou, Chiawei Chu, Weijun Dai, Ning Shen, Jia Ren and Weiping Ding**
Predicting Typhoon Flood in Macau Using Dynamic Gaussian Bayesian Network and Surface Confluence Analysis
Reprinted from: *Mathematics* 2024, *12*, 340, https://doi.org/10.3390/math12020340 . . . . . . . 82

**Han Ma, Baoyu Fan, Benjamin K. Ng, and Chan-Tong Lam**
CLG: Contrastive Label Generation with Knowledge for Few-Shot Learning
Reprinted from: *Mathematics* 2024, *12*, 472, https://doi.org/10.3390/math12030472 . . . . . . . 102

**Yuxiang He, Baisong Yang and Chiawei Chu**
GA-CatBoost-Weight Algorithm for Predicting Casualties in Terrorist Attacks: Addressing Data Imbalance and Enhancing Performance
Reprinted from: *Mathematics* 2024, *12*, 818, https://doi.org/10.3390/math12060818 . . . . . . . 123

**Zhihua Duan, Chun Wang and Wending Zhong**
SSGCL: Simple Social Recommendation with Graph Contrastive Learning
Reprinted from: *Mathematics* 2024, *12*, 1107, https://doi.org/10.3390/math12071107 . . . . . . . 136

**Yungui Chen, Li Feng, Qinglin Zhao, Liwei Tian and Lei Yang**
ARS-Chain: A Blockchain-Based Anonymous Reputation-Sharing Framework for E-Commerce Platforms
Reprinted from: *Mathematics* 2024, *12*, 1480, https://doi.org/10.3390/math12101480 . . . . . . . 156

# About the Editors

**Zhiming Cai**

   Prof. Zhiming Cai holds a bachelor's degree, master's degree, and doctoral degree in Computer Science from Hefei University of Technology, China, and is a postdoctoral fellow in Computer Science at the University of Toronto, Canada. He has worked as a teaching assistant, research associate, lecturer, associate professor, professor, and doctoral supervisor at Hefei University of Technology in China, University of Stuttgart in Germany, University of Toronto in Canada, Macao University of Science and Technology, and City University of Macau. He successively served as the deputy director of the institute of software, deputy director of the computer science department, deputy dean of the computer science school, director of the data science research center, director of the academic affairs office, and dean of the graduate school. Currently, he is a member of the Trust Committee of the Macao Science and Technology Development Fund, a member of the board of directors and the Vice President of Macau Millennium College, the President of the Macao Satellite Navigation Application Association, and the Chairman of the Macao Software Industry Association. He has been engaged in teaching and research in software engineering, operating systems, cross-border data, and system modeling for many years. He has led more than 20 scientific research projects such as the National Natural Science Foundation and the National Key Research and Development Plan, published seven books, and published more than 120 papers, of which more than 60 are SCI-indexed.

**Wencai Du**

   Professor Wencai Du is Dean of the Institute for Data Engineering and Sciences at the University of Saint Joseph, Macau. He earned his bachelor's degree in Geodynamics from Peking University and two master's degrees in Computer Sciences from Hohai University and Twente University, the Netherlands. He earned his Ph.D. in Informatics from Adelaide University and conducted postdoctoral research in Computer Science at the Israel Institute of Technology. He was Chair Professor of the Faculty of Data Sciences at the City University of Macau. Du served as Dean of the College of Information Science and Technology at Hainan University, as well as serving as Director of the Hainan Province Research Center for Ocean Communication and Network Engineering. His main research areas include computer sciences, communication and information systems, data sciences, and artificial intelligence; recently, he has taken a particular interest in social media sentiment analysis, machine learning, smart elderly care, and data analytics. He has published over 200 papers in national and international journals and international conference proceedings, 20 books, and six book chapters, and he has earned one international invention patent and fifteen national invention patents.

**Zhihai Wang**

   Dr. Zhihai Wang is a professor at the Institute of Cloud Computing and Data Science and the chair professor of Computer Majors at the School of Computer Science and Technology, Beijing Jiaotong University, China. He earned his bachelor's degree in Computer Science from Zhengzhou University, a master's degree in Computer Application from Harbin Institute of Shipbuilding Engineering, and a doctoral degree in Computer Application from Hefei University of Technology. He conducted postdoctoral research in machine learning and data mining at the School of Computer Science and Software Engineering at Monash University, Melbourne, Australia. He has also conducted research as research fellow in the School of Information Technology, Deakin University,

Geelong, Australia, as a visiting scientist in Fourier University in Grenoble, France, and at Lancaster University, Lancaster, the UK, respectively. His main research interests include machine learning and data mining, data science and technology, data warehouses and data security, and artificial intelligence and its applications. He has published over 50 research papers in reputable international journals and conference proceedings, which have mainly focused on the shapelet representation of time series and related classification learning models, the multispectral image information composite method for sparse feature identification in crop diseases, and data-flow learning technology.

**Zuobin Ying**

Dr. Zuobin Ying is an associate professor in the School of Data Science at City University of Macau. Dr. Ying graduated from Xidian University and conducted postdoctoral research at Nanyang Technological University in Singapore. He currently serves as the Director of the Doctoral Program, the Chair of the Membership Development Committee of IEEE MACAU, a Member of the Blockchain Committee of the China Society for Industrial and Applied Mathematics, a Member of the Life and Biotechnology Committee of the Guangdong–Hong Kong–Macao Greater Bay Area Standardization Innovation Alliance, and a Guangdong Provincial Entrepreneurship Mentor. Dr. Ying has specialized in research in information security, blockchain applications, and privacy computing. He has led and participated in more than 10 national- and provincial-level research projects, published over 90 academic papers, and holds two authorized patents. Dr. Ying also serves as the Technical Program Committee Co-chair for international conferences such as IEEE ICBD and EAI MobiMedia and is a reviewer for SCI journals including *IEEE TVT*, *IEEE TNSE*, *IEEE TII*, and *IEEE IoTJ*. He has guided university students in multiple innovation and entrepreneurship projects and research competition projects that have received awards.

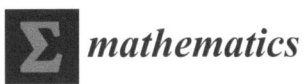 

Article

# From Replay to Regeneration: Recovery of UDP Flood Network Attack Scenario Based on SDN

Yichuan Wang [1,2], Junxia Ding [1], Tong Zhang [1,*], Yeqiu Xiao [1] and Xinhong Hei [1,2]

[1] School of Computer Science and Engineering, Xi'an University of Technology, Xi'an 710048, China; chuan@xaut.edu.cn (Y.W.); dingjunxia@stu.xaut.edu.cn (J.D.); xiaoyeqiu@xaut.edu.cn (Y.X.); heixinhong@xaut.edu.cn (X.H.)
[2] Shaanxi Key Laboratory for Network Computing and Security Technology, Xi'an 710048, China
* Correspondence: zhangtong@xaut.edu.cn; Tel.: +86-139-9186-3253

**Abstract:** In recent years, various network attacks have emerged. These attacks are often recorded in the form of Pcap data, which contains many attack details and characteristics that cannot be analyzed through traditional methods alone. Therefore, restoring the network attack scenario through scene reconstruction to achieve data regeneration has become an important entry point for detecting and defending against network attacks. However, current network attack scenarios mainly reproduce the attacker's attack steps by building a sequence collection of attack scenarios, constructing an attack behavior diagram, or simply replaying the captured network traffic. These methods still have shortcomings in terms of traffic regeneration. To address this limitation, this paper proposes an SDN-based network attack scenario recovery method. By parsing Pcap data and utilizing network topology reconstruction, probability, and packet sequence models, network traffic data can be regenerated. The experimental results show that the proposed method is closer to the real network, with a higher similarity between the reconstructed and actual attack scenarios. Additionally, this method allows for adjusting the intensity of the network attack and the generated topology nodes, which helps network defenders better understand the attackers' posture and analyze and formulate corresponding security strategies.

**Keywords:** SDN; network attack; scenario reconfiguration; probabilistic model; topology reconfiguration model

**MSC:** 68M25

## 1. Introduction

With the rapid development of computer networks and internet technologies, networks have permeated into various fields, facing increasingly complex security challenges. Network attacks are often recorded in the form of Pcap data, which contains numerous attack details and features. Traditional data processing methods often overlook many attack behavior features, leading to resource waste. Therefore, this paper proposes an SDN-based UDP flood network attack scene reconstruction method. By reconstructing network attack scenarios, the original data can be restored, and new mixed data can be generated by adjusting the intensity of network attacks, topology nodes, and other types of network attacks. This enables network defenders to better understand the attacker's posture, analyze the monitored data and information, and formulate corresponding security strategies to enhance their ability to respond to network attacks.

Due to the openness of the internet, the inherent imperfections of network protocols, and various application software, devices on the network are vulnerable to potential danger. Nowadays, the UDP protocol is widely used in networks and various applications. However, a network utilizing the UDP protocol is easily targeted in attacks since the sender does not need to establish a connection via three handshakes, while the receiver

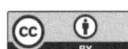

has to receive and process the packet. Therefore, it is crucial to protect the network from attacks exploiting the vulnerabilities of the UDP protocol. UDP flood is one of the most common attacks targeting the UDP protocol, which typically targets DNS servers, RADIUS authentication servers, or streaming video servers by flooding them with a large number of small UDP packets [1–3]. Such attacks are often directed towards a random port on the target, and the victim system must analyze the incoming data to determine which application service has requested it. This makes it difficult for defenders to protect the network from such attacks. In fact, a dynamic game process occurs between attackers and defenders, where defenders develop corresponding security strategies in response to changes in attackers' techniques, while attackers constantly research new techniques to evade network security protection and achieve their attack objectives. Timely detection of potential security threats to the network is crucial for defenders. Therefore, this article proposes a network attack scene reconstruction method, which lays a solid foundation for defending against network attacks from the attacker's perspective. To achieve better results in network attack scene reconstruction, this article suggests using software-defined networking (SDN) for scene reconstruction.

SDN offers dynamic programmable network configuration, which improves network performance and management efficiency, and enables network services to provide flexible customization capabilities similar to those of cloud computing. In addition, SDN decouples the forwarding plane of network devices from the control plane, enabling the controller to manage network devices, orchestrate network services, and schedule service traffic [4]. SDN overcomes the limitations of traditional networks and offers benefits such as low cost, centralized management, and flexible scheduling [5]. In SDN testing, Mininet is commonly used as a testbed as it enables easy creation of an SDN-enabled network, with each host working like a real computer. Programs can launch applications and send packets to the Ethernet ports, which are received and processed by switches and routers. SDN also supports complex network topologies, allowing the addition of new features to the network, testing, and easy deployment into real hardware environments [6]. Therefore, SDN-based attack recovery can provide a realistic scenario for a network that is under attack.

In response to the challenge of lacking the reconstruction of traffic rebirth and elasticity in existing network attack scene reconstruction, this paper proposes an SDN-based UDP flood network attack scene reconstruction method. This method can automatically create network topology and regenerate network traffic using sample Pcap packets. Additionally, this solution allows users to modify any component in the virtual network and adjust the network attack-related parameters and intensity to meet the needs of different scenarios. The main contributions of this paper are threefold:

- Existing approaches to network attack scenario recovery lack the ability to regenerate real network attack traffic, and the research in this paper is one of the first articles to fill this gap.
- The method proposed in this paper can automate the network attack scenario recovery, it is studied for packet delivery probability events, and it can simulate network attack scenarios more realistically.
- This paper can change the network topology nodes and network attack intensity based on the network attack scenario recovery, which can bring convenience to the network attack defenders to better detect and defend against malicious attacks.

The remainder of this paper is structured as follows. Section 2 provides an introduction to the definition of SDN and related research. Section 3 presents the SDN-based topology reconfiguration model for network attack scenarios and the reconfiguration probability model. Section 4 analyzes the constructed models, while Section 5 offers a comparative analysis of the experiments from both qualitative and quantitative perspectives. Finally, Section 6 concludes our work.

## 2. Related Work

Regarding the problem of network attack scene recovery, we have reviewed the relevant literature from the past 5 years and broadly divided network attack scene recovery methods into four main types. The first type is network attack scene recovery based on traffic replay. The second type involves using graph networks for network attack scene recovery. The third type uses correlation analysis for network attack scene recovery. The fourth type encompasses other methods for network attack scene recovery. Details on each category are provided below:

(1) Network attack scene recovery method based on traffic replay.

A multi-node traffic replay method was proposed by [7]. This method designs a self-selected IP mapping algorithm to construct an IP mapping between the target network and the existing network in order to reproduce the interaction between the existing network nodes. The method is effective in aggregating large flows and achieving high similarity in playback timing sequences and bandwidth and can be used to reproduce real network scenarios for network device testing and network security experiments.

A deterministic TCP replay method for performance diagnosis was proposed by [8]. This method can faithfully replay packet traces using a low-overhead timer and an efficient file access method, capturing all interactive traffic in TCP connections for all hosts and replaying selected packets to reproduce performance issues at low overhead. However, these methods can only fully reproduce the last attack and do not account for weak points, reinforcement points, or chain events. In contrast, the network attack scenario reproduction method presented in this paper can automatically create the network topology and execute the attack based on the Pcap packets, allowing for manual addition of devices such as hosts and attack relationships between devices as needed.

A virtual network traffic replay method built on a network simulation platform was proposed by [9]. This method is capable of performing IP mapping-based virtual node replay of any traffic captured or generated by one or more interfaces. However, it is unable to simulate changes in attack strength based on the original data.

A precise traffic replay method based on interaction sequences and timestamps was proposed by [10]. The method achieves high consistency in playback time, but does not regenerate the data, rather it simply replays the network traffic at the recorded time.

(2) Network attack scene recovery based on graph networks.

The graph-based fusion module (GM) to fuse all captured attack information to reconstruct a multi-step attack scenario approach was proposed by [11]. The approach uses a weighted directed graph to model the network communication and a fusion algorithm to update it. The weighted directed graph with attributes is then used to fuse the attack information and reconstruct the attack scenario. However, some manual processing is still required to reconstruct the attack scenario when dealing with fake IP addresses.

The use of graph theory to construct a system connection matrix and network path function for forming a network topology model was proposed by [12]. The method analyzed its practicality in optimal routing design and verified the feasibility of the model step by step based on its structural characteristics, laying the foundation for modeling and simulating tactical communication systems. However, further verification is needed to ensure its conformity with the characteristics of the network topology.

A reconstruction method for a big data-based attack scenario was proposed by [13], which utilizes temporal concept maps and neural networks. This method allows the reconstruction of complex attack scenarios based on large amounts of data. In addition to tracing the entire attack scenario, a temporal concept graph is used to represent the big data and the dependencies between them. The model is able to classify possible attack scenarios in real time using RBF networks and converge to the most potential attack scenarios with the support of Elman networks. However, the processing of the proposed model is initiated based on the collection of event sets generated by traditional intrusion detection systems. These systems may not be suitable to represent alerts in big data environments.

A real-time mining method for reconstructing multi-step attack scenarios was proposed by [14]. This method constructs a directed graph through association analysis by analyzing the alarm logs from intrusion detection systems to achieve the construction of attack trees. This method can combine attack patterns between different hosts and reduce false alarms. However, this method only provides an abstract description of the attack process to achieve scenario reconstruction, and does not build network topology structures and regenerate traffic. In contrast, this paper analyzes Pcap data packets and reconstructs attack scenarios by creating network topology and regenerating traffic based on the analysis results. Moreover, this method can transform the original scenario based on the reproduction.

(3) Network attack scene recovery based on correlation analysis.

A attack scenario reconstruction method based on causal knowledge and spatio-temporal correlation has been proposed by [15]. This method utilizes a causal knowledge network to conduct correlation analysis on alerts from multiple dimensions including causality, time and space, in order to restore the complete attack penetration process of the attacker and reconstruct the attack scene. This method can discover potential hidden relationships to a certain extent, but it does not regenerate network attack traffic.

A method of reconstructing attack scenarios based on association analysis was proposed by [16]. It emphasizes the temporal relationship between alerts from a holistic perspective of the network and associates aggregated alerts to build the attack scenario. This method can restore attack relationships to a certain extent but does not reproduce network attack traffic.

(4) Other methods for network attack scene recovery.

An efficient reconstruction method for advanced persistent threat (APT) attacks based on the hidden Markov model was proposed by [17]. This method describes the action sequence based on the temporal order or the conditions reached by the attack, uses data association and advanced probabilistic methods to mine the hidden APT attack phases, and finally reconstructs the attack path. However, it only provides the network attack paths and does not create any network topology.

A RouteNet model was proposed by [18]. This is a novel network model based on SDN's graph neural network (GNN). This model can accurately estimate the delay distribution and packet loss per source/destination by understanding the complex relationships between topology, routing, and incoming traffic.

A network attack probability analysis method was proposed by [19]. The model takes into account the severity of vulnerabilities, attack scenarios, and various potential participants and their motives. Based on the results obtained from the model, the most likely attack scenarios are further inferred.

SDN has been applied to combat DDoS attacks since it has logically centralized control, network programmability, and separation of control and forwarding. Reference [20] proposes a real-time DDoS detection attack method for SDN controllers. Reference [21] analyzes simulated DDoS attacks in an SDN environment. Reference [22] present a flexible SDN-based architecture, which identifies and mitigates low-rate DDoS attacks via machine learning. Although the aforementioned works show that SDN is available for the analysis of network attacks, SDN has not been fully applied to defend networks against UDP flood. Therefore, we will reconstruct UDP flood scenario with the aid of SDN in this paper.

In conclusion, the network attack scenario recovery method based on traffic replay can replay existing traffic, but it cannot generate new traffic or change network topology configuration, structure, or enhance/reduce network attack intensity. The graph-based network attack scenario recovery method can display the attack relationship of the network in a graph to some extent and restore the attack relationship, but it does not reproduce traffic. The correlation-based network attack scenario recovery method can discover potential hidden relationships to some extent but also does not reproduce traffic. Other methods for recovering network attack scenarios focus only on recovering some scenarios in the attack path, relationship, or steps without reproducing traffic. Therefore, this article proposes an SDN-based UDP flood network attack scenario recovery method, which can reconstruct the topology, reproduce traffic, scale network attack intensity, and change experimental topology in the recovered scenario.

## 3. Models

In this section, a topology reconstruction model, a probabilistic model, and an attack sequence model are established regarding the process of reconstructing a network attack scenario. The network attack scenario topology reconstruction model enables the creation of a topology that accurately and meaningfully reflects the true network topology as far as possible based on the available information. The probabilistic model and the attack sequence model are used to generate network attack commands for all events (including small sample events) to the greatest extent possible. The end result is that the regenerated data are highly similar to the sample data.

*3.1. Network Attack Scenario Topology Reconfiguration*

Due to the flexibility and programmability of SDN networks, this paper uses SDN networks for topology creation. The SDN network topology is created mainly through the Mininet platform, and the network devices are mainly selected from remote controllers, OpenFlow switches, hosts, etc. The network topology reconstruction model integrates SDN connection line attributes into the Waxman model and uses information such as IP addresses and MAC addresses from Pcap packets to configure the network. The goal is to create a topology structure that is as accurate and meaningful as possible in order to reflect the real network topology. According to the rules of network topology building, this paper abstracts the process of building network topology and forms a reconfiguration model of network attack scenarios. To better illustrate this, the following definitions are provided.

**Definition 1.** *The connection line attribute between nodes. A connection line attribute is an n-tuple $(b_1, b_2, b_3, \ldots, b_n)$, where $b_j$ $(1 \leq j \leq n)$ denotes the jth attribute of the connection line between nodes and the connection line attribute $q = (b_1, b_2, b_3, \ldots, b_n)$ between nodes of the network.*

In this paper, the connection line property between nodes is defined as a 5-tuple, $q_j = (bandwidth, delay, loss, max\ queue\ size, jitter)$. Where *bandwidth* refers to the transmission speed of the link that connects two nodes in the network topology, expressed in Mbps (megabits per second), with a default value of 10. The *"delay"* parameter represents the delay of a link in the network topology, which is the time it takes for a packet to travel from one host to another. This delay includes not only physical delay but also other factors such as buffering, queuing, and transmission delays, and is measured in milliseconds (ms). The default value is 0. The *"loss"* parameter represents the packet loss rate of the network link, which refers to the proportion of lost packets during data transmission. This parameter is often used to simulate noise, interference, and other situations in the network to more realistically simulate the network environment. The value range is from 0 to 1, with a default of 0. The *"max queue size"* parameter refers to the maximum length of the queue on a network link, which is used to control the number of packets on the link and prevent network congestion. When a packet arrives at a link, if the queue is already full, packet loss may occur. Therefore, setting an appropriate queue length is crucial for controlling network congestion and reducing packet loss. The unit is in packets and the default value is infinite. *"Jitter"* refers to the variation in delay between adjacent data packets. Normally, data packets arrive at the receiving end at regular intervals, but congestion and packet loss in the network can cause fluctuations in packet delay. Generally speaking, the smaller the jitter, the more stable the network transmission, and the larger the jitter, the less stable the network transmission. The unit is milliseconds and the default value is 0.

The construction of the network topology in this paper is based on the Waxman model, which has a core idea: all nodes are randomly (or according to the heavy-tailed distribution) placed in a plane; considering each pair of nodes, an edge is added between the node pairs $(u, v)$ with a certain probability $P(u, v)$ (also called edge probability). The Waxman model is a static model that can only simulate the number of nodes, edges, and distances between nodes in network topology. However, since network topology models are merely simulations of real network topology structures, a simplistic and fixed model cannot effectively simulate a real network as the network evolves and QoS requirements arise. Therefore, the Waxman model serves only as a reference for topology research and needs to add connection attributes, such as bandwidth, latency, cost, and packet loss rate (QoS parameters), on existing connections to better simulate a real network. Thus, improvements need to be made to the Waxman model.

According to the improved Waxman model proposed in this paper, the attribute of connecting lines between nodes of 5-tuples will be added, and the distance between any two node functions will be taken as the independent variable to calculate the probability of direct connection between two nodes. The probability function of the model is given by

$$P(u,v) = \alpha e^{-\frac{d}{L\beta}}, \tag{1}$$

where $\alpha \geq 0$, $\beta \leq 1$; $d$ is the European distance from $u$ to $v$; $L$ is the longest distance between two points. When increasing $\alpha$, the model will have more short edges, longer hop diameter and shorter length diameter. Increasing $\beta$ will increase the proportion of long edges in the model.

### 3.2. Reconstructing Probabilistic Models for Network Attack Scenarios

During the process of traffic regeneration, there are many uncertain and complex factors in the network. Introducing probability models can reduce the difficulty of traffic regeneration to some extent, decrease errors, and improve the effectiveness of traffic regeneration.

In the network attack scenario reconstruction probability model, this paper divides the behavior of each host sending packets into three categories: not sending packets, sending packets in the form of forged IPs, and sending packets with the real IPs of hosts. If there are n hosts, the probability of not sending packets from host $i$ to host $j$ (where $i$ denotes the number of the host sending packets, $j$ denotes the number of the host receiving packets, and all host numbers are unique) is $P_{ij}^1$, the probability of sending packets in the form of forged IP is $P_{ij}^2$, and the probability of sending packets with the real IP of the host probability is $P_{ij}^3$, where $P_{ij}{}^1 + P_{ij}{}^2 + P_{ij}{}^3 = 1$, but in a network attack, $P_{ij}^3$ is almost 0. In particular, for small sample events, $0 < P_{ij}{}^2 \ll P_{ij}{}^1 < 1$. According to the network scenario reconstruction probability rules proposed in this paper, the network attack sequence scenario reconstruction probability model is shown in Figure 1, where the ... in the figure indicates the label of the host.

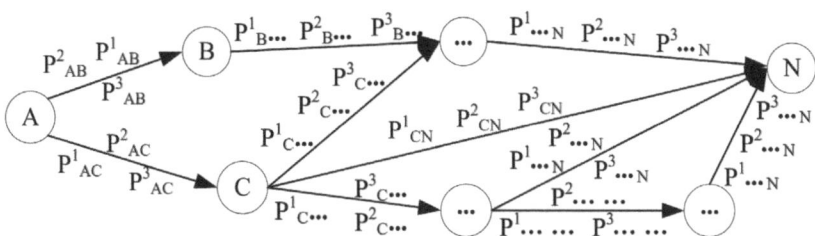

**Figure 1.** Host Probability Distribution Chart.

Additionally, for $P_{ij}^2$, there is a different case for host $i$. That is, when host $i$ sends packets by forging a different IP address or forging a different port, etc., it is considered to be a different action. This paper gives the different actions statistics of their probability of occurrence. These different actions constitute probabilities satisfying $P_{ij}{}^2 = P_{ij}{}^{21} + P_{ij}{}^{22} + \ldots + P_{ij}{}^{2n}$, where $P_{ij}{}^{2k}(1 \leq k \leq n)$ is a certain action of this host, $n$ means that there are n actions in this host, but the value of $n$ may be different for different hosts. The action probability distribution diagram of a host sending packets is shown in Figure 2.

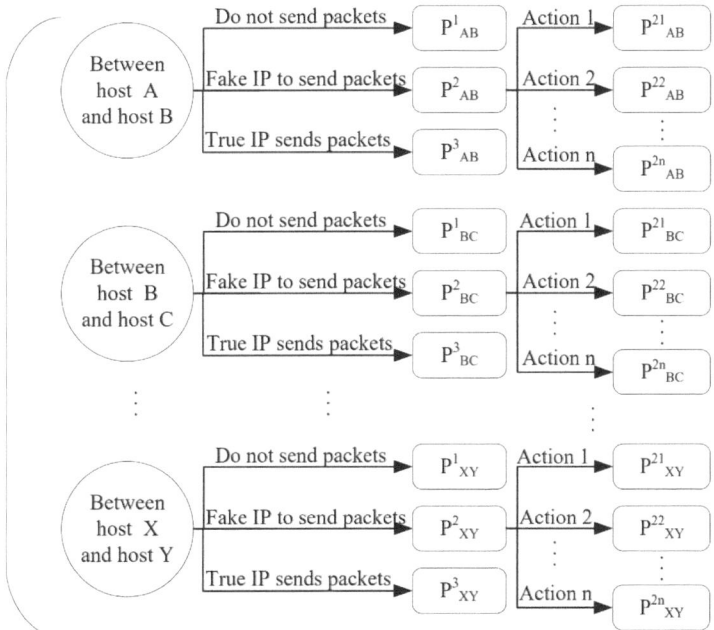

**Figure 2.** Probability diagram of contracting action event.

*3.3. Network Attack Relationship Sequence Generation*

A key point of network attack scene reconstruction is to build a set of action event attack relationship sequences, that is, from the set of action events (set if action events, $SAE$) to find all the highly relevant attack relationship sequences, constituting a set of attack scene sequence (set of attack scene sequence, $SASS$).

From the characteristics of network attacks, it is known that there are different network attack actions in network attacks. Each action has a purpose to reach the destination address of that attack, and these different action behaviors can be reflected by the preprocessing of Pcap packets. In order to get the attack corresponding attack commands from the preprocessing of Pcap packets, this paper first preprocesses the original Pcap packets, standardizes the format of the packets, and classifies and converts the data into a collection of data containing the network attack relationships. To better illustrate the content of this paper, the following definitions are given.

**Definition 2.** *Action events. An action event is an n-tuple $(c_1, c_2, c_3, \ldots, c_n)$, where $c_i(1 \leq i \leq n)$ denotes the ith attribute of the action event, and note that the action event $P = (c_1, c_2, c_3, \ldots, c_n)$.*

**Definition 3.** *Network attack relationship sequence. A set of strongly consistent action events in chronological order is called a network attack relationship sequence, denoted as $NARS$. $NARS =< e_1, e_2, e_3, \ldots, e_n >$, satisfies $e_i.timestamp < e_j.timestamp(1 \leq i < j \leq n)$ &&$e_i.srcMAC == e_j.srcMAC$&&$e_i.dstMAC == e_j.dstMAC$.*

In this paper, the action event is designed as an 8-tuple, $P_i = (timeline, srcIP, dstIP, srcMAC, dstMAC, dType, srcPort, dstPort)$. where $timeline$ denotes the timestamp of the action event; $srcIP$ and $dstIP$ denote the source and destination IP addresses of the action event, respectively; $srcMAC$ and $dstMAC$ denote the source and destination MAC addresses of the action event, respectively; $dType$ denotes the type of the attack; $srcPort$ and $dstPort$ denote the source and destination ports of the action, respectively.

The network attack relationship sequence is crucial for the reproduction of network attacks through which the attack relationship between hosts can be known and form cyber attack orders. The core of the algorithm: First, the MAC address pairs of action events are extracted through the algorithm. Then, according to the association relationship between address pairs, it iteratively judges whether the current action event belongs to a certain type of existing action event collection. If it exists, it will be directly placed in the appropriate location of the current action event collection. If it does not exist, it will create a new action event collection to place it. After all the action events are placed in the appropriate positions of the action event sets of different categories, all the action event sets have been orderly, all the action event sets are attack relationship sequences at the same time, thus finally completing the construction of network attack relationship sequence sets. The network attack relationship sequence construction algorithm is presented as Algorithm 1.

---

**Algorithm 1:** Constructing Network Attack Relationship Sequence Sets ($CNARS$) based on Action Event Sets ($SAE$)

**Input:** Collection of action events $SAE = \{e_1, e_2, \ldots, e_n\}$
**Output:** A collection of cyber attack relationship sequences
$CNARS = \{NARS_1, NARS_2, \ldots, NARS_n\}$

1  Create $CNARS = null$;
2  **while** $SAE$ is not $\varnothing$ **do**
3  $\quad$ $temp = SAE.first$ and delete $SAE.first$;
4  $\quad$ **for** $NARS_i$ in $CNRAS$ **do**
5  $\quad\quad$ **if** *(temp.srcMAC, temp.dstMAC couple is in $NARS_i.MACSet$)* **then**
6  $\quad\quad\quad$ $index = f(temp, NARS_i)$; /*This function is used to find the index of the last action event in $NARS_i$ with a MAC pair equal to $temp$.*/
7  $\quad\quad\quad$ **if** *(index == $NARS_i.size - 1$)* **then**
8  $\quad\quad\quad\quad$ add $temp$ to $NARS_i$;
9  $\quad\quad\quad\quad$ add $temp.MACnew$ couple to $NARS_i.MACSet$;/*$NARS_i.MACSet$ can be automatically de-duplicated*/
10 $\quad\quad\quad\quad$ GoTo 2;
11 $\quad\quad\quad$ **else**
12 $\quad\quad\quad\quad$ Create $NARS_{inew}$;/*Take the $NARS_i$ 0-index items and create a new attack relation sequence NARSinew derived from $NARS_i$*/
13 $\quad\quad\quad\quad$ Create $NARS_{inew}.MACSet$;
14 $\quad\quad\quad\quad$ add $temp$ to $NARS_{inew}$;
15 $\quad\quad\quad\quad$ add $temp.MAC$ couple to $NARS_{inew}.MACSet$;
16 $\quad\quad\quad\quad$ $CNARS = CNARS \cup NARS_{inew}$;
17 $\quad\quad\quad\quad$ GoTo 2;
18 $\quad$ Create $NARS_{new}$;
19 $\quad$ add $temp$ to $NARS_{new}$ and create $NARS_{new}.MACSet$;
20 $\quad$ add $temp.MAC$ couple to $NARS_{new}.MACSet$;
21 $\quad$ $CNARS = CNARS \cup NARS_{new}$;
22 Return $CNARS$

---

The main body of the algorithm is run by double layer iteration. Using induction, it can be concluded that when the size of the set of action events is n, the number of times the subject is executed in its worst case of operation is approximately $n(n-1)/2$, so the time complexity of the algorithm is $O(n^2)$. The body of the algorithm is temporarily the space complexity of the algorithm, which is $O(n)$ when the size of the set of action events is $n$.

Using the SDN-based network attack scenario topology model, nodes can be connected together in an orderly way, and with the attributes of network topology connecting lines, the network attack scenario topology reconstruction model is completed.

## 4. Model Analysis

*4.1. Relevance*

This paper uses Pearson's correlation coefficient to evaluate the quality of regenerative flows, which reflects the degree of correlation between the variables. Pearson's correlation coefficient is calculated by the product-difference method, which reflects the correlation between two variables based on the deviation of their mean values from their respective values. The higher the value of the correlation coefficient is, the higher is the correlation between the two sets of data and the higher the fidelity of the regenerative flows.

In this paper, the experimental results from Section 5.5 were subjected to similarity calculation using Pearson correlation coefficient. The results showed that the similarity score was above 90% for various experimental data such as IP frequency distribution, protocol information, and changes in attack flow over time. This indicates a high degree of similarity in the experimental data analyzed. The specific correlation coefficients are calculated in the experimental section of Section 5.

*4.2. Authenticity*

The network topology reconfiguration model proposed by this paper is not a simple, fixed network topology model. It adds the properties of connection lines based on the Waxman model, such as adding parameters such as connection bandwidth, connection delay, connection maximum queue size, and connection packet loss rate. The network topology with these connection parameters can meet the QoS requirements proposed in the network. Mininet can easily simulate the operation and architecture of networks in real environments, mainly by using the namespace mechanism of the Linux kernel. In layman's terms, the namespace mechanism is to be able to simulate a space for each virtual device in the network. The experiments conducted on Mininet can be seamlessly moved to the real environment. This satisfies the first step in reconfiguring the network attack scenario: topology reconstruction. The probabilistic model is then added, and the attack made by this model is not simply a completion of the attack event but is able to simulate a small sample of events at the time of the attack with a small sample of packet sending behavior. In this way, the network attack scenario recovery performed is no longer just a network traffic replay but a high degree of reduction in the attack scenario. The generated packets can achieve a high degree of match with the sample packets, as demonstrated in the experiments of Section 5.

*4.3. Efficiency*

Network attack scene recovery includes three steps: data preprocessing, network topology creation, attack command generation and attack implementation. Assume that the data preprocessing time is $T_1$, the network topology creation time is $T_2$, and the attack command generation and implementation time is $T_3$. Then the total time t of network attack scene recovery is given by

$$T = T_1 + T_2 + T_3. \quad (2)$$

In the whole process of network attack scene recovery, the consumption of time and space is mainly reflected in data preprocessing. Before the network topology is generated, the preprocessing part has already prepared the configuration information such as the IP address when the network topology is created, and the connection line attributes that meet the QoS requirements. Because Mininet itself has the characteristics of rapid reconfiguration and restart, it takes very little time to create the network topology. A lot of experiments show that the process is at a constant, that is, $T_2 \approx 1.5$ s. Before the attack command is generated and implemented, the data preprocessing stage will also compare the data packet information with the rule base to obtain the corresponding attack command parameters, which need to be spliced and the attack started. Once the attack is started, it only takes about 40 s, and the CPU and other occupancy rates of the network will reach 100%. So overall, the speed of network attack scene reconstruction is still very fast. The experiments in Section 5.5 show that processing 500 pieces of data takes less than 8 s, and even with 100,000 pieces of data, it only takes less than 1 min. The specific time statistics in the experiments are detailed in Section 5.

*4.4. Scalability*

The experimental approach in this paper not only enables the replication of a network attack scenario but also allows for the addition or reduction of network attack intensity, changes to network topology nodes, etc. on the basis of this experiment. Through the replication and extension of the attack scenario, it is possible to gain insight into the network attack posture view, analyze the data and information monitored during the attack, and formulate corresponding security strategies. It can bring convenience to network attack defenders to better detect and defend against malicious attack phenomena. Specific experiments are described in Section 5.

The model is implemented with the idea of high cohesion and low coupling. The necessary interfaces are reserved in the process of model implementation, which greatly improves the scalability of the model and facilitates subsequent expansion. Based on the scalability of the model, the model can be replicated for more types of network attack scenarios, thus further enhancing the compatibility of the model in the future. The model analyzes and splits the data in the process of implementation and constructs pluggable tool libraries such as custom function libraries and attack relationship libraries. They are highly reusable and lay the foundation for the subsequent expansion of the model.

## 5. Experimental Analysis

*5.1. Development Environment*

The experimental environment in this paper uses Ubuntu operating system, version 21.04; the network topology is created based on the SDN network topology of the Mininet platform; the controller used is the Ryu controller. The specific environment configuration for the intelligent reconfiguration of the SDN-based network attack scenario is shown in Table 1.

**Table 1.** Environment Configuration Details.

| Environment Matching | Usage Details |
|---|---|
| CPU | Intel(R) Core(TM) i5-10400F CPU @ 2.90 GHz 2.90 GHz |
| GPU | NVIDIA GeForce GTX 1660 SUPER |
| Operating system | Ubuntu 21.04 64-bit operating system |
| Memory | 16.0 GB |
| Debugging environment | Mininet 2.3.0, Ryu 4.34 |
| Development language | Python language |
| Packet capture tool | Wireshark |

*5.2. Introduction to the Simulation Environment*

The environment for this experiment is the SDN network simulation environment tool Mininet with Ryu.

Mininet is a process virtualisation network simulation tool developed by Stanford University based on the Linux Container architecture [23]. It can be used to create a virtual network containing hosts, switches, controllers and links with OpenFlow support for switches and highly flexible custom software-defined networks [24]. With this platform, we can easily simulate the network operation and architecture in a real environment. In addition, Mininet combines many of the advantages of emulators, hardware test beds and simulators [25]:

- Comparison with emulators: fast startup; large scalability; more bandwidth provision; easy installation and easy to use.
- Comparison with emulators: can run real code; easy to connect to real networks.
- Comparison with hardware testbeds: cheap; fast reconfiguration and restart.

There are three ways to create a network topology through Mininet. First, create a basic network topology with a quick command and then add the required nodes and node information through the command line if needed. Second, open the visualization tool MiniEdit; after opening the tool, you can select the controller, OpenFlow switch, host, and other tools as needed. The controller is usually configured as a remote controller, i.e., Ryu controller; after drawing the topology, you can export it as a .py file via File -> Export Level2 Script. Next time, you can continue to open and edit it next time. Third, write a Python script file directly through a compiler or editor to create a network topology.

Ryu is an open-source SDN controller led by Nippon Telegraph and Telephone Corporation. It provides users with a flexible and programmable network control interface while enabling simple and logical centralised control of thousands of OpenFlow switches [26]. As a platform for building SDN applications, Ryu is based on the Python language for development, so it is simple and easy to use for novices. Ryu, a rising star among SDN controllers, is now widely used in the industry [27].

The method used to create the network topology in this article is the third one, written directly by writing a Python script file. The controller used is the Ryu controller.

*5.3. Datasets*

The data used for the experiments in this paper is the 2019 Canadian Institute for Cyber Security Dataset (CIC-DDoS2019). The data contains benign and up-to-date common distributed denial-of-service (DDoS) attacks in the CICDDoS2019 dataset, which is extremely similar to real-world data (Pcap) [28]. It also includes the results of CICFlowMeter-V3 network traffic analysis using tagged flows based on timestamps, source and destination IPs, source and destination ports, protocols, and attacks (CSV files). Using their proposed B-Profile system, Sharafaldin et al. (2016) characterized the abstract behavior of human interactions and generated natural benign background traffic in the proposed testbed. The dataset is collated once a day, and the raw data, including network traffic and event logs (Windows and Ubuntu event logs) for each machine, are recorded daily. For the feature extraction process of the raw data, 80+ dimensional features were extracted using CICFlowMeter-V3 and saved as CSV files for each machine. For this dataset, abstract behaviors of 25 users were constructed based on HTTP, HTTPS, FTP, SSH, and email protocols, and the dataset is used by universities, private companies and independent researchers around the world [29].

*5.4. Experimental Results*

In this paper, recovery of UDP flood network attack scenario is based on SDN. The Ryu controller is first started and the program is run to process the Pcap packets through data preprocessing. The network attack scenario topology reconstruction model is then used to automatically compose the corresponding network topology, while information such as the type of attack and the attack relationship is derived from the inter-node information. Based on this information and the network attack scenario reconstruction probability model, corresponding attack commands are automatically generated. Finally, the automated replication of the corresponding attack scenarios is completed and a large amount of attack data is regenerated.

In this paper, we take the CICDDoS2019 dataset from the Canadian Institute for Cybersecurity Research as an example. First, a Pcap packet is selected from this dataset, the Ryu controller is opened, and the corresponding program is run, which automatically parses and preprocesses the sample Pcap packet by running it to generate the corresponding four intermediate files. These four intermediate files have a corresponding role in the subsequent creation of the network topology and the generation of the attack script. The information of the corresponding intermediate files is shown in Table 2.

**Table 2.** Description of Intermediate Documents.

| File Name | File Content | Document Description |
|---|---|---|
| Sum.txt | srcMAC,dstMAC,srcIP,dstIP | This file is used to store the source MAC address, destination Mac address, source IP address, destination IP address of the packet |
| SrcIP.txt | srcIP | This file is used to save the source IP address after de-duplication |
| DstIP.txt | dstIP | This file is used to save the destination IP address after de-duplication |
| Mac.txt | Mac | This file is used to save all Mac address information after de-duplication |
| MacRelation.txt | (srcMAC,dstMAC) | This file is used to save the source Mac address and destination Mac address as a whole after de-duplication |
| IpRelation.txt | (srcIP,dstIP) | This file is used to save the source IP address and destination IP address as a whole after de-duplication |

Based on the information files of the three intermediate files, SrcIP.txt, DstIP.txt, and Mac.txt, the number of hosts, switches, etc., are calculated. The network attack scenario topology reconstruction model is then used to automatically compose the corresponding network topology. The network topology for this sample is shown in Figure 3, where the topmost person represents the attacker, the small blue circles represent the attacker, and each dotted circle represents a different identity of the attacker. The different hosts in this experiment represent multiple IP addresses, and the small ovals represent all but one identity shared by that host.

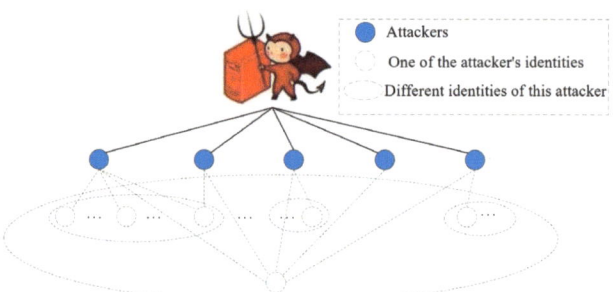

**Figure 3.** Network Topology.

After the network topology is generated, in this paper, we run the generated network attack script on the network topology to execute the attack and count the network attack traffic during the network attack. In this case, this paper counts the network attack for 60 s, and the number of sFlow bytes over time is shown in Figure 4. In the first 5 s, the attack script is executed, the attack starts to proceed, and the rate at which packets are sent begins to grow rapidly. After the attack lasts for 5 s, almost every attacker is in working condition and the rate of packets sent by the attacker increases slowly. Until 25 s, the attack rate almost reaches the set peak, and after 25 s, the packet rate is in a stable fluctuation.

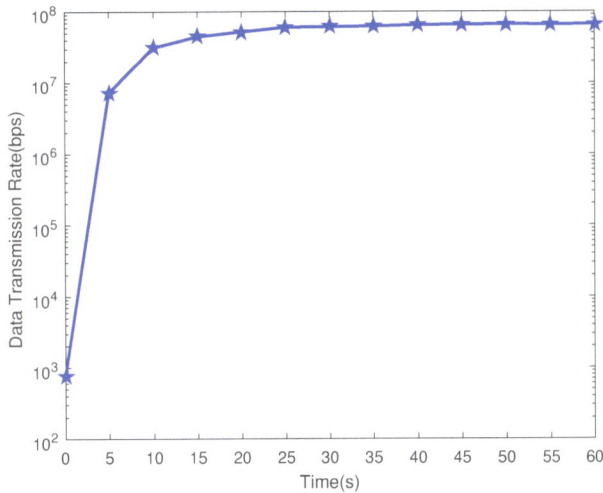

**Figure 4.** Change Diagram of sFlow Bytes in Network Attack Process.

During the attack, there is a direct correlation between sFlow bytes and network throughput rate. As the sFlow bytes increase, the network throughput rate also keeps increasing. That is, it increases rapidly from 0 to 5 s and slowly from 5 to 25 s until 25 s, when the attack rate almost reaches the set peak. After 25 s, the sFlow packets are also basically at a stable value because the packet rate is in a stable state. In this paper, we counted 60 s of network attacks, and the sFlow packet variation over time is shown in Figure 5.

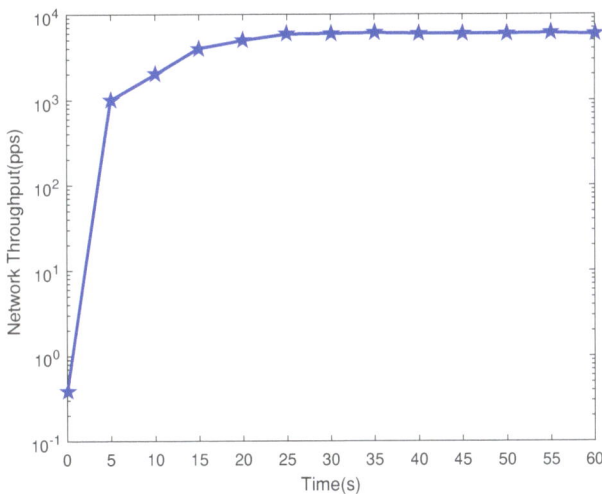

**Figure 5.** Change Diagram of SFlow Packets in Network Attack Process.

During the network attack, the rapid increase of sFlow bytes and sFlow packets make the transmission traffic grow rapidly, and the CPU occupancy and memory occupancy also increase significantly from 0 to 30 s. After that, with sFlow bytes and sFlow packets at a stable value, the attack is also at a critical moment, and the CPU occupancy reaches 100%. After 20 s, the packets are continuously sent. After 50 s, the CPU occupancy and memory occupancy reach the maximum value, and the CPU and memory change during the network attack, as in Figure 6.

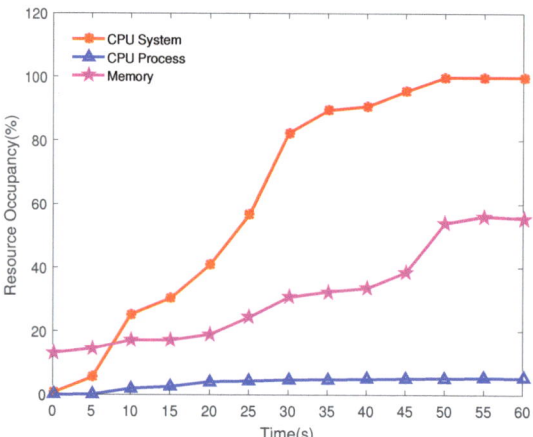

**Figure 6.** Graph of Changes in CPU, Memory, etc. During Network Attacks.

*5.5. Experimental Comparison*

When reconstructing the network attack scenario, the sample packets are first preprocessed, and the results returned from the preprocessing are some basic information for reconstructing the network topology and the attack parameters needed in the network attack. such as the packet type, the port information, the IP information of the attacker and the attacked, the length of the attacked packets, etc. Then the network topology is reconstructed and the network attack is implemented based on the preprocessed information. This reproduces the network attack scenario to achieve a high degree of matching with the sample.

To demonstrate the similarity between our proposed method and the original data, we will compare and analyze the five following aspects: IP address distribution and usage frequency, similarity calculated by Pearson algorithm, protocol proportions, packet length, and port binding services. By comparing these aspects, we can illustrate the degree of similarity between the original data and the regenerated data for attack scenarios. The specific comparisons are as follows:

(1) IP address distribution and usage frequency.

With the SDN-based network attack scenario recovery method proposed in this paper, the similarity of attack scenario recovery can be improved as much as possible. The model can fully represent the original data by adding probabilistic events, including the small sample of events present in the original data. In the raw data of this paper, each host has multiple different spoofed IP identities, and according to the statistics all attackers used a total of 28 IP addresses, but the number of packets sent by the attackers using different IPs varies. The IPs, 192.168.50.1, 192.168.50.6, 192.168.50.7, 172.217.11.2, and 172.217.9.226, are used with the highest frequency, and the remaining IPs are used with very low frequency. The statistics were also calculated in this paper, and the frequency graph of forged IPs is shown in Figure 7. The content in brackets after the IP address represents the number of times the IP appears. In the attack scenario recovery, to more clearly illustrate, the small sample events have been added. First, the main attack event IP is 172.16.0.5 for the statistics, accounting for 99.1818% of the sample and 99.2407% of the regenerated data. After that, the IP frequencies of the regenerated packets and the sample packets are compared, and the comparison graph is shown in Figure 8.

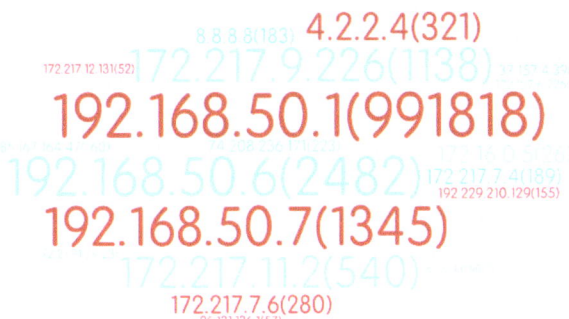

**Figure 7.** Frequency Diagram of Pseudo IP Addresses.

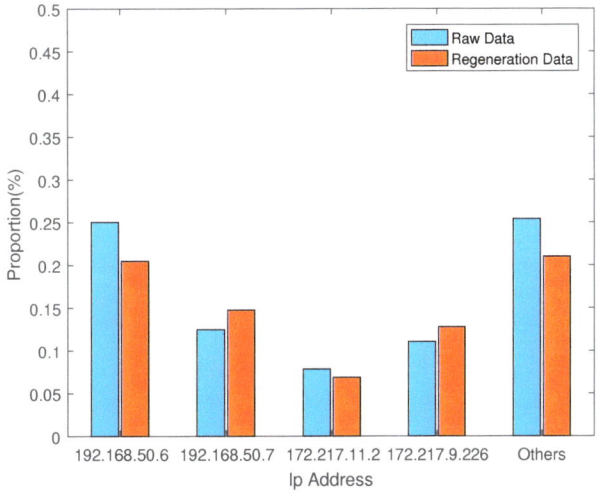

**Figure 8.** Probability Comparison Chart of Attack Packets and Sample Packets.

We can clearly see from the comparison graph in Figure 8 that there is a high degree of consistency between the original and regenerated data in terms of IP address usage frequency. Even for small sample events with very low IP usage, they can be accurately simulated due to the added probability model. Using the Pearson correlation coefficient calculation, the similarity can reach up to 99%.

(2) Similarity calculated by Pearson algorithm.

According to the network attack scenario recovery method proposed in this paper, the number of packets sent by the regenerated data and the original data in time are counted and the similarity of the attacks is compared. In this paper, we choose the time period from 0 to 5.5 s and count the total number of packets sent by the original data and the regenerated data every 0.5 s, respectively. From 0 to 2 s, the number of packets increases at a fast rate and there is a certain gap between the number of packets sent by the regenerated data and the original data. After that, as the number of sent packets slowly increases, the graph of the number of packets sent by the regenerated data floats around the graph of the number of packets sent by the original data, but the two rates are basically the same and the graphs of the changes of the two curves basically overlap together. The statistical results of the total number of packets sent during the time period from 0 to 5.5 s are shown in Figure 9.

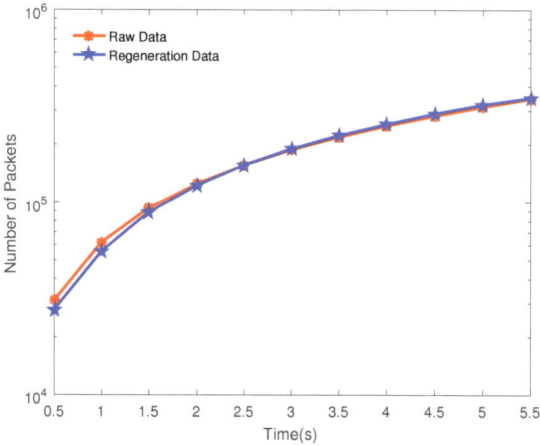

**Figure 9.** Comparison Chart of The Total Sum of Packets Sent on The Time Series.

According to the similarity calculation method mentioned in Section 4.1 using Pearson correlation coefficient: this paper has done three sets of experiments on three different Pcap packets, the first of which is the experimental result in Figure 9. The correlation coefficients were calculated for the original data and the regenerated data from the three sets of experimental results, where X is the original data, Y is the regenerated data, $\mu_X$ is the mean of X, $\mu_Y$ is the mean of Y, $\sigma_X$ is the standard deviation of the original data X, $\sigma_Y$ is the standard deviation of the regenerated data Y, and $\rho_{X,Y}$ is the correlation coefficient. In this paper, three different groups of experiments were performed. The statistics are shown in Table 3.

**Table 3.** Statistical Table of Correlation Coefficients.

| Group | Group 1 | Group 2 | Group 3 |
| --- | --- | --- | --- |
| $\mu_X$ | 172,198.0833 | 182,011.3 | 141,554.8 |
| $\mu_Y$ | 173,701.0833 | 200,759.3 | 145,845.8 |
| $\sigma_X$ | 113,199.1511 | 100,338.73414 | 78,006.45636 |
| $\sigma_Y$ | 117,431.6822 | 117,964.93129 | 77,420.57464 |
| $\rho_{X,Y}$ | 0.9998 | 0.9978 | 0.99 |

Based on the comparison described above, the Pearson correlation was calculated for the regenerated and original data for all three experiments. The three experiments showed high consistency and achieved a very high degree of similarity. As can be seen from Table 3, the method is stable, and the regenerated data traffic is essentially the same as the original traffic in terms of sending time attributes.

(3) Protocol proportions.

To demonstrate the similarity in the recovery of the network attack scenarios, the experiments were also compared statistically in terms of packet protocols, packet lengths, port binding services for sending packets, and port binding services for receiving packets. In this experiment, the protocols in the sample are mainly UDP protocols, and a few are ICMP protocols and TCP protocols, along with some other protocols, but the other protocols are almost a very small part. The results of the statistical comparison are shown in Table 4. By comparing the difference between both is not more than 0.2%. Based on the protocol distribution in Table 4 and comparison using Pearson correlation, the similarity of protocols can reach up to 98%.

Table 4. Network Packet Protocol Proportion Information.

| Protocol | Raw Data | Regeneration Data |
|---|---|---|
| UDP | 99.2815% | 99.0780% |
| TCP | 0.7028% | 0.8908% |
| ICMP | 0.0155% | 0.0269% |
| Others | 0.0002% | 0.0043% |

(4) Packet length.

In the sample data protocols are mainly UDP protocols, a small number of TCP protocols and ICMP protocols, and some other protocols because different protocols send packets of different lengths. The length of packets used to send in the UDP protocol is mainly 524, and there are a few other lengths of UDP protocol packets. The TCP and ICMP protocols themselves account for a smaller proportion, and the packet length distribution is more dispersed, so the proportion of the total number of packets is even smaller. The results of comparing the regenerated data with the native data are shown in Table 5. Using the Pearson correlation to compare the distribution of packet lengths in Table 5, the similarity can reach up to 98%.

Table 5. Packet Length Proportion Information Table.

| Packet Length | Raw Data | Regeneration Data |
|---|---|---|
| $UDP.length == 524$ | 99.1404% | 99.0768% |
| $UDP.length ! = 524$ | 0.1411% | 0.0012% |
| $TCP.length > 45$ | 0.3423% | 0.5344% |
| $TCP.length \leq 45$ | 0.3605% | 0.3564% |
| Others | 0.0157% | 0.0312% |

(5) Port-binding services.

Due to the presence of several different protocols in this sample packet, there are different services bound to the same port. For example, on port 1483 both packets of the TCP protocol and packets of the UDP protocol are sent. As the source and destination ports are spread out, the number of different services bound to the port is counted in the statistics. The statistics show that the number of different services bound to different ports is 51,350 for the original data and 52,245 for the regenerated data. In conclusion, the difference between the two is negligible.

Through the comparison from five different perspectives above, it can be concluded that the regenerated network traffic for attack scenarios shows high similarity with the original data traffic.

According to the content mentioned in Section 4.4, the experiment can not only reproduce the UDP flood attack but also control the strength of the attack on the network. For network defenders, it would be significant to be able to identify other problems in the network by modulating the intensity of the attack on top of reproducing it. Therefore, based on this experiment, this paper regenerates traffic that increases and decreases the intensity of the network attack under the same network topology. The data generated by increasing and decreasing intensity were also compared with the sample data, and the results of the comparison are shown in Figure 10.

At the same time, network topology nodes can be added to the experiment, and the addition of network topology nodes allows the experimenter to perform some other types of attacks or experiments on these nodes. In this paper, we address the addition of network topology nodes and still perform attacks on the attacking hosts in the experiment without changing the original attack parameters. The initial state of the experiment is six hosts, and the number of packets is observed from 0 to 5.5 s by gradually increasing the number of hosts. The number of packets sent by the attacker in the experiment increases with the number of hosts. The number of packets sent by the attacker varies with the number of hosts versus time, as shown in Figure 11.

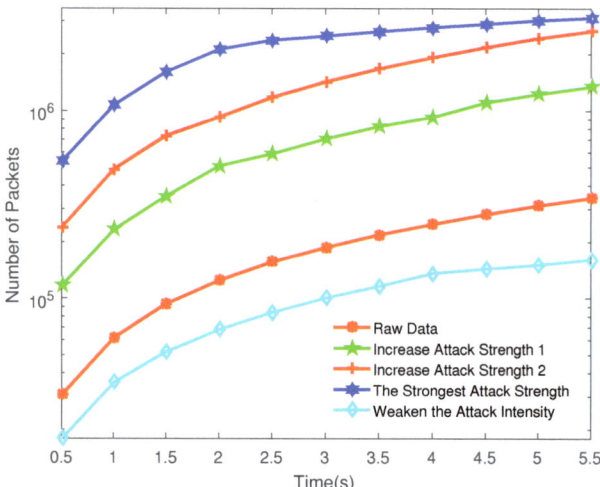

**Figure 10.** Frequency Diagram of Pseudo-IP Addresses.

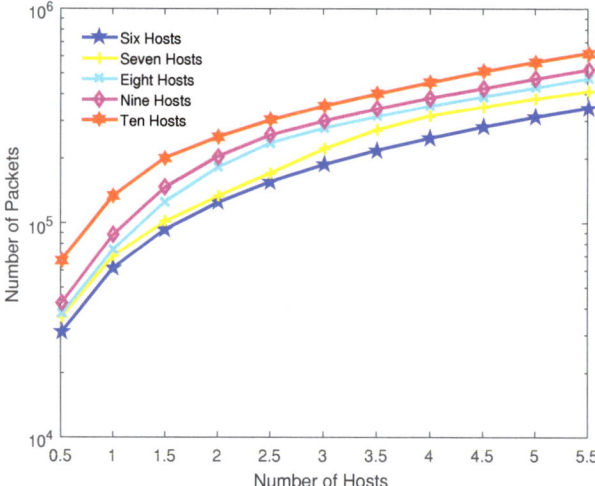

**Figure 11.** Packet change graph after increasing the number of hosts.

The network attack scenario recovery method proposed in this paper not only has a high reproduction rate and scalability, but also the attack scenario recovery is particularly fast. According to the relevant calculation methods mentioned in Section 4.3, The total time $T$ spent in network attack scenario recovery is mainly concentrated in three aspects: data preprocessing $T_1$, network topology creation $T_2$, and attack command generation and attack execution $T_3$. For different numbers of datasets, time statistics are performed separately from these three aspects. As the number of packets increases, the time increases but is still fast. The statistical results are shown in Table 6.

Table 6. Timetable Required for Network Attack Recovery.

| Time (s) | 500 | 1000 | 5000 | 10,000 | 100,000 |
|---|---|---|---|---|---|
| $T_1$ | 3.57 | 8.86 | 19.68 | 27.83 | 51.96 |
| $T_2$ | 1.46 | 1.61 | 1.55 | 1.50 | 1.53 |
| $T_3$ | 2.23 | 2.44 | 2.68 | 2.98 | 3.23 |
| $T$ | 7.26 | 12.91 | 23.91 | 32.31 | 56.72 |

There exist many network topology reconstruction models with network attack scenario reconstruction models. However, with the proposed QoS requirements in the network, the simple, fixed network topology model is not a good simulation of the real network, and it is necessary to add connection properties to the existing connections. For example, QoS parameters such as bandwidth, latency, cost, and packet loss rate are added to the network model to better simulate the real network. Currently, the network topology scenario reconstruction mainstream is expressed in the form of language and diagram and does not really create the topology. The network topology model proposed in this paper not only adds QoS parameters but also creates the real network topology.

In the process of network attack recovery, the proposed network attack scenario recovery method in this paper is qualitatively evaluated against existing network attack scenario recovery methods. Four main aspects are compared: whether the network topology is created in the network attack scenario recovery; whether the real network traffic is regenerated; whether the intensity of the attack is controllable during the network attack; and the recovery emphasis of the network attack scenario. The comparison results are shown in Table 7.

Table 7. Qualitative Analysis Table.

| Methods | Create Topology | Regenerate Real Traffic | Control the Intensity of the Attack | Restore Capability |
|---|---|---|---|---|
| H. Liu [7] | Yes | No | No | Strong |
| Y. Djemaiel [13] | No | No | No | Medium |
| Y. Zhang [14] | No | No | No | Strong |
| H. Wu [10] | Yes | No | No | Strong |
| W. Wang [15] | No | No | No | Weak |
| T. Guo [16] | No | No | No | Weak |
| Our method | Yes | Yes | Yes | Strong |

*5.6. Extra Costs and Limitations Discussion*

In this section, we will mainly discuss the possible extra costs and limitations that may be involved in our research plan. We will analyze the potential limitations of our study and the associated extra expenses and propose corresponding solutions to these issues.

5.6.1. Extra Costs

In this experiment, we utilized a publicly available dataset that had already been labeled for network attack scene recovery, so there were no significant additional costs incurred. However, in real-world network attack scenarios, the time span for packet collection can be quite long. If we obtain a raw dataset, additional costs will be incurred. We would need to spend considerable time or technical resources to calibrate the attack process and extract the proper data. The accuracy of our network attack scene recovery is dependent on the accuracy of data calibration. Only with more accurate calibration data can we recover scenes closer to reality.

5.6.2. Limitations

In this work, although the SDN-based network attack scene restoration method proposed in this paper has achieved some results, due to the complexity and diversity of network attacks, if data packets containing unknown network protocols are mixed in during scene reconstruction, these unknown network protocol packets still cannot be revived.

## 6. Conclusions

This paper proposes an SDN-based network attack scene recovery method. This method is able to regenerate the original data and integrate other network attacks into the reconstructed scene, generating new blended data. The first step of this method is to parse Pcap data of network attacks obtained from public sources. The second step is to generate the network topology by utilizing the network attack scenario topology reconfiguration model and generate corresponding attack scripts using the network attack scenario recovery probability model and attack sequence algorithm and finally, to regenerate traffic on the network topology. The experimental results show that the proposed method is closer to the actual network attack scenario, with a higher similarity of the attack scenario. Additionally, the proposed method not only enables the recovery of network attack scenarios but can also be extended to other experiments. For example, based on the restored network attack scenarios, the network topology nodes can be modified and the strength of the attack can be intensified or weakened and combined with other types of attacks.

Regarding the limitations mentioned in Section 5.6.2, for future work, we aim to investigate how to construct unknown protocol data packets and revive them, in hopes of automating adaptation and resurrection of various types of data packets. Additionally, we will enhance the accuracy and reliability of our model by introducing more data sources, optimizing algorithm design, and exploring new data analysis and modeling methods, among other approaches.

**Author Contributions:** Conceptualization, Y.W. and T.Z.; methodology, Y.W. and T.Z.; software, Y.W. and J.D.; validation, Y.W., J.D. and T.Z.; formal analysis, Y.W. and J.D.; investigation, Y.W. and J.D.; writing—original draft preparation, Y.W., J.D., Y.X. and X.H.; writing—review and editing, Y.W. and J.D. All authors have read and agreed to the published version of the manuscript.

**Funding:** This research work is supported by the National Natural Science Founds of China (62072368, U20B2050) and the Key Research and Development Program of Shaanxi Province (2021ZDLGY05-09, 2022GY-040).

**Data Availability Statement:** Sample data sets used in the experiment site: https://www.unb.ca/cic/datasets/index.html; accessed on 2 March 2023, this study generated data sets, please contact dingjunxia@stu.xaut.edu.cn.

**Acknowledgments:** The authors would like to thank the editors and the reviewers for their valuable suggestions and comments.

**Conflicts of Interest:** The authors declare no conflict of interest.

## References

1. Shen, Z.-Y.; Su, M.-W.; Cai, Y.-Z.; Tasi, M.-H. Mitigating SYN Flooding and UDP Flooding in P4-based SDN. In Proceedings of the 2021 22nd Asia-Pacific Network Operations and Management Symposium (APNOMS), Online Event, 8–10 September 2021; pp. 374–377.
2. Mladenov, B. Studying the DDoS Attack Effect over SDN Controller Southbound Channel. In Proceedings of the 2019 X National Conference with International Participation (ELECTRONICA), Sofia, Bulgaria, 16–17 May 2019; pp. 1–4.
3. Runze, C.; Fangming, R.; Yidan, L.; Lan, Y.; Yanli, C. A Simple DDoS Defense Method Based SDN. In Proceedings of the 2021 IEEE 15th International Conference on Anti-Counterfeiting, Security, and Identification (ASID), Xiamen, China, 29–31 October 2021; pp. 88–92.
4. Csikor, L.; Szalay, M.; Rétvári, G.; Pongrácz, G.; Pezaros, D.P.; Toka, L. Transition to SDN is HARMLESS: Hybrid Architecture for Migrating Legacy Ethernet Switches to SDN. *IEEE/ACM Trans. Netw.* **2020**, *28*, 275–288. [CrossRef]
5. Gedia, D.; Perigo, L. Performance Evaluation of SDN-VNF in Virtual Machine and Container. In Proceedings of the 2018 IEEE Conference on Network Function Virtualization and Software Defined Networks (NFV-SDN), Verona, Italy, 27–29 November 2018; pp. 1–7.
6. Amin, R.; Reisslein, M.; Shah, N. Hybrid SDN Networks: A Survey of Existing Approaches. *IEEE Commun. Surv. Tutor.* **2018**, *20*, 3259–3306. [CrossRef]

7. Liu, H.; An, L.; Ren, J.; Wang, B. An Interactive Traffic Replay Method in a Scaled-Down Environment. *IEEE Access* **2019**, *7*, 149373–149386. [CrossRef]
8. Li, Y.; Miao, R.; Alizadeh, M. DETER: Deterministic TCP replay for performance diagnosis. In Proceedings of the 16th USENIX Symposium on Networked Systems Design and Implementation (NSDI), Boston, MA, USA, 26–28 February 2019; pp. 437–452.
9. Li, L.; Hao, Z.; Zhang, Y.; Liu, Y.; Li, D. Modeling for Traffic Replay in Virtual Network. In Proceedings of the 2018 IEEE 20th International Conference on High Performance Computing and Communications, IEEE 16th International Conference on Smart City, IEEE 4th International Conference on Data Science and Systems (HPCC/SmartCity/DSS), Exeter, UK, 28–30 June 2018; pp. 495–502.
10. Wu, H.; Liu, H.; Wang, B.; Xin, G. Accurate traffic replay based on interactive sequence and timestamp. In Proceedings of the 2017 IEEE 9th International Conference on Communication Software and Networks (ICCSN), Guangzhou, China, 6–8 May 2017; pp. 1107–1110.
11. Mao, B.; Liu, J.; Lai, Y.; Sun, M. MIF: A multi-step attack scenario reconstruction and attack chains extraction method based on multi-information fusion. *Comput. Netw.* **2021**, *198*, 108340. [CrossRef]
12. Wei, Y.; Wu, F. Research on Network Topology Model of Tactical Communication System. In Proceedings of the 2020 IEEE 9th Joint International Information Technology and Artificial Intelligence Conference (ITAIC), Chongqing, China, 11–13 December 2020; pp. 808–811.
13. Djemaiel, Y.; Fessi, B.A.; Boudriga, N. Using Temporal Conceptual Graphs and Neural Networks for Big Data-Based Attack Scenarios Reconstruction. In Proceedings of the 2019 IEEE International Conferance on Parallel & Distributed Processing with Applications, Big Data & Cloud Computing, Sustainable Computing & Communications, Social Computing & Networking (ISPA/BDCloud/SocialCom/SustainCom), Xiamen, China, 16–18 December 2019; pp. 991–998.
14. Zhang, Y.; Zhao, S.; Zhang, J. RTMA: Real Time Mining Algorithm for Multi-Step Attack Scenarios Reconstruction. In Proceedings of the 2019 IEEE 21st International Conference on High Performance Computing and Communications, IEEE 17th International Conference on Smart City, IEEE 5th International Conference on Data Science and Systems (HPCC/SmartCity/DSS), Zhangjiajie, China, 10–12 August 2019; pp. 2103–2110.
15. Wang, W.; Du, X.; Ren, Z.; Shan, D. Reconstructing attack scenarios based on causal knowledge and spatio-temporal correlation for cloud platforms. *Comput. Sci.* **2021**, *48*, 317–323.
16. Guo, T. *Research on Attack Scene Reconstruction Algorithm Based on Correlation Analysis*; Beijing University of Posts and Telecommunications: Beijing, China, 2018.
17. Huang, Y.; Sun, Y.; Lin, K.; Xie, B.; Fan, J.; Ma, Y. An Effective Reconstruction Method of the APT Attack Based on Hidden Markov Model. *J. Circuits Syst. Comput.* **2021**, *31*, 2250108. [CrossRef]
18. Rusek, K.; Suárez-Varela, J.; Almasan, P.; Barlet-Ros, P.; Cabellos-Aparicio, A. RouteNet: Leveraging Graph Neural Networks for Network Modeling and Optimization in SDN. *IEEE J. Sel. Areas Commun.* **2020**, *38*, 2260–2270. [CrossRef]
19. Hajizadeh, M.; Phan, T.V.; Bauschert, T. Probability Analysis of Successful Cyber Attacks in SDN-based Networks. In Proceedings of the 2018 IEEE Conference on Network Function Virtualization and Software Defined Networks (NFV-SDN), Verona, Italy, 27–29 November 2018; pp. 1–6.
20. Sun, W.; Li, Y.; Guan, S. An Improved Method of DDoS Attack Detection for Controller of SDN. In Proceedings of the 2019 IEEE 2nd International Conference on Computer and Communication Engineering Technology (CCET), Beijing, China, 16–18 August 2019; pp. 249–253.
21. Naing, M.T.; Khaing, T.T.; Maw, A.H. Evaluation of TCP and UDP Traffic over Software-Defined Networking. In Proceedings of the 2019 International Conference on Advanced Information Technologies (ICAIT), Yangon, Myanmar, 6–7 November 2019; pp. 7–12.
22. Pérez-Díaz, J.A.; Valdovinos, I.A.; Choo, K.-K.R.; Zhu, D. A Flexible SDN-Based Architecture for Identifying and Mitigating Low-Rate DDoS Attacks Using Machine Learning. *IEEE Access* **2020**, *8*, 155859–155872. [CrossRef]
23. Gill, S.; Lee, B.; Qiao, Y. Containerchain: A Blockchain System Emulator based on Mininet and Containers. In Proceedings of the 2021 IEEE International Conference on Blockchain (Blockchain), Melbourne, Australia, 6–8 December 2021; pp. 1–7.
24. Zulu, L.L.; Ogudo, K.A.; Umenne, P.O. Simulating Software Defined Networking Using Mininet to Optimize Host Communication in a Realistic Programmable Network. In Proceedings of the 2018 International Conference on Advances in Big Data, Computing and Data Communication Systems (icABCD), Durban, South Africa, 6–8 August 2018; pp. 1–6.
25. Lee, S.; Ali, J.; Roh, B.-H. Performance Comparison of Software Defined Networking Simulators for Tactical Network: Mininet vs. OPNET. In Proceedings of the 2019 International Conference on Computing, Networking and Communications (ICNC), Honolulu, HI, USA, 18–21 February 2019; pp. 197–202.
26. Tivig, P.T.; Borcoci, E.; Brumaru, A.; Ciobanu, A.-I.-E. Layer 3 Forwarder Application - Implementation Experiments Based on Ryu SDN Controller. In Proceedings of the 2021 International Symposium on Networks, Computers and Communications (ISNCC), Dubai, United Arab Emirates, 1–3 June 2021; pp. 1–6.
27. Chouhan, R.K.; Atulkar, M.; Nagwani, N.K. Performance Comparison of Ryu and Floodlight Controllers in Different SDN Topologies. In Proceedings of the 2019 1st International Conference on Advanced Technologies in Intelligent Control, Environment, Computing & Communication Engineering (ICATIECE), Bangalore, India, 19–20 March 2019; pp. 188–191.

28. Elsayed, M.S.; Le-Khac, N.-A.; Dev, S.; Jurcut, A.D. DDoSNet: A Deep-Learning Model for Detecting Network Attacks. In Proceedings of the 2020 IEEE 21st International Symposium on "A World of Wireless, Mobile and Multimedia Networks" (WoWMoM), Cork, Ireland, 31 August–3 September 2020; pp. 391–396.
29. Nguyen, M.H.; Lai, Y.-K.; Chang, K.-P. An Entropy-based DDoS attack Detection and Classification with Hierarchical Temporal Memory. In Proceedings of the 2021 Asia-Pacific Signal and Information Processing Association Annual Summit and Conference (APSIPA ASC), Tokyo, Japan, 14–17 December 2021; pp. 1942–1948.

**Disclaimer/Publisher's Note:** The statements, opinions and data contained in all publications are solely those of the individual author(s) and contributor(s) and not of MDPI and/or the editor(s). MDPI and/or the editor(s) disclaim responsibility for any injury to people or property resulting from any ideas, methods, instructions or products referred to in the content.

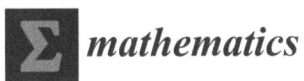 

Article

# Optimal Multi-Attribute Auctions Based on Multi-Scale Loss Network

Zefeng Zhao [1], Haohao Cai [1], Huawei Ma [2], Shujie Zou [1] and Chiawei Chu [1,*]

[1] Faculty of Data Science, City University of Macau, Macau 999078, China
[2] Institute of AI and Blockchain, Guangzhou University, Guangzhou 510006, China
\* Correspondence: cwchu@cityu.mo

**Abstract:** There is a strong demand for multi-attribute auctions in real-world scenarios for non-price attributes that allow participants to express their preferences and the item's value. However, this also makes it difficult to perform calculations with incomplete information, as a single attribute—price—no longer determines the revenue. At the same time, the mechanism must satisfy individual rationality (IR) and incentive compatibility (IC). This paper proposes an innovative dual network to solve these problems. A shared MLP module is constructed to extract bidder features, and multiple-scale loss is used to determine network status and update. The method was tested on real and extended cases, showing that the approach effectively improves the auctioneer's revenue without compromising the bidder.

**Keywords:** optimal mechanism; multi-attribute auction; multi-scale loss

**MSC:** 91-10; 68T07

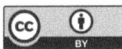

## 1. Introduction

The multi-attribute auction is a practical tool widely used on various occasions, such as government auctions of rare resources such as minerals, land, and spectra; online advertising auctions [1]; and supply chain management [2]. In a single-attribute auction, bidders only need to consider one bidding factor, such as price, to determine their bidding strategy. Such auctions lack universality. Multi-attribute auctions provide participants with more options. Bidders can consider multiple factors, such as, in the auction of transportation services, to ensure that the transported items arrive at the designated location more safely. Participants have special needs in terms of price, service quality, delivery time, etc.; this makes the formulation of bidding strategies more complex.

Myerson [3] designed a unique mechanism: the single-item optimal auction mechanism. This is in line with the pursuit of maximizing the interests of one party in the auction. For example, in the aforementioned public resource auction scenario, the optimal auction can pursue the maximization of public welfare. But the optimal mechanism design is complex. In terms of item quantity, the optimal mechanism design for a single item is easy, but it is difficult for multiple items. Dütting [4] solved the 40-year stagnation problem of multiple items using the deep learning method and subsequently derived more complex single-attribute optimal auction mechanisms.

However, the problem of multiple attributes has yet to be solved. Previous papers have proven that the multi-attribute optimal mechanism for single bidders is highly complex [5]. Furthermore, attributes contain private information belonging to participants and cannot be directly converted to one attribute. This paper proposes a new network model and a shared module in Section 4.2 to address this issue.

We noticed that maximizing expected utility implies no labels for network training. Additionally, multi-attribute optimal auctions must satisfy individual rationality (IR) and incentive compatibility (IC) [6] constraints, where IR means that individuals make decisions that they believe will lead to optimal rewards and IC means that each participant can achieve their best outcome by acting according to their true preferences. These require the network to be updated within a certain range. Therefore, a multi-scale loss network optimization method (MLN) was designed.

Then, the MLN method was tested on real reverse-auction cases. The results indicate that this method could effectively reduce auctioneers' expenses while not causing harm to bidders, ensuring the sustainability of the auction. Moreover, the method was tested with extended experiments, demonstrating its generalization performance and robustness.

## 2. Contributions

1. This paper proposes a dual network structure that includes a shared module. This module extracts multiple non-price attributes from multi-attribute optimal auctions as standard features, which can handle bidding with different preferences and settings.

2. A multi-scale loss method is proposed to optimize the networks. IR, IC, and additional constraints in special auction scenarios are mapped to multi-scale loss functions, ensuring that the auction rule satisfies all parties' interests.

## 3. Related Work

The optimal auction is a special auction mechanism and concept, with the core of maximizing revenue for one party. Myerson solved the problem of maximizing seller returns in a single-indivisible-item, multi-bidder auction while satisfying the incentive compatibility mechanism for bidders to submit true valuations, which is a great innovation. Although Myerson's method cannot achieve the mechanism design of a multi-item, multi-bidder auction, it has indeed been proven to be difficult to calculate [7,8]. With the increase in the number of bidders and items and the complexity of auction forms, especially when bidders' submissions are continuous, the design and verification of mechanisms become extremely difficult [9,10].

Machine learning methods have brought about a turnaround in this matter. For example, Duting [11] designed a simple three-layer MLP network (RochetNet) based on Rochet's idea [12], successfully solving the single-attribute optimal auction problem for multiple items and single bidders. Subsequently, the author proposed a new network structure (RegretNet) to solve the optimal auction problem of multiple items and bidders. The author designed two networks for allocation and payment, where the networks' input is the bidding of multiple bidders for multiple lots, and the output is the probability of each bidder obtaining each item and the price that should be paid. With the emergence of RegretNet, many mechanism design methods for dealing with more complex scenarios have been derived, such as considering the budget of bidders [13], coding, and classifying participants' preferences [14,15]. Meanwhile, machine learning methods have proven effective in practice. Zhe [16] applied the design of an optimal auction mechanism based on neural networks to allocate vehicular edge computing resources. Liu [1] used an optimal auction mechanism based on neural networks in advertising bidding in e-commerce.

The earliest multi-attribute mechanism, consisting of two attributes, i.e., the cost and time of the bidder, was proposed by Ellis [17] and was applied to the auction of highway contracting. Although the auction content is relatively simple and the time factors can be converted to calculate profits, it initiated formal research on multi-attribute auctions. Compared with the single-attribute mechanism, multiple attributes can better take care of the needs of participants [18,19]. Therefore, this mechanism is widely used in real life. But multiple attributes also bring more uncertainty. In 1991, Staschus et al. [20] proposed a multi-attribute auction framework, which was not verified with experiments, that converts all bid attributes of bidders into a single price attribute of the auctioneer. But this method is difficult to calculate in complex scenarios.

On the other hand, attributes and utility functions represent participants' private information. On this topic, Chen Ritzo et al. [21] proposed a multi-attribute reverse-auction mechanism with limited information feedback. Gupta et al. [22] analyzed the information disclosure mechanism in multi-attribute auctions and designed a multi-attribute auction mechanism with changeable feedback information for experiments. However, the problem of multi-attribute optimal mechanism design has not been solved. Existing research has proved that it is difficult to calculate the multi-dimension of a single bidder [5,23], let alone multiple bidders.

## 4. Methodology
### 4.1. Optimal Multi-Attribute Auction

Let us suppose a multi-attribute, multi-item, multi-bidder auction scenario: There are a set of $N$ bidders $\{1, 2, \ldots, n\}$ with additive valuations and individual rationality, and $G$ items $\{1, 2, \ldots, g\}$. Each bidder $i$ has $t$ non-price attributes requirements for each item $\{p_{ij}, q_{ij1}, \ldots, q_{ijt}\}$, where $p_{ij}$ is the price of the item and $q_{ijt}$ are non-price attributes. The bid submitted by bidder $i$ in the auction is $b_i = \{b_{i1}, b_{i2}, \ldots, b_{ig}\}$, where $b_{ij} = \{p_{ij}, q_{ij1}, \ldots, q_{ijt}\}$ and $b_i : 2^G \to \mathbb{R} \geq 0$.

After receiving bids from all bidders, the auctioneer decides the probability of each person winning each item and the fee. Then, the bidder's expected utility ($u_i$) can be expressed as

$$u_i = \sum_j Pr_{ij}(b_{ij}) p_{ij} - Pay_{ij} \qquad (1)$$

where the formula indicates that the expected return of the bidder is calculated by subtracting the actual expenditure from the expected expenditure.

In this simple scenario, let us assume that the auctioneer has $t$ reserved attributes $R = (r_{j1}, \ldots r_{jt})$ for item $j$. If the submitted attribute $q_i$ exceeds the reserved attribute, it harms the auctioneers' revenue, and the weight is $W_{jk}$. Then, the auctioneer's expected utility ($u_0$) can be expressed as follows:

$$u_0 = \sum_i \sum_j Pr_{ij}(b_j) Pay_{ij} - \sum_k^t W_{ijk}\left(r_{jk} - q_{ijk}\right) \qquad (2)$$

where the formula states that the auctioneer's expected utility is calculated by subtracting the expected revenue from the loss due to the non-price attributes being lower than the reserved attributes.

Due to IR, which also conforms to the characteristics of the economic behavior of the auction, the bidders' purpose must be to maximize profit, at least not to cause losses to themselves. It is foreseeable that if there are no conditional restrictions, the bidder obtains extra income $e_i$ by submitting an untrue bid $b'_i$.

$$e_i = \sum_j \sum_k \varphi_{ijk}\left(q'_{ijk} - q_{ijk}\right) \qquad (3)$$

where $\varphi$ represents the weight of lying and $q$ are untrue non-price attributes. Then, the bidder's expected utility ($u_i$) is

$$u_i = \sum_j Pr_{ij}(b_{ij}) p_{ij} + e_{ij} - Pay_{ij} \qquad (4)$$

The purpose of the optimal mechanism is to maximize the auctioneer's expected utility; hence, the most direct way to satisfy this purpose is to let bidders submit their actual values. In order to satisfy this condition and make the mechanism sustainable, IC must be satisfied, whereby bidder $i$'s income from submitting a true bid must not be lower than that from submitting an untrue one.

$$u_i(b_i, b_{-i}) \geq u'_i(b'_i, b_{-i}) \qquad (5)$$

At the same time, the mechanism needs to satisfy IR, whereby it cannot damage the participants' benefits.
$$u_i(b_i, b_{-i}) \geq 0 \tag{6}$$

### 4.2. Network Design

Since the design of the multi-attribute optimal mechanism mainly consists of payment rules and allocation rules, this paper designed a dual network with reference to Dütting [4]. The Allocation Network and Payment Network were constructed to determine the probability of bidders obtaining items and the proportion of their payments, respectively (Figure 1). The Allocation Network is denoted by $A^\gamma$, and the Payment Network is denoted by $P^\delta$. Among them, $\gamma$ and $\delta$ represent the parameters of the network. These two networks together constitute our optimal mechanism or rules $(A^\gamma, P^\delta)$. The input multi-attribute bidding data are extracted into one feature using shared modules. The extracted features are then processed by the Allocation Network and the Payment Network to obtain allocation and payment results, respectively. The two results are used for the computerized status and for updating the networks.

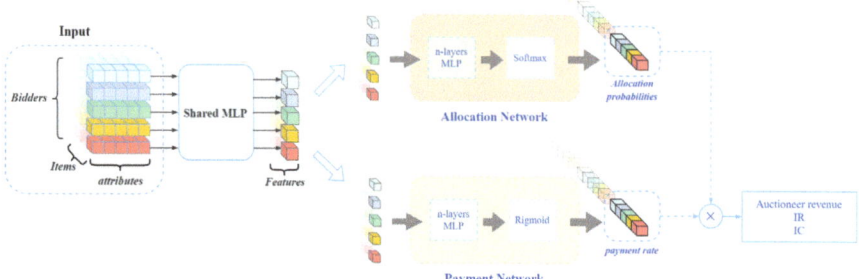

**Figure 1.** Figure of network structure.

The purpose of the optimal auction is to maximize the auctioneer's expected utility ($u_0$) (Formula (7)) while satisfying the IR and IC conditions. Usually, the artificially designed mechanism considers the participation enthusiasm of bidders and the sustainability of the auction by restricting rules based on IC, such as adjusting payment prices based on ranking or bidding content to satisfy IC constraints.

$$\max u_0 = A^\gamma(b) \times P^\delta(b) \times (\text{price} + W(q-r)) \tag{7}$$

Without constraints, the payment rules would cause significant losses to bidders for deep learning networks. If there were only the IC constraint, it would only make misreporting lose meaning for bidders, as the auctioneer could infinitely increase the payment ratio without considering true and untrue bids. Therefore, Formulas (8) and (9) are used to measure whether the degrees of incentive compatibility and individual rationality are satisfied, respectively. Then, these two parameters are used to assist in network optimization.

$$IC = A^\gamma(b'_i, b_i) \times P^\delta(b'_i, b_i) \times (\text{price}'_i + \varphi_i(q'_i - q_i)) - A^\gamma(b_i) \times P^\delta(b_i) \times \text{price}_i \tag{8}$$

$$IR = A^\gamma(b_i, b_{-i}) \times P^\delta(b_i, b_{-i}) \times \text{price}_i - A^\gamma(b_i) \times \text{price}_i \tag{9}$$

$$\begin{aligned} \max \quad & A^\gamma(b) \times P^\delta(b) \times (\text{price} + W(q-r)) \\ s.t \quad & IR \geq 0 \\ & IC = 0 \end{aligned} \tag{10}$$

In previous mechanism design research based on deep learning, researchers commonly used a sigmoid function as the activation function of the Payment Network to convert the specific payment price into a payment proportion between 0 and 1, which increases the generalization performance and robustness of the model. However, due to the limitations of sigmoid functions, the network does not generate a penalty or incentive payment ratio exceeding 100%.

To solve this problem, this paper introduces the Rigmoid function.

$$Rigmoid = \frac{1}{0.5 + e^{-x}}. \tag{11}$$

Although this expands the payment ratio to between 0 and 2, the payment ratio does not reach an astonishing 200% due to the limitation of IR. It is even possible to create a "win-win space" without infringing the interests of both parties when the utility functions of bidders and auctioneers are significantly different.

As for the output of the Allocation Network, since the allocated probability of an item is at most 1 and there is no case where all bidders are unqualified, we use a simple SoftMax function as the activation function of the output layer of the Allocation Network.

In addition, compared with single-attribute auction research, this paper faces the problem of mapping multiple attributes. As noted above, the auctioneer does not know the bidders' true bids or utility function. It would violate the rule to suppose that multiple attributes are mapped as a single attribute by directly using the utility function of the bidder in the data pre-processing stage. If all the attributes submitted by all bidders were added in the hidden layer without processing, in that case, it would result in (1) slow training due to the increase in network parameters and (2) possible over-fitting.

In order to solve the above two foreseeable problems, this paper created a shared encoder to extract the characteristics of bidders' bids and then output the allocation and payment results that satisfy each bidder of Formulas (5) and (6) with the Allocation Network and Payment Network. Finally, the network is used for optimization according to the feedback of Formulas (5) and (6), and the auctioneer's income. In this paper, the multi-attribute bidding of each bidder has the same nature, so it can be processed by sharing weights. A four-layer MLP (Multi-Layer Perceptron) module was built. This module was placed before the Allocation and Payment Networks to extract the original $\{G\ items, N\ bids, t+1\ attributes\}$ data into the features of $\{G\ items, N\ bidders\}$.

*4.3. Model Adjustment*

Multi-attribute auctions are complex. To demonstrate the effectiveness of the MLN method, we chose the "Yili" case with rich parameters for the experiments [24]. It is an auction of about 100 units of dairy transportation rights with detailed information on the auctioneer (shipper) and bidders (carriers) (carrier's shipping cost ($cost_i$), shipping time ($time_i$), damage rate during shipping ($det_i$), and carrier's shipping capacity ($cap_i$)) (Table 1); three preferences for bidding attributes (cases 1, 2, 3); and two preferences for time requirements (cases A, B) (Table 2). The shipper expects that shipping time $t_a$ is completed within 5 days, and the deterioration rate ($m_a$) of shipping dairy products is less than 5%. The bidders' delivery performance impacts the auctioneer's costs, and the revised cost is

$$S = \sum_i cost_i + \Delta t \times t_i + \Delta m \times m_i \tag{12}$$

where $\Delta m_i = m_i - m_a$. The revised costs are subsequently deemed to be the auctioneer's costs.

**Table 1.** Bidders' information.

| Attribute | a1 | a2 | a3 | a4 | a5 | a6 | a7 | a8 | a9 |
|---|---|---|---|---|---|---|---|---|---|
| Cost (USD 100) | 9.5 | 9 | 10 | 10 | 7 | 8 | 9.5 | 9 | 8.5 |
| Transportation time (day) | 5 | 4 | 2 | 3 | 6 | 8 | 6 | 4 | 7 |
| Deteriorate rate (percent) | 5 | 6 | 4 | 2 | 7 | 6 | 3 | 1 | 7 |
| Capacity (truckload) | 30 | 25 | 20 | 30 | 35 | 20 | 25 | 30 | 30 |

**Table 2.** Auction settings based on auctioneer's preference.

| Case A | $\Delta ti = 2 \times (\max\{0, (ti - ta)\}) - 2 \times (\max\{0, (ta - ti)\})$ (focus on speed) |
|---|---|
| Case B | $\Delta ti = |ti - ta|^{0.5}$ (focus on punctuality) |
| Case 1 | $W_{\text{time}} = 0.1, W_{\text{Deteriorate rate}} = 0.1$ (focus on cost) |
| Case 2 | $W_{\text{time}} = 2, W_{\text{Deteriorate rate}} = 0.1$ (focus on time) |
| Case 3 | $W_{\text{time}} = 0.1, W_{\text{Deteriorate rate}} = 2$ (focus on service quality) |

As mentioned above, the model's loss function should be composed of three constraints, auctioneer expenditure, IC, and IR, which is different from the conventional model training process. In addition, in the "YILI" case, each bidder has transportation capacity limitations. Using the SoftMax function in the output layer of the Allocation Network is likely to output results that exceed the capabilities of bidders.

Constructing several loss functions can solve these problems. In this case, the higher the payment ratio of the bidder, the higher the auctioneer's expenses. Therefore, maximizing the expected revenue is changed to minimizing the expected fees ($p_0$) (Formula (13)).

$$\min p_0 = A^\gamma(b) \times P^\delta(b) \times S_i \tag{13}$$

$ext_i$ stands for the extra benefits that bidders obtain by misreporting (Formula (14)). $ext_i$ is used to limit the motivation of bidders to "lie" and ensure that bidders do not lose money in the auction as much as possible.

$$ext_i = \text{ReLu}\left(A^\gamma(b'_i, b_i) \times P^\delta(b'_i, b_i) \times \text{price}'_i - A^\gamma(b_i) \times P^\delta(b_i) \times \text{price}_i\right) \tag{14}$$

$def_i$ is a new IR constraint, which means that the deficit calculation function of the profit part is weakened (Formula (15)).

$$def_i = \text{LeakyReLu}\left(A^\gamma(b'_i) \times \text{price}'_i - A^\gamma(b'_i) \times P^\delta(b'_i) \times \text{price}'_i\right) \tag{15}$$

$rev_i$ measures whether the allocation result is over-allocate (OA). Then, it is necessary to determine which loss function to use to optimize the model based on the priority of OA = IR = IC > goal (Figure 2).

$$rev_i = \text{ReLu}(A^\gamma(b_i) \times 100 - \text{Capacity}) \tag{16}$$

Bidders explore how to adjust misreport $b'_i$ under the rules during the auction process to pursue higher profits. The problem is solved by calculating the gradient of the bidding content based on the earnings from misreports.

$$\nabla_{b'_i} A^\gamma(b'_i, b_i) \times P^\delta(b'_i, b_i) \times \text{price}_i \tag{17}$$

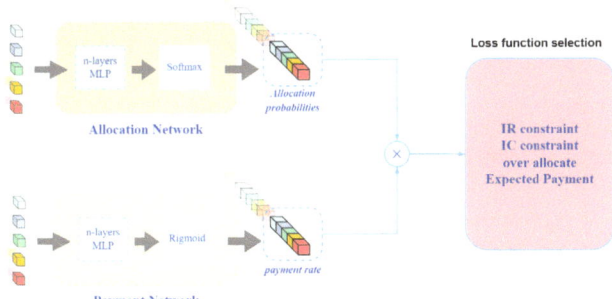

**Figure 2.** The network state is judged according to the loss function; then, the corresponding loss function is selected to optimize the network.

The training process of the MLN model is described below.

| Training Process |
|---|
| **hyper-parameters:** learning rate of the Network $\eta = 0.0001$, learning rate of updating misreport $\xi = 0.01$, batch size = 20, Penalty weight $\rho > 0$ |
| **Initialize:** Lagrange multipliers $\lambda, \mu, \nu \in \{R\}$, network parameters $\gamma, \delta \in \{R\}$ |
| For 0 to data size/batch size: |
|     Batch B = $\{b^1, b^2, \ldots, b^{20}\}$ |
|     For 0 to B |
|         Input true bid $b_i$ into Allocation and Payment Network $\rightarrow A^\gamma(b), P$ |
|         Update misreport $b'_i$ by calculating $b_i$ gradient: |
|         $b'_i = b'_i - \xi \nabla_{b'_i} A^\gamma(b'_i, b_i) \times P^\delta(b'_i, b_i) \times \text{price}_i$ |
|         Input misreport $b'_i$ into Allocation and Payment Network $\rightarrow A^\gamma(b'_i), P^\delta(b'_i)$ |
|         Calculate revised cost: $S = \sum_i \cos_i + \Delta t \times t_i + \Delta m \times m_i$<br>        Calculate the bidder's deficit $def$ (15).<br>        Calculate the additional benefit bidders gain by misrepresenting $ext$ (14).<br>        Calculate the degree to which the allocation results exceed the bidder's transportation capacity $rev$ (16). |
|         loss function judgment: |
|             if $def > 0$: $loss = def$ |
|             else if $ext > 0$: $loss = ext$ |
|             else if $rev > 0$: $loss = rev$ |
|             else: $loss = p_0$ (13) |
|         loss.backward() |
|         Updating model |

## 5. Experiments

The range of data attributes was determined with reference to Table 1:

$$\text{cost}_i \sim \frac{1}{2} \times U_{\text{cost}}[7, 10] \in \mathbb{Z} \tag{18}$$

$$\text{time}_i \sim U_{\text{time}}[2, 8] \in \mathbb{Z} \tag{19}$$

$$\det_i \sim U_{det}[1,7] \in \mathbb{Z} \tag{20}$$

$$\text{cap}_i \sim 4 \times U_{cap}[4,8] \in \mathbb{Z} \tag{21}$$

Then, auction datasets (1), (2), and (3) were generated with uniform distribution, and three experiments were conducted on each dataset corresponding to the same cases (A1, A2, A3) of auction preferences as the original.

(1) One item, nine bidders.

Randomly generated bidder data were used for model training. Then, we used the same information as Zhang as the input data for the model during validation and compared the results of testing with other methods.

Figure 3 and Table 3 show that the performance of the rules generated with the MLN method in terms of time and deterioration rate was similar to that of the method by Zhang and was subject to IC constraints. In case A1, the auctioneer had a low weight of 0.1 for both time and deterioration rate, which had little impact on the correction cost function. MLN maintained a good level of time and deterioration rate and reduced expenses for auctioneers by approximately 55 (USD 100) without causing deficits to bidders.

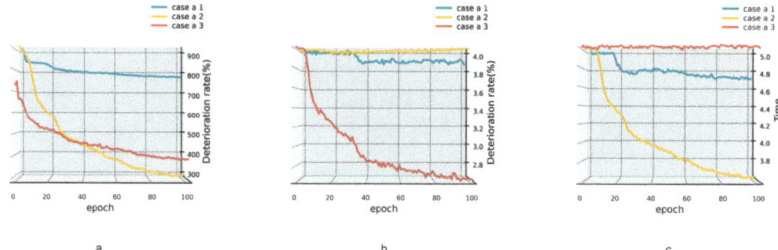

**Figure 3.** Experimental results. (**a**) Auctioneer's expenditure results caused by the model's output rules during training under three case settings. (**b**) Time results. (**c**) Deterioration rate results.

**Table 3.** Results of experiment (1).

|  | A1 | | | A2 | | | A3 | | |
| --- | --- | --- | --- | --- | --- | --- | --- | --- | --- |
|  | Ours | Zhang | P-VCG [25] | Ours | Zhang | P-VCG | Ours | Zhang | P-VCG |
| Time (day) | 5.64 | 5.5 | 6.25 | 3.78 | 3.25 | 6.25 | 4.24 | 3.75 | 6.25 |
| Deterioration (%) | 5.6 | 5 | 5.25 | 3.6 | 3.25 | 5.25 | 2.7 | 2.5 | 5.25 |
| Cost | 848.50 | 904 | 937 | 441.86 | 884 | 1469 | 483.72 | 918.5 | 1108 |
| IC | 0 | 0 | None | 0 | 0 | None | 0 | 0 | None |

In case A2, the time and deterioration rate weights were 2 and 0.1, respectively, due to the auctioneer's preference for time being "faster is better" and four out of nine bidders having transportation times shorter than $ta = 5$ days, which could create more revenue for the auctioneer. This gave the MLN method a better chance at improving performance, ultimately resulting in a reduction of more than half in the revised cost of the auctioneer. In case A3, the time and deterioration rate weights were 0.1 and 2, respectively. The revised cost was higher than that in case A2, for the magnification of $\Delta mi$ was smaller than $\Delta ti$, but our method still made significant progress.

The MLN method could achieve good time and deterioration rates and reduce expenses for auctioneers under all three preferences. The reason is that it did not transfer the profits obtained thanks to the bidder's good performance to the bidder, and it can be seen that the bidder had no deficit in the auction and received an higher average price than the bid. Overall, the auction rules generated by the model are sustainable and can significantly reduce auctioneers' expenses.

The mechanism design of multi-attribute, multi-item auctions is complex. To further expand the experiment, the original numbers of items and participants were modified to demonstrate the robustness of the MLN model and its contribution to multi-attribute, multi-item auctions.

(2) Three items, nine bidders.

The number of items was increased to three. The experiment used randomly generated data that followed the data distribution for model training (Figure 4) and testing and presented the last epoch's results (Table 4).

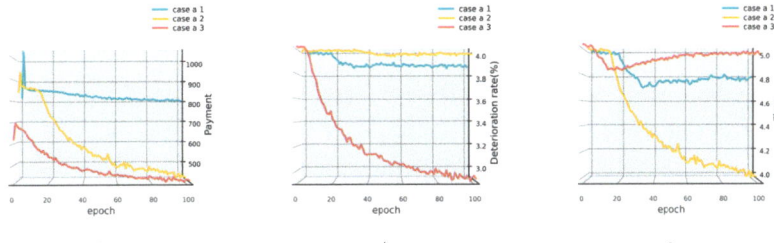

**Figure 4.** Experimental results. (**a**) Auctioneer's expenditure results caused by the model's output rules during training under three case settings. (**b**) Time results. (**c**) Deterioration rate results.

**Table 4.** Results of experiment (2).

|  | A1 | A2 | A3 |
| --- | --- | --- | --- |
| Time | 4.79 | 3.89 | 4.92 |
| Deterioration rate (%) | 3.90 | 3.96 | 2.96 |
| Payment (USD 100) | 804.86 | 385.15 | 450.85 |
| IR | −13.2 | −15.3 | −37.3 |
| IC | 0 | 0 | 0 |

Similar to experiment (1), the average expenditure of auctioneers under the three cases was the same as the trend in (1) due to the weights of time and damage rate preferences. After increasing the number of items, MLN also achieved good results. It was found that the average cost of testing results was relatively lower than that obtained using nine-bidder original data because there was a strong correlation between the transportation time and damage rate of bidders in the original dataset, unlike in random bidding generated based on the distribution.

(3) Four items, seven bidders.

To further test the generalization performance of MLN, this paper conducted experiments on four items and seven bidders. The bidder data were still random, followed the same distribution, and were used during testing.

It was noticed that compared with the setting of nine bidders, the experimental performance of seven bidders was slightly inferior (Table 5), especially in cases A2 and A3, where the average payment of the auctioneer in experiment (3) increased compared with experiment (2) (Figure 5). The reason is that as the number of bidders increases, the bidding base conducive to auctioneers also increases relatively.

**Table 5.** Results of experiment (3).

|  | A1 | A2 | A3 |
|---|---|---|---|
| Time | 4.81 | 4.36 | 4.93 |
| Deterioration rate (%) | 3.91 | 3.99 | 3.32 |
| Payment (USD 100) | 817.76 | 595.60 | 508.24 |
| IR | −19.26 | −24.04 | −6.22 |
| IC | 0 | 0 | 0 |

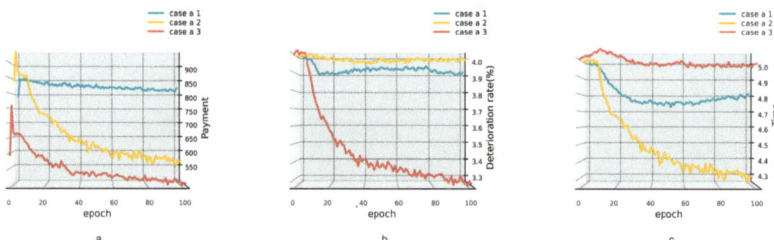

**Figure 5.** Experimental results. (**a**) Auctioneer's expenditure results caused by the model's output rules during training under three case settings. (**b**) Time results. (**c**) Deterioration rate results.

## 6. Conclusions

This paper proposes a dual network based on multi-scale loss and shared modules that encodes the inputs of multiple attributes of bidders into a single feature, solving the problem of incomplete information and computation in designing multi-attribute mechanisms. The scene settings for multi-attribute auctions are complex and diverse. In the experimental phase, the post-paid "YILI" case was used. The loss function of the network was adjusted according to the limit of the number of bidders allocated, and the model significantly reduced the expenditure of the auctioneer. Subsequently, in the expansion experiment, the model also performed well when dealing with different combinations of bidders, and numbers of bidders and items, demonstrating its generalization performance and robustness.

**Author Contributions:** Conceptualization, Z.Z. and C.C.; methodology, Z.Z.; software, Z.Z.; validation, S.Z. and H.C.; formal analysis, H.M.; investigation, H.M.; resources, H.M.; data curation, Z.Z.; writing—original draft preparation, Z.Z.; writing—review and editing, C.C.; visualization, H.C. and H.M.; supervision, C.C.; project administration, C.C.; funding acquisition, S.Z. and H.M. All authors have read and agreed to the published version of the manuscript.

**Funding:** This research was funded by (1) OST-FDCT projects 0058/2019/AMJ Research and Application of Cooperative Multi-Agent Platform for Zhuhai-Macau Manufacturing Service, and (2) Research and Development fund by Wuyi University, Hong Kong and Macau (2019WGAlH21).

**Conflicts of Interest:** We declare that we have no financial and personal relationships with other people or organizations that can inappropriately influence our work, and there are no professional or other personal interests of any nature or kind in any product, service, and/or company.

## References

1. Liu, X.; Yu, C.; Zhang, Z.; Zheng, Z.; Rong, Y.; Lv, H.; Huo, D.; Wang, Y.; Chen, D.; Xu, J.; et al. Neural auction: End-to-end learning of auction mechanisms for e-commerce advertising. In Proceedings of the 27th ACM SIGKDD Conference on Knowledge Discovery & Data Mining, Singapore, 14–18 August 2021; pp. 3354–3364.
2. Pham, L.; Teich, J.; Wallenius, H.; Wallenius, J. Multi-attribute online reverse auctions: Recent research trends. *Eur. J. Oper. Res.* **2015**, *242*, 1–9. [CrossRef]
3. Myerson, R.B. Optimal auction design. *Math. Oper. Res.* **1981**, *6*, 58–73. [CrossRef]

4. Dütting, P.; Feng, Z.; Narasimhan, H.; Parkes, D.; Ravindranath, S.S. Optimal auctions through deep learning. In Proceedings of the International Conference on Machine Learning, Long Beach, CA, USA, 10–15 June 2019; pp. 1706–1715.
5. Chen, X.; Diakonikolas, I.; Paparas, D.; Sun, X.; Yannakakis, M. The complexity of optimal multidimensional pricing. In Proceedings of the Twenty-Fifth Annual ACM-SIAM Symposium on Discrete Algorithms, Portland, OR, USA, 5–7 January 2014; pp. 1319–1328.
6. Jap, S.D. The impact of online reverse auction design on buyer–supplier relationships. *J. Mark.* **2007**, *71*, 146–159. [CrossRef]
7. Daskalakis, C.; Deckelbaum, A.; Tzamos, C. The complexity of optimal mechanism design. In Proceedings of the Twenty-Fifth Annual ACM-SIAM Symposium on Discrete Algorithms, Portland, OR, USA, 5–7 January 2014; pp. 1302–1318.
8. Haghpanah, N.; Immorlica, N.; Mirrokni, V.; Munagala, K. Optimal auctions with positive network externalities. *ACM Trans. Econ. Comput. (TEAC)* **2013**, *1*, 1–24. [CrossRef]
9. Conitzer, V.; Sandholm, T. Complexity of mechanism design. *arXiv* **2002**, arXiv:1408.1486.
10. Bai, Y.; Zhou, Z.; Xiao, H.; Gao, R. A Stackelberg reinsurance–investment game with asymmetric information and delay. *Optimization* **2021**, *70*, 2131–2168. [CrossRef]
11. Feng, Z. Machine Learning-Aided Economic Design. Ph.D. Thesis, Harvard University, Cambridge, MA, USA, 2021.
12. Rochet, J.C. A necessary and sufficient condition for rationalizability in a quasi-linear context. *J. Math. Econ.* **1987**, *16*, 191–200. [CrossRef]
13. Feng, Z.; Narasimhan, H.; Parkes, D.C. Deep learning for revenue-optimal auctions with budgets. In Proceedings of the 17th International Conference on Autonomous Agents and Multiagent Systems, Stockholm, Sweden, 10–15 July 2018; pp. 354–362.
14. Peri, N.; Curry, M.; Dooley, S.; Dickerson, J. Preferencenet: Encoding human preferences in auction design with deep learning. *Adv. Neural Inf. Process. Syst.* **2021**, *34*, 17532–17542.
15. Shen, W.; Peng, B.; Liu, H.; Zhang, M.; Qian, R.; Hong, Y.; Guo, Z.; Ding, Z.; Lu, P.; Tang, P. Reinforcement mechanism design: With applications to dynamic pricing in sponsored search auctions. In Proceedings of the AAAI Conference on Artificial Intelligence, New York, NY, USA, 7–12 February 2020; Volume 34, pp. 2236–2243.
16. Zhe, Y.; Ziyuan, Z.; Peng, N. A Deep-Learning-Based Optimal Auction for Vehicular Edge Computing Resource Allocation. In Proceedings of the 2022 IEEE 7th International Conference on Smart Cloud (SmartCloud), Shanghai, China, 8–10 October 2022; pp. 39–46.
17. Ellis, R.D., Jr.; Herbsman, Z.J. *Cost-Time Bidding Concept: An Innovative Approach*; Transportation Research Record: Washington, DC, USA, 1990.
18. Bachrach, Y.; Ceppi, S.; Kash, I.A.; Key, P.; Kurokawa, D. Optimising trade-offs among stakeholders in ad auctions. In Proceedings of the Fifteenth ACM Conference on Economics and Computation, Palo Alto, CA, USA, 8–12 June 2014; pp. 75–92.
19. Zhang, Z.; Liu, X.; Zheng, Z.; Zhang, C.; Xu, M.; Pan, J.; Yu, C.; Wu, F.; Xu, J.; Gai, K. Optimizing Multiple Performance Metrics with Deep GSP Auctions for E-commerce Advertising. In Proceedings of the P14th ACM International Conference on Web Search and Data Mining, Virtual Event, 8–12 March 2021; pp. 993–1001.
20. Staschus, K.; Davidson, J.; Gross, G.; Logan, D.; Perone, S.; Shirmohammadi, D.; Vojdani, A. A multi-attribute evaluation framework for electric resource acquisition in California. *Int. J. Electr. Power Energy Syst.* **1991**, *13*, 73–80. [CrossRef]
21. Chen-Ritzo, C.H.; Harrison, T.P.; Kwasnica, A.M.; Thomas, D.J. Better, faster, cheaper: An experimental analysis of a multiattribute reverse auction mechanism with restricted information feedback. *Manag. Sci.* **2005**, *51*, 1753–1762. [CrossRef]
22. Gupta, A.; Parente, S.T.; Sanyal, P. Competitive bidding for health insurance contracts: Lessons from the online HMO auctions. *Int. J. Health Care Financ. Econ.* **2012**, *12*, 303–322. [CrossRef] [PubMed]
23. Weinberg, S.M.; Zhou, Z. Optimal Multi-Dimensional Mechanisms are not Locally-Implementable. In Proceedings of the 23rd ACM Conference on Economics and Computation, Boulder, CO, USA, 11–15 July 2022; pp. 875–896.
24. Zhang, J.; Xiang, J.; Cheng, T.E.; Hua, G.; Chen, C. An optimal efficient multi-attribute auction for transportation procurement with carriers having multi-unit supplies. *Omega* **2019**, *83*, 249–260. [CrossRef]
25. Parkes, D.C.; Kalagnanam, J. Models for iterative multiattribute procurement auctions. *Manag. Sci.* **2005**, *51*, 435–451. [CrossRef]

**Disclaimer/Publisher's Note:** The statements, opinions and data contained in all publications are solely those of the individual author(s) and contributor(s) and not of MDPI and/or the editor(s). MDPI and/or the editor(s) disclaim responsibility for any injury to people or property resulting from any ideas, methods, instructions or products referred to in the content.

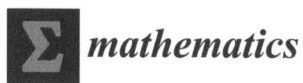 *mathematics*

Article

# Parallel Dense Video Caption Generation with Multi-Modal Features

Xuefei Huang [1], Ka-Hou Chan [1,2], Wei Ke [1,2,*] and Hao Sheng [1,3,4]

1. Faculty of Applied Sciences, Macao Polytechnic University, Macau 999078, China; xuefei.huang@mpu.edu.mo (X.H.); chankahou@mpu.edu.mo (K.-H.C.); shenghao@buaa.edu.cn (H.S.)
2. Engineering Research Centre of Applied Technology on Machine Translation and Artificial Intelligence of Ministry of Education, Macao Polytechnic University, Macau 999078, China
3. State Key Laboratory of Virtual Reality Technology and Systems, School of Computer Science and Engineering, Beihang University, Beijing 100191, China
4. Zhongfa Aviation Institute of Beihang University, 166 Shuanghongqiao Street, Pingyao Town, Yuhang District, Hangzhou 311115, China
* Correspondence: wke@mpu.edu.mo

**Citation:** Huang, X.; Chan, K.-H.; Ke, W.; Sheng, H. Parallel Dense Video Caption Generation with Multi-Modal Features. *Mathematics* 2023, 11, 3685. https://doi.org/10.3390/math11173685

Academic Editor: Zhiming Cai, Wencai Du, Zhihai Wang, Zuobin Ying

Received: 27 July 2023
Revised: 22 August 2023
Accepted: 23 August 2023
Published: 26 August 2023

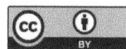

**Copyright:** © 2023 by the authors. Licensee MDPI, Basel, Switzerland. This article is an open access article distributed under the terms and conditions of the Creative Commons Attribution (CC BY) license (https://creativecommons.org/licenses/by/4.0/).

**Abstract:** The task of dense video captioning is to generate detailed natural-language descriptions for an original video, which requires deep analysis and mining of semantic captions to identify events in the video. Existing methods typically follow a localisation-then-captioning sequence within given frame sequences, resulting in caption generation that is highly dependent on which objects have been detected. This work proposes a parallel-based dense video captioning method that can simultaneously address the mutual constraint between event proposals and captions. Additionally, a deformable Transformer framework is introduced to reduce or free manual threshold of hyperparameters in such methods. An information transfer station is also added as a representation organisation, which receives the hidden features extracted from a frame and implicitly generates multiple event proposals. The proposed method also adopts LSTM (Long short-term memory) with deformable attention as the main layer for caption generation. Experimental results show that the proposed method outperforms other methods in this area to a certain degree on the ActivityNet Caption dataset, providing competitive results.

**Keywords:** dense video caption; video captioning; multimodal feature fusion; feature extraction; neural network

**MSC:** 68T45

## 1. Introduction

With the widespread use of video as an information transmission medium, recordings for playback and live broadcasting have become increasingly popular today. Video processing has gradually become a hot research topic in computer vision [1,2]. Video caption generation is an important task that provides understanding and representation of videos between two media: frame-to-text. This task has also involved critical artificial intelligence (AI) technologies [3,4]. Such technologies have potential applications in the development of smart glasses to assist the visually impaired, intelligent commentary on sports events, early childhood education, and the generation of video surveillance reports [5–7].

Dense video captioning tasks mostly use datasets directly crawled from online sources such as YouTube, whose videos typically consist of long content without pruning [8]. Unlike traditional video captioning, which uses concise sentences to explain the video content, dense video captioning requires not only dividing long videos into various events, but also describing the behaviours in a series of events as accurate as possible. The objective of dense video captioning is to generate as detailed and general description for videos clearly.

A cross domain method is required to perform such video analysis and comprehension, so as to represent the events as sentences. In practice, the video is always based on a sequence of frames of fast-playing images that also contain important audio information usable in the captioning. Therefore, the computer needs to perform a high-level understanding of the video content, aiming to localise/categorise the interesting objects, then represent their motion and behaviour in detail.

Reviewing previous achievements, the process of generating dense video captions can be summarised into two main procedures: dividing event regions and generating descriptive sentences, as shown in Figure 1a. There are different orders to arrange the video localisation and description, mostly following a sequential top-down or bottom-up structure. Inevitably, this makes the generation of captions more dependent on the quality of the previous steps [9–12]. In other words, the performance of the generated descriptions can decrease if the former module does not perform well, and the complexity of the module design is less relevant. Moreover, these methods are not trained end-to-end in the traditional sense and require additional steps for extensive and complicated training, which also affects the results to a certain extent. The parallel method shown in Figure 1b defines dense video caption generation as a set of prediction tasks and decodes the divided events and sentences simultaneously, which solves the problem of dependence on previous results [13]. Although this type of method has produced good results, there are still bottlenecks in the decoding branch that limit the fine-grained description of the video. Therefore, further improvement is necessary.

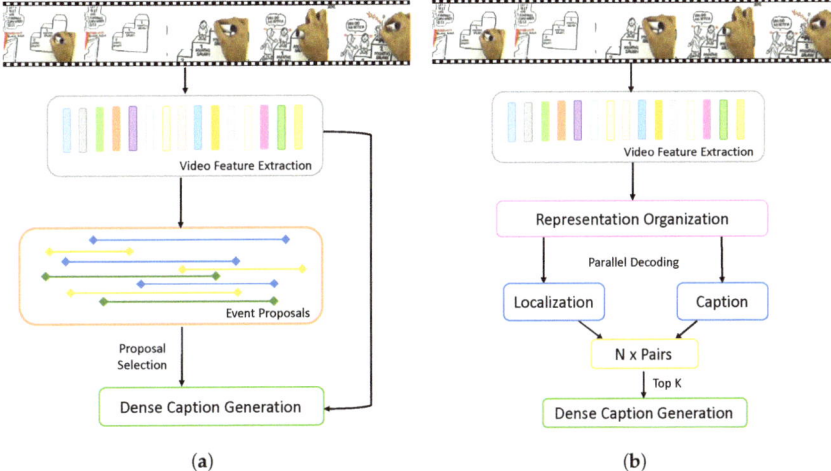

**Figure 1.** Comparison between existing methods and the parallel method. (**a**) Localise-then-describe method. (**b**) Parallel method.

This work builds on previous research and further explores the techniques to alleviate the fine-grained bottleneck that arises when generating dense video captions in parallel. Additionally, this approach fully exploits the multi-modal features of videos. The main contributions are summarised below:

- A novel model for video caption generation is proposed, which effectively utilises the visual–audio features. Unlike the common conventional sequential mechanism of localise-then-describe approach, the proposed model reasonably associates the proposal and caption modules through parallel paths, which enhances the comprehensiveness of the textual expression.
- In addition, a simplified method is proposed to eliminate the redundancy generated by the anchor mechanism on which the maximum suppression algorithm relies and to reduce the steps of manually setting hyperparameters for end-to-end training of the model.

- The decoding side introduces the representation organisation module as intermediate information for event localisation and description and extracts temporal boundary information from the video to generate all potential events.

## 2. Related Work

In early years of video captioning, the main approach was to use template matching to generate logical and specific sentences through keyword sorting or selection. However, this approach only supported simple sentence structures and was inflexible for complex event representation, making it poor for understanding multiple scenes in long videos [14]. With the development of powerful neural networks, deep learning approaches using artificial intelligence (AI) have become possible for extracting multimedia information, marking a milestone in the field of video captioning [15]. Inspired by image captioning methods, such technology can be directly extended to video captioning, enabling the discovery of correlations between image sequences [16–18]. For dense video captioning tasks, significant breakthroughs have been made in the generation of detailed and rich descriptive sentences for event representation. Deep learning in image processing has shown that the Sequence-to-Sequence (Seq2Seq) framework can be applied to video captioning [3,19]. This framework consists of two neural network models over an encoder and a decoder. Most of the input videos use CNN-based network models such as VGGNet [20], VGGreNet [21], or ResNet [22] for the encoder. Conversely, the decoder uses RNN-based network models to generate native sentences for the final output. This encoder–decoder design projects visual features into text sentences, extracting important abstract information and discarding noise in the application [23].

In recent years, attention mechanisms have shown outstanding performance when integrated into various neural models. They have the potential to play a prominent role in image captioning and are increasingly used to address the problem of video captioning [24,25]. Dense video captioning involves visual understanding processes that locate different events in a video and generate descriptive captions for each interesting object. This approach represents video content in detail by transforming frame sequences into multiple descriptive sentences among multiple clips in a long video [26–28]. In the research of Shen et al. [29], dense image captioning is migrated to the video field by combining the multi-scale suggestion module and a visual context perception mechanism. Additionally, Huang et al. in their work [30] divide the long video into several different regional sequences and comprehensively express the video content. However, the feature extraction of regions within the frame sequence is a complicated process in the Seq2Seq framework. It is not an end-to-end method in the traditional sense, and extensive hyperparameters may be required for the input of a non-fixed length video. Furthermore, if too many small regions are split within a shot, it becomes difficult to represent the entire video and to categorise objects within specific regions, making it difficult to discover their correlations.

Since a video can be considered as a sequence of images with an additional time dimension, multiple scene events can occur, and objects can appear and perform actions within a range of frames. To address the neglected time series problem in video more comprehensively, Tran et al. [5] introduced a 3D CNN approach for extracting video features. An advanced model, C3D, was developed based on the 3D CNN, which can handle more complex cases in terms of various scenes [1,31–33]. In addition, Carreira et al. [34] added optical flow features in the encoder part, combined with C3D to form a new Inflated 3D ConvNet (I3D) model, which enhanced the quality of the extracted video features to a certain extent. Qiu et al. [35] and others took advantages of the residual connection's ability to deepen the convolutional network, decomposed the 3D video features into a 2D spatial convolution and a 1D temporal convolution, and constructed a Pseudo-3D Residual Network (P3D) that greatly reduced the need for labelled video data, increased the network's depth, and reduced the amount of convolutional computation.

To enhance the capability of feature extraction, it is important to improve the caption generation module. Caption generation methods use advanced NLP technology such as

LSTM [36], BERT [37], Transformer [38], and other variants [39], which have been applied to video captioning with competitive results [40]. In the approach of Pasunuru et al. [41], a multi-task learning method is proposed that uses LSTM to share parameters between different tasks and improve model performance with more data. Additionally, Shetty et al. [42] used an improved deep LSTM in the decoding section, trained on two different video features, and used an evaluation network to judge video features and generated sentence keywords to improve sentence quality. The EEDVC model, the first to encode video features using Transformer, solves the problem of long-term dependence in LSTM [43]. It converts each extracted proposal into a mask, combines it with video features, and completes the end-to-end training of the model.

In addition, Yao et al. [44] applied the attention mechanism in NLP to the video captioning task. They introduced the attention weight $\alpha$ based on the codec structure. It is different from the attention to region in image captioning but is used to compute different features of a video along the time sequence. This approach allows the decoder to automatically select a more relevant time period when generating words, helping the model filter out irrelevant information and reduce the workload, ultimately improving the evaluation index.

The captioning and event generation modules in the method described above can only be trained independently. However, the results of the captioning module can theoretically be used to train the proposal process. In order to improve the localise-then-describe scheme and fully exploit the two subtasks of event localisation and caption generation, Li et al. [11] proposed a bridging idea using desperation regression to link the two subtasks. This approach allows the prediction of description complexity in the proposal module. The caption module captures video features and achieves the goal of jointly training the two subtasks. However, since many generated sentences are redundant and produce inconsistent results, it is necessary to use Non-Maximum Suppression (NMS) [45] or an Event Sequence Generation Network (ESGN) [9] to select the proposal. These modules introduce many hyperparameters and are highly dependent on manual thresholding strategies, which can affect the model results. The PDVC model [46] proposed a parallel decoding method to address these issues. By designing two parallel prediction heads (localisation head and caption head), both the scope and text description of the event query are predicted. This approach allows the PDVC to directly use the video features to match the split target events, thus providing more unique features. Experiments have shown that the parallel design can make the loss of the caption module improve the performance of event localisation. Furthermore, the absence of thresholding and NMS mechanisms makes model training more efficient. Li et al. proposed a transfer learning method that can simultaneously utilise knowledge from two types of source domains, spatial appearance and temporal motion, and transfer them to the target domain [47]. The core of the CMG-AAL [48] model is a cross-modal foundation module that is composed of two complementary attention mechanisms, which can effectively establish correspondence between text and vision, thereby improving the model's understanding and generation capabilities.

Furthermore, existing methods for analysing and understanding video content mostly rely on visual features, without taking into account clues provided by other modalities such as sound or subtitles [49]. However, incorporating other modalities can help computers understand video content and produce more detailed text descriptions. For instance, in a video of a female announcer broadcasting, the content of the broadcast may not be clear without sound. To address this issue, Jin et al. [50] developed a model that combined multiple types of features by extracting them separately, weighting the average, and, finally, fusing them together as the input for LSTM. This model aims to make full use of more comprehensive feature information to represent videos and proposes a new approach to using multi-modal features to improve the quality of video captions. Other models, such as EMVC [51] and BMT [52], have also proposed methods for incorporating audio features. The EMVC model integrates audio features to support visual cues in event generation, while the BMT model extracts feature vectors for both video and audio using I3D and

VGGish, respectively, and uses a Transformer framework to improve the quality of the generated text.

Having reviewed the existing work, it suggests that there is still room for improvement in the relationship between video event localisation and text description. Currently, there are bottlenecks in the branch of parallel decoding methods, and the auxiliary function of multi-modal features is equally important. However, due to the challenge of unifying different video lengths, the calculation of the number of contained events remains difficult. Therefore, developing a method for the computer to use the characteristics of multi-modal data in the video and to fully consider the connection between the two subtasks of event localisation and caption generation is still a challenging task.

## 3. Methodology

For an unedited video, the task of dense video captioning is to divide multiple events in the video and generate corresponding description sentences. In order to fully exploit the correlation between caption and event proposals, as well as the multi-modal features of the video to improve the efficiency of text description generation, we design a parallel multi-modal dense video caption generation model.

### 3.1. Model Overview

The entire framework and the data flow between the various parts in the schematic diagram are shown in Figure 2.

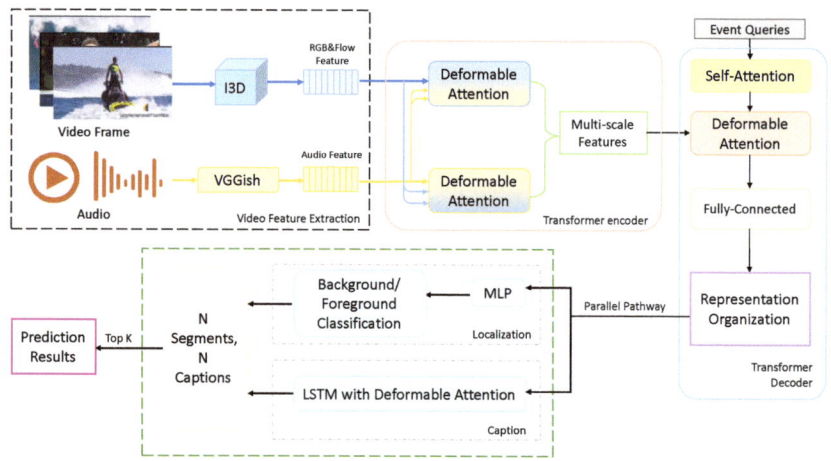

**Figure 2.** Overall framework of the proposed model.

The proposed model uses pre-trained I3D and VGGish to extract the visual and audio features of the video, respectively. It then merges the encoded multi-scale video features into a more characteristic feature set based on the deformable Transformer encoder and decoder framework [53]. Such a representation organisation allows for a more intuitive understanding of the core context of the video. In addition, the model inputs the video features into the captioning and positioning modules in parallel, rather than directly performing proposal localisation and generating captions from the video features in sequence. Finally, the model selects multiple sets of proposal-caption pairs with higher confidence to ensure content integrity and produces more logical and detailed video captions.

### 3.2. Video Encoder

The video encoding process consists of two parts: a multi-modal feature extraction component and a position encoder. The convolutional network is responsible for extracting feature information from the video, while a sequence data encoder based on the Transformer framework is used to understand the information association between contexts.

### 3.2.1. Feature Extraction

In order to enhance the use of multi-modal information in videos, the work decided to incorporate audio features based on the findings of visual modality research. To extract the features of each modality separately, the work used the proven pre-trained combination of I3D and VGGish.

For the visual modality feature extraction, the work chose the I3D network, which can solve the problem of 2D CNN not being able to extract spatial features in videos and adapt to video inputs of different lengths and resolutions by adjusting the network structure and output characteristics accordingly. I3D is constructed by expanding 2D CNN into 3D CNN, which can inherit the knowledge and parameters learned by 2D cellular neural networks in image classification and recognition tasks, without the need for training from scratch. Compared with some other models (such as C3D with only 8 layers), the 20 layers of I3D have a deeper and more complex network structure, including a multi-branch structure composed of multiple convolutional kernels of different sizes, which can capture features at different scales and reduce the number of parameters and computational costs. The I3D network can not only process RGB features, but also optical flow features and average the outputs of the two networks during testing, thus integrating colour information and motion information. Therefore, it can extract spatial features present in videos better than other options.

For audio modality feature selection, we use VGGish to extract the features, which has a strong generalisation ability with pre-trained parameters and can effectively transform audio features into feature vectors that conform to natural language logic. In our work, VGGish converts audio into 128-dimensional semantic feature vectors, which have stronger expressiveness with high-level feature vectors.

### 3.2.2. Feature Encoding

Previous methods have attempted to concatenate features with common weights, but this has proven to be insufficient. It is not possible to fuse them together because the visual and audio features have different dimensions extracted form a video. To address this issue, the work introduced the deformable Transformer as a novel component in the proposed model. The deformable Transformer can distinguish different attention heads in the framework, thereby improving the model expressive and generalisation abilities. Among them, deformable sampling locations are introduced into the pre-filtering mechanism to reduce computational complexity and memory consumption, while maintaining efficient information transmission. The deformable Transformer uses deformable attention to replace the self-attention module in the encoding part of traditional Transformers, as well as the cross-attention class module in the decoding part. This allows the model to better capture long-distance dependencies and local details in the sequence, thereby improving performance. This process can be thought of as converting video features from a video sequence to a set sequence, which is essentially a learnable positional coding. The deformable Transformer encodes the position of the extracted multi-modal video features, unfolds pixels into a one-dimensional sequence, and computes the correlation between pixels; thus, the global information of the video is fully learned. To better exploit the multi-scale features in event prediction, the work added $L$ timescale convolutional layers to obtain feature sequences spanning multiple resolutions. The multi-scale deformable attention module helps alleviate the convergence problem of self-attention by focusing on the sparse space near the reference point.

Let $X$ be the set of feature maps, given by

$$X = \left\{ x^l \right\}_{l=1}^{L}, \tag{1}$$

where each multi-scale feature map $x^l$, with size $x^l$ is $C \times H^l \times W^l$, is extracted from the feature map output in the previous stage for $1 \leq l \leq L$. A projection matrix $H_{milt}$ is used to project the sample offset into the features. The $H_{milt}$ matrix is associated with a linear operator, expressed as the offset of the $t$-th sampling point of the $i$-th query element on the $l$-th scale in the $m$-th attention head,

$$H_{milt} = \phi_l(\hat{p}_i) + \Delta p_{milt}, \qquad (2)$$

where $\hat{p}_i$ is the coordinate of the reference point of each query element $q_i$ in the $[0,1]^2$ space, $\phi_l$ is a function that converts the normalised reference point to the input feature map at the $l$-th layer, and $\Delta p_{milt}$ is a sampling offset that is derived from a linear transformation on the query element.

Then, the deformable Transformer is used to understand the long-distance associations of different segments in long videos and output multi-scale video features. The Multi-Scale Deformable Attention (MSDAttn) dynamically adjusts sampling positions and attention weights by using learnable offsets, allowing for adaptive allocation of attention resources based on the characteristics and needs of the data. MSDAttn can also reduce computational complexity and memory consumption by sampling sparsity, improving the running speed and performance of the model. The traditional attention mechanism requires fully connected operations on all input features, which leads to an exponential increase in computational and storage capacity as the input features increase. This uses deformable convolutional kernels to sparsely sample input features, selecting only a portion of important features for attention calculation, greatly reducing computational and storage costs.

$$\text{MSDAttn}(q_i, \hat{p}_i, X) = \sum_{m=1}^{M} W_m \left( \sum_{l=1}^{L} \sum_{t=1}^{T} A_{milt} \cdot W'_m X H_{milt} \right), \qquad (3)$$

where, the MSDAttn module samples $L$ points from multi-scale feature maps, instead of sampling $T$ points from single-scale feature maps. The $m$ denotes attention heads, $M$ is the number of heads, $t$ denotes sampling keys, and $T$ is the total number of sampling keys ($T \leq HW$), and $A_{milt}$ represents the attention weight of the $t$-th sampling point in the $m$-th attention head, which is calculated by using *softmax* on the query feature $q_i$.

### 3.3. Video Decoder

In the decoder section, the work used the deformable Transformer to decode video features at multiple scales. These features are then fed in parallel to the localisation and captioning modules. As an intermediate information hub, the work also constructed a representation organisation module that receives video temporal features and implicitly generates multiple event proposals.

#### 3.3.1. Feature Decoding

The work incorporated the query mechanism and set prediction loss from the DETR framework for object detection into the video captioning domain during the decoding phase. The input query is a learnable vector or parameter that represents an initial estimate of the event location at the input layer, which is then updated and optimised by attention at each decoding layer. The output queries are considered as the representations of $N$ events, with each output token from the decoder corresponding to a potential event. Therefore, all tokens predict a set of events without changing the meaning of the original text. Moreover, the work also included a module for organising representations prior to the parallel method. This module serves as intermediate information for event localisation and sentence generation. Representation organisation uses a feed-forward neural network to identify the most important features in a spatio-temporal context and generate all the possible proposal representations. Each representation becomes the central information of the event, including the timestamps and sentences.

It is important to note that the input event query is used to replace the anchor. This method is learnable and allows the model to automatically identify regions in the image that may contain objects, with a capacity of up to 100 such regions. Then, using a bipartite graph matching method, valid prediction boxes are filtered from the 100 prediction boxes, and the loss function is calculated. Therefore, the event query is equivalent to replacing the anchor with a learnable method that avoids generating a large number of invalid boxes that result from using the anchor.

The number of input event queries can be controlled, which limits the maximum number of proposals the model can generate. This may result in a low recall rate if the number of queries is set too low, which may affect the accuracy of the subsequent positioning module and result in the loss of important information. In turn, although it may improve the recall rate to some extent if the number of queries is set too high, it reduces the accuracy rate of the title generation module, resulting in repeated words or unnatural language logic. Therefore, the number of event queries must be carefully considered and counted to ensure the best possible results.

$$N_{set} = argmax(v_{len}), \qquad (4)$$

where the $v_{len}$ represents a fixed-size feature vector for prediction. By using the deformable Transformer in combination with the event query during decoding, this work can more accurately divide the extreme point regions of object boundaries, resulting in more precise event edge detection and can accelerate the network training by focusing on sparse spatial locations and combining multi-scale feature representations.

### 3.3.2. Parallel Pathway

The query features and reference enhanced by the representation organisation are sent to the localisation and captioning proposal modules in parallel. This is followed by a one-to-one matching process and filtering to select the combination that best matches the actual video content to achieve dense video captioning.

Localisation Module

The primary objective of this module is to match the output of the representation organisation module to the video on a one-to-one basis and to determine the centre and timestamp of the event proposal. The work used a multi-layer perceptron for box prediction, which involves regression of the event boundary and binary classification of foreground and background. In box prediction, the work calculates the relative offset of the reference point from the actual ground and determines the centre and duration of the event. The purpose of binary classification is to generate a confidence score for the foreground of each event proposal. The final output time proposal consists of the start time $t_i^{star}$, the end time $t_i^{end}$, and the confidence of the location proposal $c_i^{loc}$.

Caption Module

The captioning module allows the model to focus on video frames that are highly correlated with the output words. This helps mine fine-grained interactions between words and video frames. Most traditional methods rely on LSTM with soft attention to generate captions. This allows the importance of each element to be dynamically determined by restricting the attentional field to event proposals and ensures that the generated words are all contained in the same event for sentence and video matching. However, the work wants to use a parallel method for this task and cannot rely directly on the information from the positioning module. If the work used the above method, the association between the reference text and the video would be lost. Therefore, the work proposed to use deformable soft attention combined with LSTM to generate captions, as shown in Figure 3.

By using deformable soft attention, a reference point can be predicted for each input query as the reference position of the centre point of the event proposal, and the weight of the sampling point can be calculated to limit the event to a more precise region. Specifically, the hidden state $h_{it}$ of LSTM at the $t$-th moment is given by

$$h_{it} = \text{LSTM}\left(w_{i,t-1}, h_{i,t-1}, \widetilde{q}_{i,t-1}\right), \quad (5)$$

where $w_{i,t-1}$ is the word generated at the previous moment, and $\widetilde{q}_{i,t-1}$ is the event query output by the representation organisation. Then, take $[h_{it}, \widetilde{q}_i]$ as the query in deformable soft attention to obtain the context feature $z_{it}$,

$$z_{it} = \text{DSAttn}([h_{it}, \widetilde{q}_i]), \quad (6)$$

and the output features $z_{it}$ are restricted to a relatively small region to narrow down the scope of event proposals. Next, LSTM takes $z_{it}$, $w_{i,t-1}$, and $\widetilde{q}_i$ in series as input to obtain the generated $t$-th word $w_{it}$ and calculates the probability distribution $p$ of the word $w_{it}$ in the entire vocabulary,

$$p(w_{it} \mid w_{i,t-1}) = \text{Softmax}(w_{i,t-1}, z_{it}, \widetilde{q}_i). \quad (7)$$

According to the probability distribution $p$, the embedded word sequence can be continuously sampled until an End-of-Sentence (<EOS>) symbol is encountered, resulting in a complete sentence.

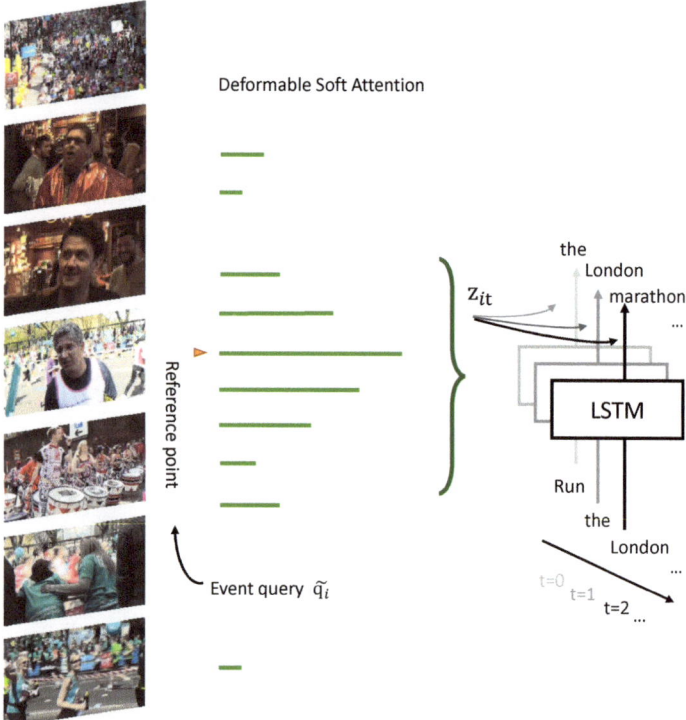

**Figure 3.** LSTM with deformable attention.

### 3.3.3. Caption Generation

The localisation information and captions obtained by the parallel method are combined into a proposal set. This set also requires checking for proposal-caption pairs, similar to the number of event queries introduced in Section 3.2.2. However, too many features for output can lead to redundancy and poor readability, while too few features can lead to missing of important information from the video. To avoid these problems, we perform a bipartite match between $N$ proposals in the proposal set and $K$ captions in the Ground Truth (GT), and measure the difference between the predicted foreground and background regions of the model and the actual annotated regions through the cross-entropy loss function, to obtain proposal-caption pairs. To ensure consistency in semantic information and size, we use the set prediction loss for the calculation, which is the weighted sum of the individual module losses,

$$L = \mu \left( L_{giou} + L_{cls} + L_{cr-e} + L_{cap} \right), \tag{8}$$

where $L_{giou}$ represents the generalised IOU between the generated timestamps and the GT, $L_{cls}$ means the focal loss of binary matching, $L_{cr-e}$ represents the cross-entropy loss between the generated number of event proposals and the GT number, and $L_{cap}$ is the cross-entropy loss between the generated words and the GT words. Based on the calculation result, the work keeps use of the prediction frame with a confidence level higher than the threshold as the final output and obtains a text description that is more suitable for the video content and has an accurate time stamp.

## 4. Experiment

In order to evaluate our newly proposed method for dense video caption generation, this work verifies the performance on the ActivityNet Caption dataset and compares the results with those from the state-of-the-art methods.

### 4.1. Dataset and Data Pre-Processing

The ActivityNet Caption dataset is a publicly available dataset that is widely used for dense video captioning tasks. It covers several domains relevant to our method. The dataset consists of 20 K video clips, each with an average duration of 2 min. Each clip is annotated with the events, including the start and end time of each event, along with a human-written textual description of the event content. The dataset is derived from YouTube videos, but some videos have been removed or altered by their original authors and are not available for direct download. The work used an alternative approach provided by the authors to retrieve the missing videos and obtain a complete dataset. Like most researchers, here, we split the dataset into training, validation, and test sets. The training set contains 10 K clips, the validation set contains 4 K clips, and the test set contains 5 K clips. However, the labels for the test set have not yet been released, so this work used the validation set for experimentation and comparison purposes.

Before training the model, the work preprocessed the reference sentences by converting all letters to lowercase, removing non-text characters, and adding special markers <BOS> and <EOS> at the beginning and end of each sentence. To reduce the impact of large vocabularies and low-frequency words, the work replaced words occurring less than five times with <UNK>. However, this replacement resulted in the loss of some semantic information, also known as the out-of-bag error. This work also added a start token to the decoder input, which allowed the caption to be generated word-by-word until the end marker was reached.

### 4.2. Implementation

Our model was trained on an Ubuntu 20.04 system using two NVIDIA GeForce RTX 3070 GPUs, and the work used PyTorch [54] as the neural network engine. For multi-modal feature extraction, the work followed the approach of BMT [52]. This work used I3D to extract 64 RGB features and 64 optical flow features at 25.0 fps with a size of 224, producing feature vectors with a dimension of 1024. We also used VGGish to extract audio features. The learning rate was set to $1e-4$, and the batch size was 32. The work used a multi-scale deformable attention of size 4 and applied a two-layer deformable Transformer to encode and decode the video features. The hidden layer size of the feed-forward network was set to 2048, and we set the number of event queries to 10. In the caption module, the work set the hidden layer dimension of the LSTM to 512 and the word embedding size to 468.

The work used a dynamic learning rate and set the warm-up steps to 10 epochs, gradually increasing from 0 to $5e-5$. We trained the relation detection with fixed prediction loss and set the learning rate to $5e-4$. This work used the Adam optimiser [55] for the loss function.

*4.3. Results and Analysis*

The work tested our framework by following the implementation details above and performing experiments on the ActivityNet Caption dataset. We compared the results with those obtained by the state-of-the-art methods. This work also performed an ablation study to investigate how different modules in our framework affected the experimental results. Finally, the work presents the results of the qualitative analysis in a visualisation, which provides a clearer picture of the benefits of our proposed framework.

4.3.1. Comparison to the State-of-the-Art

This work contrasted our proposed model with the state-of-the-art methods for the dense video captioning task, consisting of EEDVC [43], DCE [8], MFT [26], WLT [27], SDVC [9], EHVC [31], MDVC [28], BMT [52], EMVC [51], PPVC [13], and PDVC [46]. The contrast results are displayed in Table 1.

**Table 1.** Comparison of the performance of our proposed method with the state-of-the-art methods on the ActivityNet Captions dataset.

| Models | B@1 | B@2 | B@3 | B@4 | METEOR | CIDEr |
|---|---|---|---|---|---|---|
| EEDVC [43] | 9.96 | 4.81 | 2.91 | 1.44 | 6.91 | 9.25 |
| DCE [8] | 10.81 | 4.57 | 1.90 | 0.71 | 5.69 | 12.43 |
| MFT [26] | 13.31 | 6.13 | 2.84 | 1.24 | 7.08 | 21.00 |
| WLT [27] | 10.00 | 4.20 | 1.85 | 0.90 | 4.93 | 13.79 |
| SDVC [9] | **17.92** | 7.99 | 2.94 | 0.93 | 8.82 | - |
| EHVC [31] | - | - | - | 1.29 | 7.19 | 14.71 |
| MDVC [28] | 12.59 | 5.76 | 2.53 | 1.01 | 7.46 | 7.38 |
| BMT [52] | 13.75 | 7.21 | 3.84 | 1.88 | 8.44 | 11.35 |
| EMVC [51] | 14.65 | 7.10 | 3.23 | 1.39 | 9.64 | 13.29 |
| PPVC [13] | 14.93 | 7.40 | 3.58 | 1.68 | 7.91 | 23.02 |
| PDVC [46] | - | - | - | **1.96** | 8.08 | 28.59 |
| **Proposed** | 15.23 | **8.02** | **3.91** | 1.75 | **9.68** | **29.17** |

Bold font indicates the highest result.

As reported in Table 1, $B@N$ is an evaluation metric known as BLEU [56], which measures the quality of translations by comparing the matching degree of $N$-grams in the candidate and reference translations. BLEU is commonly used for text generation tasks in NLP. METEOR [57] is based on BLEU and uses the F-value as the final evaluation metric, taking into account both recall and precision. CIDEr [58] calculates the similarity between candidate and reference sentences, making it suitable for image and video captioning evaluation tasks. Higher quality text descriptions receive higher scores on these evaluation metrics.

The work thoroughly analysed the comparative results based on the evaluation metrics mentioned above. Our proposed method performed slightly worse in $B@1$ and $B@4$, but outperformed other methods in terms of METEOR and CIDEr. The SDVC uses reinforcement learning to train the model, resulting in a higher $B@1$ score compared to all other methods. Furthermore, all our metrics are higher than those of BMT and EMVC, which also use multi-modal features as inputs. This demonstrates the feasibility of using parallel paths to generate textual descriptions. When compared to the two parallel decoding methods of PPVC and PDVC, it can be seen that most of our metrics are slightly higher. It is worth noting that PDVC's input also includes visual and audio features, indicating that our method is still competitive.

### 4.3.2. Ablation Study

The work conducted several comparative experiments to analyse the impact of different components of our proposed model on the output results. This includes comparing the performance of the localisation module, investigating the effect of LSTM with deformable attention on the caption module, and assessing the influence of multi-modal features as inputs on model generation.

Table 2 shows the quality of event localisation on the ActivityNet Captions dataset. Our method achieves a higher F1 score compared to MFT and SDVC. It outperforms the traditional localise-then-describe methods and uses event proposal networks to generate event proposals. Meanwhile, our method uses a representation organisation to filter better quality events and overlays a localisation module to accurately locate event proposals. As a result, our method significantly outperforms MFT on various metrics and achieves better overall results compared to other models. These metrics demonstrate the effectiveness of our proposed localisation module. The @$tIoU$ represents the temporal intersection of the unions, with 4 thresholds of $\{0.3, 0.5, 0.7, 0.9\}$.

**Table 2.** Performance comparison of the localisation module.

| Models | Proposal Network | Recall (@$tIoU$) | | | | | Precision (@$tIoU$) | | | | | F1 |
|---|---|---|---|---|---|---|---|---|---|---|---|---|
| | | 0.3 | 0.5 | 0.7 | 0.9 | avg | 0.3 | 0.5 | 0.7 | 0.9 | avg | |
| MFT [26] | ✓ | 46.18 | 29.76 | 15.54 | 5.77 | 24.31 | 86.34 | 68.79 | 38.30 | 12.19 | 51.41 | 33.01 |
| SDVC [9] | ✓ | **93.41** | 76.40 | 42.42 | 10.10 | 55.58 | 96.71 | 77.73 | **44.84** | 10.99 | 57.57 | 56.56 |
| PPVC [13] | - | 91.71 | 78.90 | **56.73** | 20.60 | 61.98 | 96.23 | 73.80 | 37.66 | 12.31 | 55.07 | 58.33 |
| PDVC [46] | - | 89.47 | 81.91 | 44.63 | 15.67 | 55.42 | **97.16** | 78.09 | 42.68 | 14.40 | 58.07 | 56.71 |
| Ours | - | 90.25 | **81.97** | 48.39 | **20.77** | **63.08** | 95.51 | **79.31** | 39.60 | **15.72** | **59.10** | **58.43** |

Bold font indicates the highest result.

The work compared different methods for the caption module of our model: Vanilla LSTM, LSTM with Soft Attention (SA), and LSTM with Deformable Soft Attention (DSA). The results are shown in Table 3. When generating event proposals and captions in parallel, using Vanilla LSTM results in a lack of interaction between text and features. SA training does not allow all attention weights to be concentrated on a fixed area. Therefore, using DSA as our proposed method effectively addresses the issue of parallel methods not directly accessing event proposals and achieves better results.

**Table 3.** The effect of LSTM with deformable attention on the caption module.

| Method | B@1 | B@2 | B@3 | B@4 | METEOR | CIDEr |
|---|---|---|---|---|---|---|
| Vanilla LSTM | 14.88 | 7.15 | 3.84 | 1.70 | 8.91 | 27.39 |
| LSTM with SA | **15.44** | 7.61 | 3.70 | 1.68 | 9.23 | 28.85 |
| **LSTM with DSA(Ours)** | 15.23 | **8.02** | **3.91** | **1.75** | **9.68** | **29.17** |

Bold font indicates the highest result.

The work also confirmed that combining different types of features can help improve the quality of the text generated by the model. The comparison of the results is shown in Table 4. Experimental results also report that using only audio features is not sufficient to improve the quality of the text and can even have a negative impact on the performance of the model. Using only visual features can produce good results, but is still not as effective as using multi-modal features. By supplementing visual features with audio features, the generated text can be significantly improved.

**Table 4.** The impact of multi-modal features on the quality of generated captions.

| Method | B@1 | B@2 | B@3 | B@4 | METEOR | CIDEr |
|---|---|---|---|---|---|---|
| Visual-only | 13.66 | 7.43 | 3.11 | 1.27 | 8.35 | 23.58 |
| Audio-only | 13.07 | 6.69 | 2.94 | 1.13 | 6.81 | 16.20 |
| **Proposed** | **15.23** | **8.02** | **3.91** | **1.75** | **9.68** | **29.17** |

Bold font indicates the highest result.

4.3.3. Qualitative Analysis

This work demonstrates the proposed method on the act dataset. The generated text descriptions can be seen in Figure 4. The GT is also included for reference.

As shown in Figure 4, the proposed method divides a 2 min video into 4 proposals event and generates logical text descriptions. Compared to GT, our method accurately separates the video based on its content and scenes and avoids the event redundancy. The generated captions fully describe the content of each event. However, GT clearly identifies the name of the male protagonist as "Mr. Bean", which our method does not. This difference may be due to the fact that the video clip is from a popular TV series and GT's captions are manually marked, whereas the protagonist is relatively well known. This comparison shows that our method has not yet successfully identified the protagonist and matched his name in a complex scene.

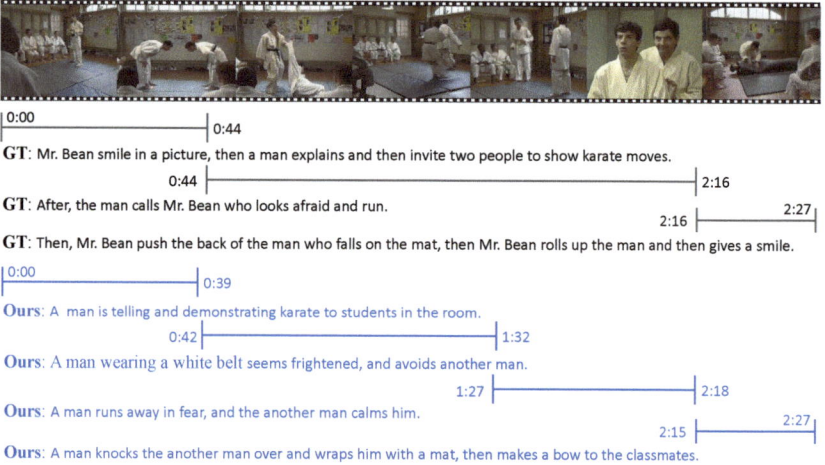

**Figure 4.** Results of a qualitative analysis of a video from the ActivityNet Caption dataset. The predicted results of the proposed model are compared with the GT reference.

## 5. Conclusions

The paper has proposed a new model for dense video captioning that achieves competitive results on the ActivityNet Caption dataset, with the following particular improvements.

- The approach was able to effectively exploit the multi-modal features of video and highlights the potential of the audio modality to enhance video details.
- A deformable Transformer was used to encode and decode features, which eliminated the need for complex anchor mechanisms and hyperparameter constraints in non-maxima suppression.
- A representation organisation module was introduced to improve the link between features and context.
- The parallel method for the two subtasks of localisation and captioning was enhanced, allowing fine-grained interaction between the submodules and improving the comprehensiveness and accuracy of the text descriptions generated by the model.

Based on the experimental results, it is evident that our method excels in event localisation and generates text descriptions that follow linguistic logic, while presenting video content from multiple perspectives. Compared to other dense video captioning methods, our proposed method has clear advantages. In the future, we will aim to overcome the branch bottleneck of existing parallel methods, improve the computer's ability to understand and represent video content, and ultimately achieve the beautiful vision of artificial intelligence.

**Author Contributions:** Conceptualisation, X.H., K.-H.C., W.K. and H.S.; methodology, X.H., K.-H.C., W.K. and H.S.; software, W.K. and H.S.; validation, X.H., K.-H.C., W.K. and H.S.; formal analysis, X.H., W.K. and H.S.; investigation, X.H.; resources, K.-H.C., W.K. and H.S.; data curation, X.H., K.-H.C., W.K. and H.S.; writing—original draft preparation, X.H., K.-H.C., W.K. and H.S.; writing—review and editing, X.H., K.-H.C., W.K. and H.S.; visualisation, X.H., W.K. and H.S.; supervision, W.K. and H.S.; project administration, W.K. and H.S.; funding acquisition, W.K. and H.S. All authors have read and agreed to the published version of the manuscript.

**Funding:** This work is partially supported by the National Key R&D Program of China (No. 2019YFB21 01600), the National Natural Science Foundation of China (No. 61872025), the Macao Polytechnic University (RP/FCA-06/2023, RP/ESCA-03/2020), and the Open Fund of the State Key Laboratory of Software Development Environment (No. SKLSDE-2021ZX-03).

**Institutional Review Board Statement:** Not applicable.

**Informed Consent Statement:** Not applicable.

**Data Availability Statement:** Not applicable.

**Acknowledgments:** Thanks for the support from Macao Polytechnic University and HAWKEYE Group.

**Conflicts of Interest:** The authors declare no conflict of interest.

# References

1. Hara, K.; Kataoka, H.; Satoh, Y. Can Spatiotemporal 3D CNNs Retrace the History of 2D CNNs and ImageNet? In Proceedings of the 2018 IEEE/CVF Conference on Computer Vision and Pattern Recognition, Salt Lake City, UT, USA, 18–23 June 2018; IEEE: Piscataway, NJ, USA, 2018. [CrossRef]
2. Sighencea, B.I.; Stanciu, R.I.; Căleanu, C.D. A Review of Deep Learning-Based Methods for Pedestrian Trajectory Prediction. *Sensors* **2021**, *21*, 7543. [CrossRef]
3. Venugopalan, S.; Rohrbach, M.; Donahue, J.; Mooney, R.; Darrell, T.; Saenko, K. Sequence to Sequence—Video to Text. In Proceedings of the 2015 IEEE International Conference on Computer Vision (ICCV), Santiago, Chile, 7–13 December 2015; IEEE: Piscataway, NJ, USA, 2015. [CrossRef]
4. Tang, M.; Wang, Z.; Liu, Z.; Rao, F.; Li, D.; Li, X. CLIP4Caption: CLIP for Video Caption. In Proceedings of the 29th ACM International Conference on Multimedia, Virtual Online, 20–24 October 2021; ACM: New York, NY, USA, 2021. [CrossRef]
5. Tran, D.; Bourdev, L.; Fergus, R.; Torresani, L.; Paluri, M. Learning Spatiotemporal Features with 3D Convolutional Networks. In Proceedings of the 2015 IEEE International Conference on Computer Vision (ICCV), Santiago, Chile, 7–13 December 2015; IEEE: Piscataway, NJ, USA, 2015. [CrossRef]
6. Wu, Y.; Sheng, H.; Zhang, Y.; Wang, S.; Xiong, Z.; Ke, W. Hybrid Motion Model for Multiple Object Tracking in Mobile Devices. *IEEE Internet Things J.* **2023**, *10*, 4735–4748. [CrossRef]
7. Wang, S.; Sheng, H.; Yang, D.; Zhang, Y.; Wu, Y.; Wang, S. Extendable Multiple Nodes Recurrent Tracking Framework with RTU++. *IEEE Trans. Image Process.* **2022**, *31*, 5257–5271. [CrossRef]
8. Krishna, R.; Hata, K.; Ren, F.; Fei-Fei, L.; Niebles, J.C. Dense-Captioning Events in Videos. In Proceedings of the 2017 IEEE International Conference on Computer Vision (ICCV), Venice, Italy, 22–29 October 2017; IEEE: Piscataway, NJ, USA, 2017. [CrossRef]
9. Mun, J.; Yang, L.; Ren, Z.; Xu, N.; Han, B. Streamlined Dense Video Captioning. In Proceedings of the 2019 IEEE/CVF Conference on Computer Vision and Pattern Recognition (CVPR), Long Beach, CA, USA, 15–20 June 2019; IEEE: Piscataway, NJ, USA, 2019. [CrossRef]
10. Wang, J.; Jiang, W.; Ma, L.; Liu, W.; Xu, Y. Bidirectional Attentive Fusion with Context Gating for Dense Video Captioning. In Proceedings of the 2018 IEEE/CVF Conference on Computer Vision and Pattern Recognition, Salt Lake City, UT, USA, 18–23 June 2018; IEEE: Piscataway, NJ, USA, 2018. [CrossRef]
11. Li, Y.; Yao, T.; Pan, Y.; Chao, H.; Mei, T. Jointly Localizing and Describing Events for Dense Video Captioning. In Proceedings of the 2018 IEEE/CVF Conference on Computer Vision and Pattern Recognition, Salt Lake City, UT, USA, 18–23 June 2018; IEEE: Piscataway, NJ, USA, 2018. [CrossRef]

12. Zhang, W.; Ke, W.; Yang, D.; Sheng, H.; Xiong, Z. Light field super-resolution using complementary-view feature attention. *Comput. Vis. Media* **2023**, *9*, 843–858. [CrossRef]
13. Choi, W.; Chen, J.; Yoon, J. Parallel Pathway Dense Video Captioning With Deformable Transformer. *IEEE Access* **2022**, *10*, 129899–129910. [CrossRef]
14. Venugopalan, S.; Xu, H.; Donahue, J.; Rohrbach, M.; Mooney, R.; Saenko, K. Translating Videos to Natural Language Using Deep Recurrent Neural Networks. In Proceedings of the 2015 Conference of the North American Chapter of the Association for Computational Linguistics: Human Language Technologies, Denver, CO, USA, 31 May–5 June 2015; Association for Computational Linguistics: Stroudsburg, PA, USA, 2015. [CrossRef]
15. LeCun, Y.; Bengio, Y.; Hinton, G. Deep learning. *Nature* **2015**, *521*, 436–444. [CrossRef]
16. Huang, L.; Wang, W.; Chen, J.; Wei, X.Y. Attention on attention for image captioning. In Proceedings of the 2019 IEEE/CVF International Conference on Computer Vision (ICCV), Seoul, Republic of Korea, 27 October–2 November 2019; IEEE: Piscataway, NJ, USA, 2019; pp. 4634–4643. [CrossRef]
17. Huang, X.; Ke, W.; Sheng, H. Enhancing Efficiency and Quality of Image Caption Generation with CARU. In *Wireless Algorithms, Systems, and Applications*; Springer Nature: Cham, Switzerland, 2022; pp. 450–459. [CrossRef]
18. Wang, S.; Yang, D.; Wu, Y.; Liu, Y.; Sheng, H. Tracking Game: Self-adaptative Agent based Multi-object Tracking. In Proceedings of the 30th ACM International Conference on Multimedia, Lisbon, Portugal, 10–14 October 2022; ACM: New York, NY, USA, 2022. [CrossRef]
19. Caspi, Y.; Simakov, D.; Irani, M. Feature-Based Sequence-to-Sequence Matching. *Int. J. Comput. Vis.* **2006**, *68*, 53–64. [CrossRef]
20. Simonyan, K.; Zisserman, A. Very Deep Convolutional Networks for Large-Scale Image Recognition. *arXiv* **2014**, arXiv:1409.1556.
21. Chan, K.H.; Im, S.K.; Ke, W. VGGreNet: A Light-Weight VGGNet with Reused Convolutional Set. In Proceedings of the 2020 IEEE/ACM 13th International Conference on Utility and Cloud Computing (UCC), Leicester, UK, 7–10 December 2020; IEEE: Piscataway, NJ, USA, 2020. [CrossRef]
22. He, K.; Zhang, X.; Ren, S.; Sun, J. Deep Residual Learning for Image Recognition. In Proceedings of the 2016 IEEE Conference on Computer Vision and Pattern Recognition (CVPR), Las Vegas, NV, USA, 27–30 June 2016; IEEE: Piscataway, NJ, USA, 2016. [CrossRef]
23. Zhao, B.; Li, X.; Lu, X. CAM-RNN: Co-Attention Model Based RNN for Video Captioning. *IEEE Trans. Image Process.* **2019**, *28*, 5552–5565. [CrossRef]
24. Sawarn, A.; Srivastava, S.; Gupta, M.; Srivastava, S. BeamAtt: Generating Medical Diagnosis from Chest X-Rays Using Sampling-Based Intelligence. In *EAI/Springer Innovations in Communication and Computing*; Springer International Publishing: Cham, Switzerland, 2021; pp. 135–150. [CrossRef]
25. Deng, J.; Li, L.; Zhang, B.; Wang, S.; Zha, Z.; Huang, Q. Syntax-Guided Hierarchical Attention Network for Video Captioning. *IEEE Trans. Circuits Syst. Video Technol.* **2022**, *32*, 880–892. [CrossRef]
26. Xiong, Y.; Dai, B.; Lin, D. Move Forward and Tell: A Progressive Generator of Video Descriptions. In *Computer Vision—ECCV 2018*; Springer International Publishing: Cham, Switzerland, 2018; pp. 489–505. [CrossRef]
27. Rahman, T.; Xu, B.; Sigal, L. Watch, Listen and Tell: Multi-Modal Weakly Supervised Dense Event Captioning. In Proceedings of the 2019 IEEE/CVF International Conference on Computer Vision (ICCV), Seoul, Republic of Korea, 27 October–2 November 2019; IEEE: Piscataway, NJ, USA, 2019. [CrossRef]
28. Rafiq, G.; Rafiq, M.; Choi, G.S. Video description: A comprehensive survey of deep learning approaches. *Artif. Intell. Rev.* **2023**. [CrossRef]
29. Shen, Z.; Li, J.; Su, Z.; Li, M.; Chen, Y.; Jiang, Y.G.; Xue, X. Weakly Supervised Dense Video Captioning. In Proceedings of the 2017 IEEE Conference on Computer Vision and Pattern Recognition (CVPR), Honolulu, HI, USA, 21–16 July 2017; IEEE: Piscataway, NJ, USA, 2017. [CrossRef]
30. Huang, X.; Chan, K.H.; Wu, W.; Sheng, H.; Ke, W. Fusion of Multi-Modal Features to Enhance Dense Video Caption. *Sensors* **2023**, *23*, 5565. [CrossRef]
31. Wang, T.; Zheng, H.; Yu, M.; Tian, Q.; Hu, H. Event-Centric Hierarchical Representation for Dense Video Captioning. *IEEE Trans. Circuits Syst. Video Technol.* **2021**, *31*, 1890–1900. [CrossRef]
32. Zeng, R.; Xu, H.; Huang, W.; Chen, P.; Tan, M.; Gan, C. Dense Regression Network for Video Grounding. In Proceedings of the 2020 IEEE/CVF Conference on Computer Vision and Pattern Recognition (CVPR), Seattle, WA, USA, 14–19 June 2020; IEEE: Piscataway, NJ, USA, 2020. [CrossRef]
33. Li, K.; Guo, D.; Wang, M. Proposal-Free Video Grounding with Contextual Pyramid Network. *Proc. AAAI Conf. Artif. Intell.* **2021**, *35*, 1902–1910. [CrossRef]
34. Carreira, J.; Zisserman, A. Quo Vadis, Action Recognition? A New Model and the Kinetics Dataset. In Proceedings of the 2017 IEEE Conference on Computer Vision and Pattern Recognition (CVPR), Honolulu, HI, USA, 21–16 July 2017; IEEE: Piscataway, NJ, USA, 2017. [CrossRef]
35. Qiu, Z.; Yao, T.; Mei, T. Learning Spatio-Temporal Representation with Pseudo-3D Residual Networks. In Proceedings of the 2017 IEEE International Conference on Computer Vision (ICCV), Venice, Italy, 22–29 October 2017; IEEE: Piscataway, NJ, USA, 2017. [CrossRef]
36. Hochreiter, S.; Schmidhuber, J. Long Short-Term Memory. *Neural Comput.* **1997**, *9*, 1735–1780. [CrossRef]

37. Devlin, J.; Chang, M.W.; Lee, K.; Toutanova, K. BERT: Pre-training of Deep Bidirectional Transformers for Language Understanding. *arXiv* **2018**, arXiv:1810.04805.
38. Vaswani, A.; Shazeer, N.; Parmar, N.; Uszkoreit, J.; Jones, L.; Gomez, A.N.; Kaiser, L.; Polosukhin, I. Attention Is All You Need. *arXiv* **2017**, arXiv:1706.03762.
39. Carion, N.; Massa, F.; Synnaeve, G.; Usunier, N.; Kirillov, A.; Zagoruyko, S. End-to-End Object Detection with Transformers. In *Computer Vision—ECCV 2020*; Springer International Publishing: Cham, Switzerland, 2020; pp. 213–229. [CrossRef]
40. Park, J.S.; Darrell, T.; Rohrbach, A. Identity-Aware Multi-sentence Video Description. In *Computer Vision—ECCV 2020*; Springer International Publishing: Cham, Switzerland, 2020; pp. 360–378. [CrossRef]
41. Pasunuru, R.; Bansal, M. Multi-Task Video Captioning with Video and Entailment Generation. In Proceedings of the 55th Annual Meeting of the Association for Computational Linguistics, Vancouver, BC, Canada, 30 July–4 August 2017; Association for Computational Linguistics: Stroudsburg, PA, USA, 2017; Volume 1. [CrossRef]
42. Shetty, R.; Laaksonen, J. Frame- and Segment-Level Features and Candidate Pool Evaluation for Video Caption Generation. In Proceedings of the 24th ACM International Conference on Multimedia, Amsterdam, The Netherlands, 15–19 October 2016; ACM: New York, NY, USA, 2016. [CrossRef]
43. Zhou, L.; Zhou, Y.; Corso, J.J.; Socher, R.; Xiong, C. End-to-End Dense Video Captioning with Masked Transformer. In Proceedings of the 2018 IEEE/CVF Conference on Computer Vision and Pattern Recognition, Salt Lake City, UT, USA, 18–23 June 2018; IEEE: Piscataway, NJ, USA, 2018. [CrossRef]
44. Yao, L.; Torabi, A.; Cho, K.; Ballas, N.; Pal, C.; Larochelle, H.; Courville, A. Describing Videos by Exploiting Temporal Structure. In Proceedings of the 2015 IEEE International Conference on Computer Vision (ICCV), Santiago, Chile, 7–13 December 2015; IEEE: Piscataway, NJ, USA, 2015. [CrossRef]
45. Neubeck, A.; Gool, L.V. Efficient Non-Maximum Suppression. In Proceedings of the 18th International Conference on Pattern Recognition (ICPR '06), Hong Kong, China, 20–24 August 2006; IEEE: Piscataway, NJ, USA, 2006. [CrossRef]
46. Wang, T.; Zhang, R.; Lu, Z.; Zheng, F.; Cheng, R.; Luo, P. End-to-End Dense Video Captioning with Parallel Decoding. In Proceedings of the 2021 IEEE/CVF International Conference on Computer Vision (ICCV), Montreal, BC, Canada, 11–17 October 2021; IEEE: Piscataway, NJ, USA, 2021. [CrossRef]
47. Li, B.; Zhang, W.; Tian, M.; Zhai, G.; Wang, X. Blindly assess quality of in-the-wild videos via quality-aware pre-training and motion perception. *IEEE Trans. Circuits Syst. Video Technol.* **2022**, *32*, 5944–5958. [CrossRef]
48. Zhang, W.; Ma, C.; Wu, Q.; Yang, X. Language-guided navigation via cross-modal grounding and alternate adversarial learning. *IEEE Trans. Circuits Syst. Video Technol.* **2020**, *31*, 3469–3481. [CrossRef]
49. Hao, W.; Zhang, Z.; Guan, H. Integrating Both Visual and Audio Cues for Enhanced Video Caption. In Proceedings of the AAAI Conference on Artificial Intelligence, New Orleans, LA, USA, 2–7 February 2018; Volume 32. [CrossRef]
50. Jin, Q.; Chen, J.; Chen, S.; Xiong, Y.; Hauptmann, A. Describing Videos using Multi-modal Fusion. In Proceedings of the 24th ACM International Conference on Multimedia, Amsterdam, The Netherlands, 15–19 October 2016; ACM: New York, NY, USA, 2016. [CrossRef]
51. Chang, Z.; Zhao, D.; Chen, H.; Li, J.; Liu, P. Event-centric multi-modal fusion method for dense video captioning. *Neural Netw.* **2022**, *146*, 120–129. [CrossRef]
52. Iashin, V.; Rahtu, E. A Better Use of Audio-Visual Cues: Dense Video Captioning with Bi-modal Transformer. *arXiv* **2020**, arXiv:2005.08271.
53. Zhu, X.; Su, W.; Lu, L.; Li, B.; Wang, X.; Dai, J. Deformable detr: Deformable transformers for end-to-end object detection. *arXiv* **2020**, arXiv:2010.04159.
54. Paszke, A.; Gross, S.; Massa, F.; Lerer, A.; Bradbury, J.; Chanan, G.; Killeen, T.; Lin, Z.; Gimelshein, N.; Antiga, L.; et al. PyTorch: An Imperative Style, High-Performance Deep Learning Library. *arXiv* **2019**, arXiv:1912.01703.
55. Kingma, D.P.; Ba, J. Adam: A Method for Stochastic Optimization. *arXiv* **2014**, arXiv:1412.6980.
56. Papineni, K.; Roukos, S.; Ward, T.; Zhu, W.J. BLEU: A method for automatic evaluation of machine translation. In Proceedings of the 40th Annual Meeting on Association for Computational Linguistics—ACL '02, Association for Computational Linguistics, Philadelphia, PA, USA, 7–12 July 2002. [CrossRef]
57. Lavie, A.; Denkowski, M.J. The Meteor metric for automatic evaluation of machine translation. *Mach. Transl.* **2009**, *23*, 105–115. [CrossRef]
58. Vedantam, R.; Zitnick, C.L.; Parikh, D. CIDEr: Consensus-based image description evaluation. In Proceedings of the 2015 IEEE Conference on Computer Vision and Pattern Recognition (CVPR), Boston, MA, USA, 7–12 June 2015; IEEE: Piscataway, NJ, USA, 2015. [CrossRef]

**Disclaimer/Publisher's Note:** The statements, opinions and data contained in all publications are solely those of the individual author(s) and contributor(s) and not of MDPI and/or the editor(s). MDPI and/or the editor(s) disclaim responsibility for any injury to people or property resulting from any ideas, methods, instructions or products referred to in the content.

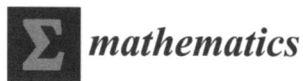

Article

# Enhancing the Security and Privacy in the IoT Supply Chain Using Blockchain and Federated Learning with Trusted Execution Environment

Linkai Zhu [1,†], Shanwen Hu [2,*,†], Xiaolian Zhu [1], Changpu Meng [3,4] and Maoyi Huang [5]

[1] Information Technology School, Hebei University of Economics and Business, Shijiazhuang 050061, China; linkai@hueb.edu.cn (L.Z.); xiaolianzhu@hueb.edu.cn (X.Z.)
[2] Faculty of Data Science, City University of Macau, Macau 999078, China
[3] iFLYTEK Co., Ltd., Hefei 230088, China; cpmeng@iflytek.com
[4] School of Computing and Information Technology, Faculty of Engineering and Information Sciences, University of Wollongong, Wollongong 2522, Australia
[5] Product Development, Ericsson, 41756 Gothenburg, Sweden; maoyi.huang@ericsson.com
* Correspondence: d21091100159@cityu.mo
† These authors contributed equally to this work.

**Citation:** Zhu, L.; Hu, S.; Zhu, X.; Meng, C.; Huang, M. Enhancing the Security and Privacy in the IoT Supply Chain Using Blockchain and Federated Learning with Trusted Execution Environment. *Mathematics* **2023**, *11*, 3759. https://doi.org/10.3390/math11173759

Academic Editor: Cheng-Chi Lee

Received: 18 July 2023
Revised: 24 August 2023
Accepted: 29 August 2023
Published: 1 September 2023

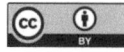

**Copyright:** © 2023 by the authors. Licensee MDPI, Basel, Switzerland. This article is an open access article distributed under the terms and conditions of the Creative Commons Attribution (CC BY) license (https://creativecommons.org/licenses/by/4.0/).

**Abstract:** Federated learning has emerged as a promising technique for the Internet of Things (IoT) in various domains, including supply chain management. It enables IoT devices to collaboratively learn without exposing their raw data, ensuring data privacy. However, federated learning faces the threats of local data tampering and upload process attacks. This paper proposes an innovative framework that leverages Trusted Execution Environment (TEE) and blockchain technology to address the data security and privacy challenges in federated learning for IoT supply chain management. Our framework achieves the security of local data computation and the tampering resistance of data update uploads using TEE and the blockchain. We adopt Intel Software Guard Extensions (SGXs) as the specific implementation of TEE, which can guarantee the secure execution of local models on SGX-enabled processors. We also use consortium blockchain technology to build a verification network and consensus mechanism, ensuring the security and tamper resistance of the data upload and aggregation process. Finally, each cluster can obtain the aggregated parameters from the blockchain. To evaluate the performance of our proposed framework, we conducted several experiments with different numbers of participants and different datasets and validated the effectiveness of our scheme. We tested the final global model obtained from federated training on a test dataset and found that increasing both the number of iterations and the number of participants improves its accuracy. For instance, it reaches 94% accuracy with one participant and five iterations and 98.5% accuracy with ten participants and thirty iterations.

**Keywords:** federated learning; Trusted Execution Environment (TEE); blockchain; supply chain; Internet of Things (IoT)

**MSC:** 68M25

## 1. Introduction

The exponential growth of Internet of Things (IoT) applications in supply chain management has introduced both opportunities and challenges. IoT devices play a crucial role in enabling intelligent control, automated operations, optimized scheduling, quality testing, and efficient delivery within production lines [1]. They also facilitate the intelligent positioning, monitoring, and management of transportation vehicles, distribution centers, and warehouses while providing real-time tracking and traceability of goods [2]. In the supply chain, enterprises rely heavily on suppliers for diverse raw materials or services necessary for manufacturing their products. IoT devices assist in the smart selection, management, and evaluation of suppliers, as well as the real-time monitoring of raw material quality, quantity, and location [3]. Although generating substantial data, the need to share and coordinate data among participants in real time arises to enhance efficiency and reduce costs. However, concerns surrounding data leakage, potential misuse, and exposure to competitors pose significant challenges concerning data privacy and trust. Moreover, the process of data sharing in the supply chain complicates the establishment of the consensus on data value and quality, as sharing parties may intentionally provide low-quality or even falsified data to benefit themselves [4]. Hence, addressing the challenge of achieving data collaboration and intelligent analysis while ensuring data security and privacy within the supply chain is of utmost importance.

Federated learning is a distributed machine learning technique that enables multiple participants to train models locally and share model parameters or updates with a central server for aggregation [5]. This approach allows each participant to improve their model's performance by leveraging data from other participants without directly sharing their raw data [6]. Federated learning offers advantages in terms of data privacy protection and reduced communication overhead, making it well suited for supply-chain-management scenarios [7–9]. Nevertheless, existing federated learning techniques still encounter security and privacy challenges. For instance, the central server could be vulnerable to hacking or tampering by internal personnel, resulting in the leakage or corruption of model parameters or updates [10,11]. Dishonest or malicious behavior among participants, such as transmitting erroneous or malicious model parameters or updates, can significantly impact the quality of the models [12]. Additionally, participants' join or exit events may lead to an unstable or inconsistent model training process [13]. To address these issues, robust and reliable security and privacy-protection mechanisms need to be introduced.

Figure 1 illustrates a typical cross-border data-sharing use case within a global supply chain, where various IoT devices' data are stored in the cloud, accessible from different regions or countries involved in the supply chain. However, this scenario exposes sensitive data to potential harm from malicious users. This paper presents a novel federated learning framework that leverages the blockchain and the Trusted Execution Environment (TEE) to enhance the security and privacy of supply chain data. Our contributions are as follows.

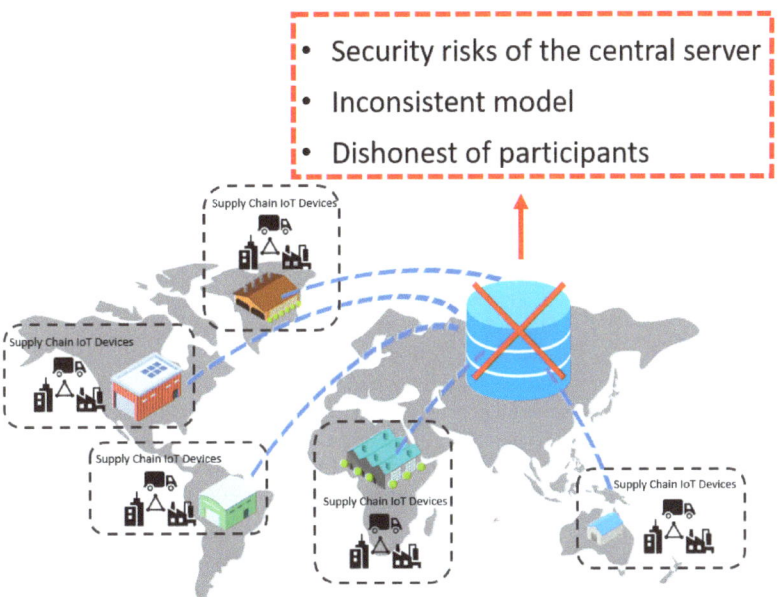

**Figure 1.** Possible challenges of traditional centralized global supply chain scenario.

(1) The framework introduces a consortium blockchain-based federated learning protocol that capitalizes on the decentralized, tamper-resistant, and traceable characteristics of blockchain technology to enable secure transmission, storage, and verification of model parameters or updates.

(2) We utilize TEE to safeguard local participant data and computation processes from leakage or tampering. We introduce a distributed local federated learning architecture based on TEE to further enhance data privacy while ensuring the quality of local client models.

(3) We conduct experimental evaluations using datasets, and the results demonstrate that our framework effectively enhances data security and privacy while achieving high model accuracy and maintaining low communication overhead.

The rest of this paper is organized as follows. Section 2 presents the related work. Section 3 introduces the proposed framework. Section 4 gives the security analysis. Section 5 presents the experimental results and evaluates various performance aspects of the proposed framework. Section 6 concludes this paper.

## 2. Related Work

(1) Trusted Execution Environment

Intel SGX [14] is a hardware-based security architecture technology that enables the creation of TEEs on Intel processors for cloud platforms and server environments. A TEE is a secure region of memory that isolates the execution of sensitive code and data from any untrusted system components, such as the operating system or the hypervisor. SGX extends CPU instructions to encapsulate the secure operations of legitimate software in an enclave, which is the basic unit of protection in SGX. Unlike other TEE technologies, such as TrustZone, SGX can run multiple secure enclaves on the same processor, each equivalent to a TEE. SGX also provides mechanisms for the attestation and sealing of enclaves, which allow for proving the integrity and confidentiality of the enclave's execution and data. SGX has been widely used to achieve privacy-preserving machine learning [15–19] by running the machine learning algorithms inside enclaves and protecting the data and models from unauthorized access.

(2) Federated Learning

Federated learning is a machine learning technique that enables distributed model training on multiple local data sources without sharing the raw data [5,20,21]. This technique leverages local model parameters, which do not reveal the original data, to construct a global model that captures the data value while preserving data privacy and security. Federated learning realizes a novel paradigm of "data available but not visible", which empowers decentralized data to be utilized for more accurate model training without violating data protection. In contrast to conventional centralized machine learning approaches, federated learning enables the collaboration of multiple parties on a shared model without exposing their private data, augmenting privacy and security [22]. It also mitigates the communication overhead and computational costs associated with centralized machine learning, as only the updates to the local model are transmitted to the central server instead of the whole dataset. Federated learning can be divided into three types: vertical federated learning, horizontal federated learning, and federated transfer learning [23]. Vertical federated learning is applicable to scenarios where data features are highly correlated but data samples are disjoint, and it can achieve cross-domain knowledge sharing. Horizontal federated learning is applicable for scenarios where data samples are highly correlated but data features are disjoint, and it can achieve cross-institutional knowledge fusion. Federated transfer learning is applicable to scenarios where data samples and data features are both disjoint but have some correlation, and it can achieve cross-domain knowledge transfer.

FedAvg is a federated learning algorithm that was introduced in a 2016 paper by Google researchers [24]. Federated learning exists to train deep neural networks on many devices, such as smartphones or tablets. These devices may have different types of data, and their users may not want to share their data with others for privacy reasons. FedAvg allows these devices to train a local model on their own data without sending the data to a central server [25]. Instead, the device only sends the model parameters, which are numbers that represent how the model learns from the data. The central server then combines the parameters from all the devices by taking their weighted average, where the weights depend on how many data each device has. The server then sends the averaged parameters back to all the devices, which update their local models with the new parameters. This cycle of local training and global averaging continues until the global model reaches a good performance. FedAvg has some benefits over traditional learning methods that require all the data to be sent to a central server, such as saving communication bandwidth, handling diverse data sources, and improving model accuracy and generalization ability.

(3) Blockchain

Blockchain technology is a novel form of distributed ledger technology that employs cryptographic techniques and consensus protocols to maintain a shared record of transactions across multiple nodes, creating a sequential chain of data blocks. This technology exhibits several distinctive features, such as decentralization, immutability, distributed storage, anonymity, transparency, and smart contracts [26,27]. Decentralization refers to the absence of a central authority or intermediary institution that governs or regulates the blockchain. All participants have equal rights to join the blockchain network and contribute to its security through consensus protocols [28]. Immutability implies that the data stored on the blockchain are permanent and irreversible. Distributed storage indicates that the blockchain data are not located on a centralized server but dispersed across multiple nodes. This enhances the reliability and security of blockchain technology, making it resilient to attacks or tampering and having high fault tolerance. Anonymity and transparency denote that blockchain technology utilizes public keys and private keys to encrypt and decrypt data, safeguarding the privacy and security of users, while all transaction records are publicly available on the blockchain, and anyone can access the blockchain data [29]. Smart contracts are a type of self-executing code based on blockchain technology that can automatically perform under predefined conditions.

Based on the various features of blockchain technology, many interesting and valuable applications have emerged in various fields. Power Ledger is a blockchain-based energy-trading platform that allows consumers to sell their excess solar energy to other consumers and verify the source and quality of the renewable energy they purchase. IBM Food Trust is a blockchain-based food-traceability platform that connects farmers, processors, distributors, and retailers. It enables data sharing and traceability along the food supply chain and improves food safety, quality, and efficiency. Medicalchain is a blockchain-based platform that aims to create a decentralized electronic health record system, where patients can securely store and share their health data with authorized medical professionals and access remote healthcare services. Estonia, as a pioneer in the field of e-government, has implemented digital identity, e-residency, e-voting, e-health, and e-justice based on the blockchain, improving the security, transparency, and efficiency of public information processes [30–33].

The consortium blockchain is a special form of blockchain that allows only authorized nodes to join its network, which usually represents different physical organizations or enterprises that need to collaborate or share a task or resource [34]. Consortium blockchain typically uses specific consensus agreements to ensure that all nodes agree on the validity and sequence of transactions while providing a high degree of control and customizability [35]. The consortium blockchain is transparent, decentralized, highly controllable, and customizable. The consortium blockchain is suitable for applications that require sharing and collaboration among multiple organizations, such as cross-organizational transactions and collaborative operations.

A brief comparison of related works of literature with respect to various methodologies is shown in Table 1. Bonawitz [36] adopted federated learning, but their research does not incorporate the use of TEE (Trusted Execution Environment) or blockchain methodologies. A significant limitation of this work is its inability to fully guarantee data security and privacy during the federated learning process. Chen et al. [37] integrates both federated learning and TEE but does not utilize the blockchain. Its limitation lies in only being able to guarantee data security and privacy during the data-aggregation process to a certain degree, implying there may be vulnerabilities or scenarios where data could be at risk. Li et al. [38] utilize federated learning and the blockchain but not TEE. This can only ensure data security and privacy within the local model to a certain extent. This might indicate potential challenges or vulnerabilities when scaling or in more complex scenarios.

**Table 1.** Comparison of related works of literature with respect to various methodologies.

| Paper | Federated Learning | TEE | Blockchain | Features |
|---|---|---|---|---|
| [36] | Yes | No | No | Cannot fully guarantee the data security and privacy in the federated learning process. |
| [37] | Yes | Yes | No | Can guarantee data security and privacy in the data aggregation process to a certain extent. |
| [38] | Yes | No | Yes | Can guarantee data security and privacy in the local model to a certain extent. |
| Ours | Yes | Yes | Yes | Can fully guarantee data security locally and privacy in the data-aggregation process. |

## 3. Proposed Framework

The summary of notations used in the methodology can be seen in Table 2.

**Table 2.** Description of notations.

| Notations | Description |
|---|---|
| $D_i$ | Local data for device $i$ |
| $E$ | Number of training epochs |
| $\alpha$ | Learning rate |
| $p, g$ | Diffie–Hellman parameters |
| $SK_i$ | Private key for Diffie–Hellman of device $i$ |
| $PK_i$ | Public key for Diffie–Hellman of device $i$ |
| $N$ | Nonce generated by TEE |
| $T$ | Attestation token generated by TEE |
| $SK_{TEE}$ | Private key for Diffie–Hellman of TEE |
| $PK_{TEE}$ | Public key for Diffie–Hellman of TEE |
| $w$ | Model weights |
| $\hat{y}$ | Model prediction |
| $y$ | True label |
| $\nabla$ | Gradient |
| $E_{weight}$ | Encrypted weight |
| $\mathcal{D}$ | Device sets |
| $K$ | Number of global iterations |
| $\eta$ | FedAvg learning rate |
| $\{w_i\}_{i \in \mathcal{D}}$ | Local model weight for each device in $\mathcal{D}$ |
| $H_{ID,i}$ | Device identity hash value for device $i$ |
| $w_0$ | Initial global weight |
| $B_t$ | Block containing verified local model weights |
| $a_{t'}$ | Aggregated update at iteration $t'$ |
| $\nabla f(a_{t'}, \mathcal{D})$ | Gradient of objective function |
| $w_{t'}$ | Global weight at iteration $t'$ |

### 3.1. System Overview

In this paper, we propose a secure and efficient federated learning framework based on a Trusted Execution Environment (TEE) and the blockchain for industrial Internet of Things (IoT) supply chain applications. Our framework aims to address the challenges of data privacy, model security, and model verifiability in federated learning, which is a promising technique to enable collaborative learning among multiple parties without sharing raw data. We consider an IoT supply chain scenario where $N$ stakeholders (e.g., manufacturers, warehouses, logistics providers, and retailers) collect data $\mathcal{D}_i = \{(\mathbf{x}_i^j, y_i^j)\}_{j=1}^{n_i}$ from various sensors installed on products, equipment, or vehicles along supply chain stages. These data are used to train local models on each stakeholder's device using TEE technology, which provides hardware-level isolation and protection for local model parameters $\mathbf{w}_i$ from being exposed to aggregation servers or malicious attackers during the training process. The local models are then aggregated by a central server using a federated averaging (FedAvg) algorithm over a blockchain network, which ensures secure aggregation and tamper-resistant storage of model parameters among distributed nodes. The server updates global model parameters $\mathbf{w}$ by computing the weighted average of local model parameters, where $n = \sum_{i=1}^{N} n_i$ is the total number of data points. The server sends the updated global model parameters $\mathbf{w}$ back to stakeholders via the blockchain consensus mechanism, which allows stakeholders to verify the correctness and integrity of global model updates. The stakeholders can use the updated global model to perform product recognition and classification tasks on their own data without revealing sensitive information to others. The framework iterates until the convergence criterion is reached or a predefined number of communication rounds are completed. Figure 2 illustrates the overview of our proposed framework.

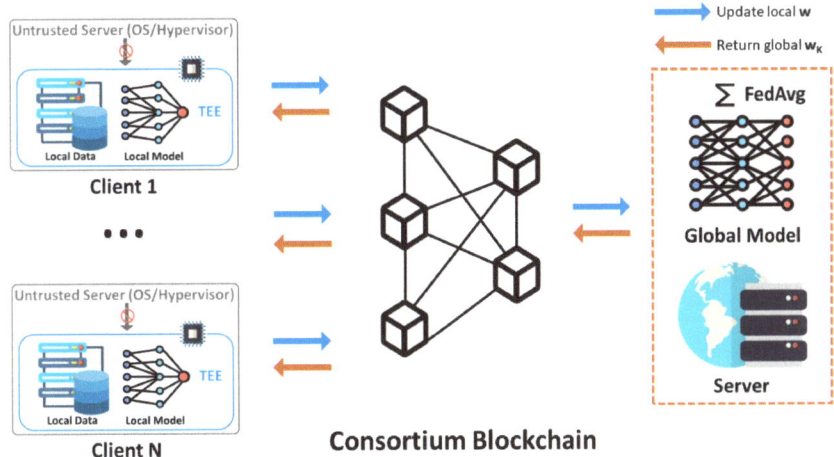

**Figure 2.** Overview of the proposed framework.

*3.2. Threat Model*

This paper investigates a federated learning system that consists of a central server and multiple clients. Each client has its own local dataset that is hidden from others. The server starts the model training by distributing the initial parameters to the clients and then receives and aggregates their updates after each round. The server is assumed to be honest and will not reveal or change the data or parameters. The communication between the clients is also assumed to be secure and will not be eavesdropped on or tampered with. Side-channel attacks are ignored when using SGX. However, some clients may be malicious and have motives to sabotage the federated learning system. Three types of attack objectives for malicious clients are identified: robustness attacks, privacy attacks, and free-riding attacks. Robustness attacks aim to impair the model's accuracy or availability, making it unsuitable or untrustworthy for its intended tasks. Privacy attacks aim to infer other clients' private data or model parameters, obtaining sensitive information or competitive advantage. Free-riding attacks aim to exploit other clients' contributions to improve their own model performance without paying the corresponding cost.

*3.3. Local Model in TEE for Federated Learning*

In order to address the problem of the security of the local model, we implement the CNN model training inside the enclave. The algorithm details a local model in a TEE for federated learning. Federated learning is a distributed machine learning technique that allows multiple parties to collaboratively train a model without sharing their raw data. A TEE is a secure area of a processor that protects the code and data from being tampered with or leaked by other processes. The overview is shown in Figure 3.

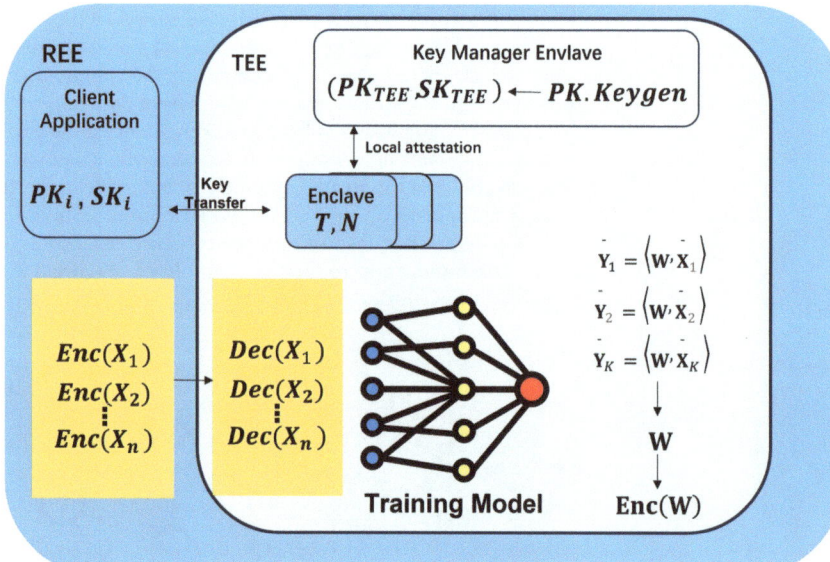

**Figure 3.** The architecture of the local model in a trusted execution environment.

Diffie–Hellman key exchange is based on the property of modular exponentiation that $(a^b)^c \mod p = a^{bc} \mod p$. Since $PK_i = g^{SK_i} \mod p$ and $PK_{TEE} = g^{SK_{TEE}} \mod p$, we have

$$
\begin{aligned}
S &= PK_i^{SK_{TEE}} \mod p \\
&= (g^{SK_i} \mod p)^{SK_{TEE}} \mod p \\
&= g^{SK_i SK_{TEE}} \mod p \\
&= (g^{SK_{TEE}} \mod p)^{SK_i} \mod p \\
&= PK_{TEE}^{SK_i} \mod p
\end{aligned}
\quad (1)
$$

Gradient descent update is based on the idea of finding the minimum of a function by moving in the opposite direction of its gradient. The gradient is the vector of partial derivatives that points to the steepest ascent of the function. The learning rate $\alpha$ controls the step size of the update. The loss function Loss measures the discrepancy between the model prediction $\hat{y}$ and the true label $y$. The model prediction $\hat{y}$ is a function of the model weights $w$ and the input $x$. The update rule can be derived as follows:

$$
\begin{aligned}
w &\leftarrow w - \alpha \cdot \nabla \mathrm{Loss}(\hat{y}, y) \\
&= w - \alpha \cdot \frac{\partial}{\partial w} \mathrm{Loss}(\hat{y}, y) \\
&= w - \alpha \cdot \frac{\partial}{\partial w} \mathrm{Loss}(\mathrm{Model}(w, x), y) \\
&= w - \alpha \cdot \frac{\partial}{\partial w} L(w)
\end{aligned}
\quad (2)
$$

where $L(w)$ is a shorthand notation for $\text{Loss}(\text{Model}(w,x),y)$.

Encryption and decryption in TEE are based on the assumption that there exists an encryption function Encrypt and a decryption function Decrypt that have the following properties:

- For any message m and key kk, $\text{Decrypt}(k, \text{Encrypt}(k,m)) = m$.
- For any ciphertext cc and key kk, $\text{Encrypt}(k, \text{Decrypt}(k,c)) = c$.
- It is computationally infeasible to recover $m$ from $\text{Encrypt}(k,m)$ without knowing $k$.

The encryption equation uses the public key of the rich execution environment (REE) as the key to encrypt the weight: $E_{\text{weight}} = \text{Encrypt}(PK_i, w)$. The decryption equation uses the shared secret key as the key to decrypt the encrypted weight: $w = \text{Decrypt}(S, E_{\text{weight}})$. Since $S = PK_i^{SK_{\text{TEE}}} = PK_{\text{TEE}}^{SK_i}$, we have:

$$\begin{aligned} w &= \text{Decrypt}(S, E_{\text{weight}}) \\ &= \text{Decrypt}(PK_i^{SK_{\text{TEE}}}, E_{\text{weight}}) \\ &= \text{Decrypt}(PK_i^{SK_{\text{TEE}}}, \text{Encrypt}(PK_i, w)) \\ &= w \end{aligned} \quad (3)$$

Algorithm 1 consists of four main parts:

- Input and output: The input includes the local data $D_i$, the number of training epochs $E$, the learning rate $\alpha$, and the Diffie–Hellman parameters $p$ and $g$. The output is the weight $w$ of the local model.
- Interaction between REE and TEE: The REE is the normal operating system that runs outside the TEE. The REE and TEE communicate through a secure channel to exchange public keys for Diffie–Hellman key exchange, which is a method to generate a shared secret key without revealing it to an eavesdropper. The public key of the REE is $PK_i = g^{SK_i} \mod p$, where $SK_i$ is the private key of the REE. The public key of the TEE is $PK_{\text{TEE}} = g^{SK_{\text{TEE}}} \mod p$, where $SK_{\text{TEE}}$ is the private key of the TEE. The shared secret key is $S = PK_i^{SK_{\text{TEE}}} \mod p = PK_{\text{TEE}}^{SK_i} \mod p$.
- Local attestation process in TEE: The TEE generates a nonce $N$ and an attestation token $T$, which is a digital signature that proves the identity and integrity of the TEE. The signature uses the private key of the TEE, denoted by $SK_{\text{TEE}}$, and can be verified by anyone who knows the public key of the TEE, denoted by $PK_{\text{TEE}}$. The nonce prevents replay attacks by ensuring that the token is fresh and unique. The TEE sends $N$ and $T$ to the REE, which verifies the token by checking if $\text{Verify}(PK_{\text{TEE}}, N, T)$ returns true.
- Local model in TEE: The TEE initializes the model weights $w$ and trains them for $E$ epochs using gradient descent on the local data $D_i$. For each sample $(x,y)$ in $D_i$, the model computes the prediction $\hat{y} = \text{Model}(w, x)$ and the gradient $\nabla = \nabla \text{Loss}(\hat{y}, y)$, where Loss is a loss function that measures the discrepancy between $\hat{y}$ and $y$. The model updates the weights by subtracting a fraction of the gradient: $w \leftarrow w - \alpha \cdot \nabla$, where $\alpha$ is the learning rate. After training, the TEE encrypts the weight using the public key of the REE: $E_{\text{weight}} = \text{Encrypt}(PK_i, w)$, where Encrypt is an encryption function. The encrypted weight is sent to the REE, which decrypts it using the shared secret key $w = \text{Decrypt}(S, E_{\text{weight}})$, where Decrypt is a decryption function. The decrypted weight is returned as the output of the algorithm.

The weight "w" is expected to improve with each iteration. The improvement here is in the context of minimizing the loss function specific to the local dataset $D_i$. Each iteration updates the weight based on the gradient of the loss, directing it toward an optimal value for those specific data.

The algorithm assumes that some functions are predefined, such as ModelModel, LossLoss, SignSign, VerifyVerify, EncryptEncrypt, and Decrypt. These functions may vary depending on the specific implementation of federated learning and TEE.

**Algorithm 1** Local Model in TEE for Federated Learning

**Input**:
  Local data: $D_i$
  Number of training epochs: $E$
  Learning rate: $\alpha$
  Diffie–Hellman parameters: $p, g$
**Output**: weight $w$

1: Generate private key for Diffie–Hellman: $SK_i$
2: Compute public key for Diffie–Hellman: $PK_i \leftarrow g^{SK_i} \mod p$
3: **Interaction between REE and TEE:**
4: REE: Send $PK_i$ to TEE
5: TEE: Receive $PK_i$ from REE
6: **Local Attestation Process in TEE:**
7: TEE: Generate nonce: $N$
8: TEE: Compute attestation token: $T = \text{Sign}(SK_{\text{TEE}}, N)$
9: TEE: Send $N$ and $T$ to REE
10: REE: Receive $N$ and $T$ from TEE
11: REE: Verify attestation token: $\text{Verify}(PK_{\text{TEE}}, N, T)$
12: **In TEE:**
13: TEE: Generate fresh private key for Diffie–Hellman: $SK_{\text{TEE}}$
14: TEE: Compute public key for Diffie–Hellman: $PK_{\text{TEE}} \leftarrow g^{SK_{\text{TEE}}} \mod p$
15: **Local Model in TEE:**
16: Initialize model weights: $w$
17: **for** $e = 1$ to $E$ **do**
18:   **for** each sample $(x, y)$ in $D_i$ **do**
19:     Compute model prediction: $\hat{y} = \text{Model}(w, x)$
20:     Compute gradient: $\nabla = \nabla \text{Loss}(\hat{y}, y)$
21:     Update model weights: $w \leftarrow w - \alpha \cdot \nabla$
22: **Interaction between REE and TEE:**
23: TEE: Send encrypted weight: $E_{\text{weight}} = \text{Encrypt}(PK_i, w)$ to REE
24: REE: Receive encrypted weight: $E_{\text{weight}}$ from TEE
25: REE: Decrypt weight using Diffie–Hellman: $w = \text{Decrypt}(SK_i, E_{\text{weight}})$
26: **return**: $w$

*3.4. Federated Averaging on Blockchain*

Federal learning involves data exchange among multiple parties. To ensure the security and integrity of the data, this paper adopts the FedAvg algorithm combined with the consortium blockchain to achieve secure data transmission. The consortium blockchain is a distributed ledger system based on blockchain technology that can improve the security and credibility of data-sharing and interaction among multiple parties. The FedAvg algorithm uses the average of the model parameters to achieve collaborative learning among participants. An overview of this process is shown in Figure 4. And the flow of reaching consensus on the blockchain is shown in Figure 5.

FedAvg is a communication-efficient algorithm for distributed training with many clients who keep their data locally for privacy. A central server communicates the global model parameter to each client and aggregates the updated local model parameters from clients. The core formula of FedAvg is

$$w^{(t+1)} = \sum_{k=1}^{K} \frac{n_k}{n} w_k^{(t+1)} \quad (4)$$

where $w^{(t+1)}$ is the global model parameter at round $t+1$, $K$ is the number of clients, $n_k$ is the number of local data samples on client $k$, $n$ is the total number of data samples across all clients, and $w_k^{(t+1)}$ is the local model parameter updated by client $k$ on round $t+1$. The formula is derived by having each selected client perform SGD on its local data using the global model parameter as the initial value and having the server take a weighted average of the received local model parameters. FedAvg can reduce communication costs and improve privacy compared to centralized methods that require sending raw data or gradients to the server.

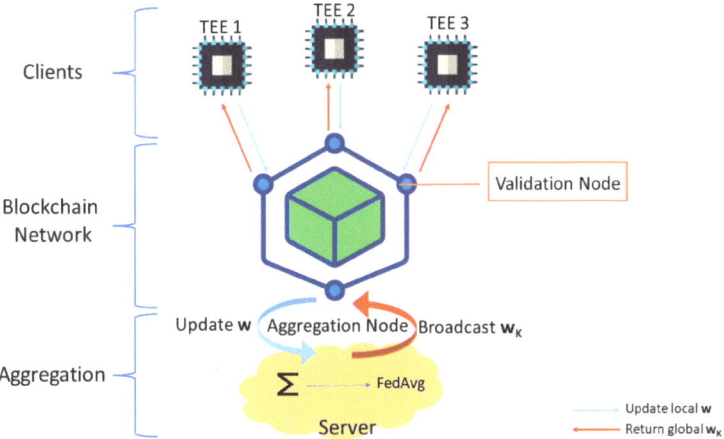

**Figure 4.** FedAvg on the blockchain.

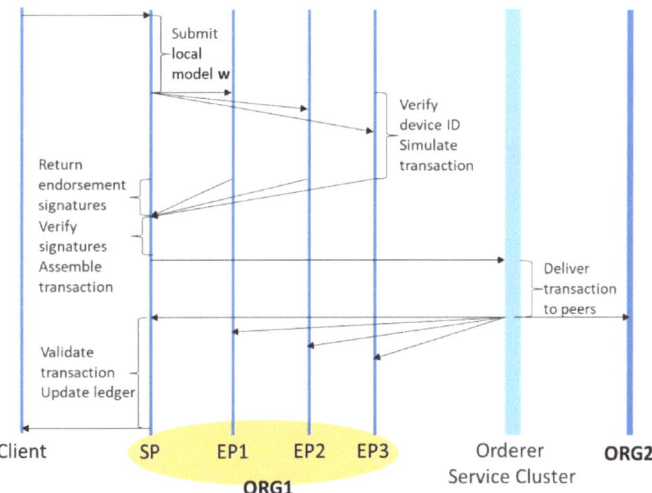

**Figure 5.** Flow of reaching consensus on the blockchain.

Algorithm 2 consists of four main parts:

- Input and output: The algorithm takes the following input, the set of devices $\mathcal{D}$, the number of global iterations $K$, the FedAvg learning rate $\eta$, the local model weight $\{\mathbf{w}_i\}_{i \in \mathcal{D}}$, and the device identity hash value $H_{ID,i}$ for all devices $i \in \mathcal{D}$. The output of the algorithm is the global weight $\mathbf{w}_K$ after global training.
- Hash Value Verification: To verify the identity information of each device, the algorithm reads the corresponding smart contract from the blockchain. If the device's identity hash value $H_{ID,i}$ matches the verified hash value, the corresponding local model weight $\mathbf{w}_i$ is stored in a list; otherwise, the local model weight $\mathbf{w}_i$ is discarded.
- Blockchain Uploading: All verified local model weights are stored in a block, which is then transmitted to the Fabric blockchain network. The algorithm waits for the

consensus result from the Raft network. If consensus is reached, the accepted block is received at all replicas, and the local model weights of the verified devices are extracted for use in the aggregation step.
- Aggregation: The local model weights of all verified devices are aggregated. The average value of these verified local model weights $\mathbf{a}_{t'}$ is computed and used to update the global model weight $\mathbf{w}_{t'}$. Here, $\mathbf{w}_{t'-1}$ represents the global model weight from the previous iteration. The FedAvg strategy is used to update the global model weight $\mathbf{w}_{t'} \leftarrow \mathbf{w}_{t'-1} - \eta \nabla f(\mathbf{a}_{t'}, \mathcal{D})$, where $f(\cdot)$ is the objective function and $\mathcal{D}$ is the global dataset.

---

**Algorithm 2** FederatedAveraging on Blockchain

---

**Input:**
  Device sets: $\mathcal{D}$
  Number of global iterations: $K$
  FedAvg learning rate: $\eta$
  Local model weight: $\{\mathbf{w}_i\}_{i \in \mathcal{D}}$ and device identity hash value: $H_{ID,i}$ for all $i \in \mathcal{D}$
**Output:** global weight $\mathbf{w}_K$

1: **procedure** FEDAVG($\mathcal{D}, K, \eta, \{\mathbf{w}_i\}_{i \in \mathcal{D}}, \{H_{ID,i}\}_{i \in \mathcal{D}}$)
2:   Initialize the global weight $\mathbf{w}_0$
3:   **for** $t = 1, 2, \ldots, K$ **do**
4:     **for** $i \in \mathcal{D}$ **do**
5:       **if** the device ID hash value in $H_{ID,i}$ is validated by the corresponding smart contract **then**
6:         Store the verified local model weight in a list: $\{\mathbf{w}_i\}_{i \in \mathcal{D}, \text{verified}}$.
7:       **else**
8:         Discard the local model weight $\mathbf{w}_i$ of device $i$ due to mismatched ID hash value.
9:     Form a block $B_t$ containing all verified local model weights $\{\mathbf{w}_i\}_{i \in \mathcal{D}, \text{verified}}$.
10:    Upload the block $B_t$ to the Fabric blockchain: $B_t \rightarrow Upload$
11:    Wait for the consensus result from the Raft network: $Consensus \rightarrow Wait$
12:    **if** consensus achieved **then**
13:      Receive the accepted block at all replicas, extract the local model weights of verified devices
14:      **Aggregate the received updates using FedAvg:** $\mathbf{a}_{t'} \leftarrow \frac{1}{C} \sum_{i=1}^{C} \mathbf{w}_i$, where $\{\mathbf{w}_i\}_{i=1}^{C}$ are the verified local model weights in the accepted block.
15:      Update the global weight using FedAvg: $\mathbf{w}_{t'} \leftarrow \mathbf{w}_{t'-1} - \eta \nabla f(\mathbf{a}_{t'}, \mathcal{D})$, where $f(\cdot)$ is the objective function and $\mathcal{D}$ is the global dataset.
16:  **return** $\mathbf{w}_K$

---

## 4. Security Analysis

Federated learning is a distributed collaborative learning technique that enables training a global model using local data from multiple clients without sharing the data. However, federated learning faces various security and privacy threats, such as data poisoning by malicious clients, model poisoning, inference attacks, free-riding attacks, and robustness attacks. To address these threats, we propose an algorithm for training a local model in TEE.

### 4.1. Local Training Model in TEE

TEE is a hardware-isolation technology that ensures that the code and data running within it are protected from external interference or leakage. The algorithm presented in this paper leverages TEE to provide the following security assurances. The proposed algorithm incorporates several security measures to mitigate security and privacy threats in federated learning. These measures include secure communication using the Diffie–Hellman key exchange protocol, local attestation, encryption and decryption mechanisms, and local model training within the TEE.

Secure communication between the REE and TEE is achieved through the utilization of the Diffie–Hellman key-exchange protocol. This protocol, based on mathematical principles, enables the two parties to negotiate a shared key over a public channel without directly sharing the key itself. By relying on the computational hardness of the discrete logarithm problem, the protocol ensures that computing the private key from the public parameters is a challenging task. As a result, this approach prevents potential man-in-the-middle attacks and replay attacks, bolstering the security of the communication channel.

To verify the identity and integrity of the TEE, a local attestation process is implemented. In this process, the TEE generates a random number (nonce) and an attestation token, which are then transmitted to the REE. Upon receiving these parameters, the REE employs the TEE's public key to verify the authenticity of the attestation token and its correspondence to the received nonce. The successful verification of these parameters establishes trust in the TEE, effectively preventing impersonation or tampering attacks. To protect the confidentiality of the model weights, encryption and decryption mechanisms are employed. The TEE utilizes the Diffie–Hellman public key received from the REE to encrypt the model weights. Subsequently, the encrypted weights are securely transmitted to the REE, which possesses the corresponding Diffie–Hellman private key required for decryption. As only the REE holds the private key, unauthorized entities are unable to decrypt or modify the weights, safeguarding against theft or unauthorized manipulation. Furthermore, local model training within the TEE ensures privacy and prevents inference attacks or GAN attacks. This process involves the initialization of model parameters using locally generated Diffie–Hellman public and private keys. Multiple rounds of training are then conducted on the local dataset, enabling the TEE to update the model weights accordingly. Since only the TEE possesses knowledge of its private key and the weights, external entities are unable to infer any sensitive information about the data or weights, reinforcing privacy and thwarting potential attacks.

By leveraging the TEE and integrating mechanisms for secure communication, local attestation, encryption, and local model training, the proposed algorithm establishes robust security measures. These measures collectively mitigate various security and privacy threats in the context of federated learning. The combination of secure communication, trust establishment, data encryption, and local training within the TEE ensures the confidentiality, integrity, and authenticity of the communication and data, bolstering the overall security of the federated learning process.

*4.2. Aggregate Security*

Federated learning also faces various security and privacy challenges, such as malicious client attacks, local weight leakage or tampering, etc. To address these challenges, this paper optimizes the aggregation part of federated learning and proposes a scheme that combines aggregation algorithms with blockchain technology, thereby improving the security and efficiency of federated learning. The scheme proposed in this paper mainly includes two steps: consortium chain-based verification and consortium chain-based transmission.

In the consortium chain-based verification step, each participant needs to upload their local weights to the chain and attach their own identity digital signature after completing the local model training. A smart contract is deployed on the consortium chain to verify whether the local weights come from legitimate clients, i.e., whether they match the identity digital signature. Only local weights that pass the verification can be recorded on the blockchain and used for subsequent global model updates. Otherwise, local weights will be rejected and discarded. This verification mechanism can effectively prevent malicious clients from forging or tampering with local weights, thereby ensuring the quality and accuracy of the global model. At the same time, this verification mechanism can also solve the trust and attack problems that exist in traditional federated learning and improve the security and reliability of federated learning. Through the consortium-chain-based verification mechanism, we can enhance trust and collaboration among participants and prevent data pollution and model poisoning attacks.

In the consortium-chain-based transmission step, each participant no longer needs to send their local weights to the aggregation server after uploading them to the chain; instead, the aggregation server obtains all participants' local weights from the blockchain and performs centralized aggregation. This transmission mechanism can effectively ensure the anti-tampering and security of local weights, prevent local weights being maliciously modified or stolen during transmission, and ensure the traceability and immutability of local weights. At the same time, this transmission mechanism can also reduce communication overhead and improve efficiency, solving the communication and efficiency problems that exist in traditional federated learning and improving the performance and effect of federated learning. Through the consortium-chain-based transmission mechanism, we can protect participants' data privacy and model knowledge and prevent data leakage and model theft attacks.

### 4.3. Adaptability

Our framework leverages Trusted Execution Environment (TEE) and blockchain technology to address data security and privacy challenges in federated learning, especially within the IoT supply chain management domain. However, our approach is general and can be extended to various contexts where data security and privacy are paramount. The core principles of our framework are ensuring data security, data integrity, and user privacy. These principles are applicable across various domains where federated learning and data security concerns overlap, such as healthcare, smart cities, or industrial IoT. Moreover, any collaborative machine learning or data analytics scenario where data privacy is a concern can potentially benefit from our framework. Examples include finance, healthcare, and e-commerce, where transactional data, patient records, and user purchase history need to be protected. The combination of TEE and blockchain ensures not only data security but also the traceability and accountability of computations, making it suitable for any scenario requiring trustworthiness and auditability. Furthermore, our system is modular and adaptable. Different components (e.g., a different blockchain or a different TEE) can be integrated based on the specific requirements of another context, allowing for flexibility in deployment. Therefore, our framework has a wide range of potential applications beyond IoT supply chain management.

## 5. Results

In this section, we provide an overview of the implementation and evaluation of our proposed framework.

### 5.1. Experimental Methodology

We present the experimental results of our proposed scheme for privacy-preserving federated learning based on TEE and the blockchain. We first evaluated the performance of the local model training in TEE for federated learning. Then, we conducted experiments to compare the performance of federated learning with blockchain-based parameter updates with different numbers of nodes and transactions. We collected a dataset from real-world IoT devices of a supply chain, which includes production data from multiple suppliers, sales data from retailers, and product data. The detailed configuration of the experimental environment is presented in Table 3.

**Table 3.** Experiments setup.

| Experiments Setup | Specification |
| --- | --- |
| CPU | Intel Xeon Processor 2695 CPU 2.40 GHz |
| Ram | 64 GB |
| Operating System | Ubuntu 18.04 |
| Implementation | Python 3.7.0 |
| Libraries | Pytroch 1.6.0 |
| System Setup | Hyperledger Fabric 2.0, Docker 20.10.7 |

*5.2. Performance Evaluation*

We conducted an experiment to evaluate our framework's performance in local clients using federated learning from Figure 6. We compared the time costs of local training and aggregated three models (LeNet, VGG16, and ResNet) with 200 data samples each on two datasets (Fashion MNIST and MNIST) under two scenarios: using TEE in Intel SGX or using REE. We varied the number of local nodes from 5 to 30 and measured the total time required for each scenario. Figure 6 shows the results of our experiment. We observed that ResNet had similar trends on both datasets, as shown in Figure 6a,d. The training and aggregation time remained stable until 15 local nodes but increased when reaching 20 local nodes or more. The increase was about 1.6 s for both scenarios. Figure 6b,c show the results for LeNet and VGG on the MNIST dataset. We found that using TEE increased the time cost by about 1.57 s compared to using REE when using 30 local nodes for VGG model. However, this was only 1.7 s slower than not using SGX at all for aggregation. The other models had similar results. The main reason for the increased time cost in TEE was the memory limitation of Intel SGX, which affected the efficiency of federated learning.

We evaluated our framework's accuracy by testing the final global model obtained from federated training on a test dataset. We varied the number of participants and the number of iterations in our experiment. We considered four scenarios with different numbers of iterations: 5, 10, 20, and 30. We also varied the number of participants from 1 to 30. Figure 7 shows our accuracy results for each scenario. We found that increasing the number of both iterations and participants improved the accuracy of our global model. For example, when using only one participant and five iterations, our model achieved an accuracy of 94%. However, when using ten participants and thirty iterations, our model reached an accuracy of 98.5%. This indicates that more iterations and participants allow our framework to capture more features from the training data and generate a better classifier. The main reason for this improvement is that each participant randomly selects samples from their local data for each iteration. When there are few participants or iterations, some samples may not be used for training at all, which reduces the diversity and representativeness of our global model. By increasing both factors, we can ensure that our framework covers more samples from different distributions and learns a more accurate model.

For the evaluation of the system throughput, we mainly measured the overall scale of the system in recording verification and data acquisition in the blockchain. We constructed three experimental scenarios with different numbers of participants joining, where the transaction number was set to 500, 1000, and 2000. Figure 8 shows the relationship between different numbers of participants and system throughput under the condition of completing the transaction number of the three experimental scenarios. When the number of participants was two, the system throughput performance showed a significant upward trend as the set's transaction number increased, rising from about 20 TPS to about 34 TPS. However, as the number of participants increased, the system throughput decreased. Under normal circumstances, the increase in participants would have a positive effect on system throughput. The reason for this, we believe, is that the transaction number was set too high, resulting in too many data generated by participants, causing data-congestion problems for the system and a performance bottleneck. We also conducted throughput experiments for four and six participants in different stages of the FedAvg on Chain process, such as local weight upload, verification, and aggregation, as shown in Figure 9. Figure 9a is a graph of the relationship between transaction volume and throughput for four participants and Figure 9b is for six participants. A common point for four and six participants is that the throughput of local weight uploaded to the blockchain stage is lower than that of the other two stages, and as the transaction volume increases, the throughput performance of four participants is better than that of six participants, for the same reason that too much data generation leads to performance bottlenecks. Only when the transaction volume is too large will it cause a decline in the throughput performance. FedAvg on Chain does not have thousands of iterations, ensuring that the system can run normally with multiple participants.

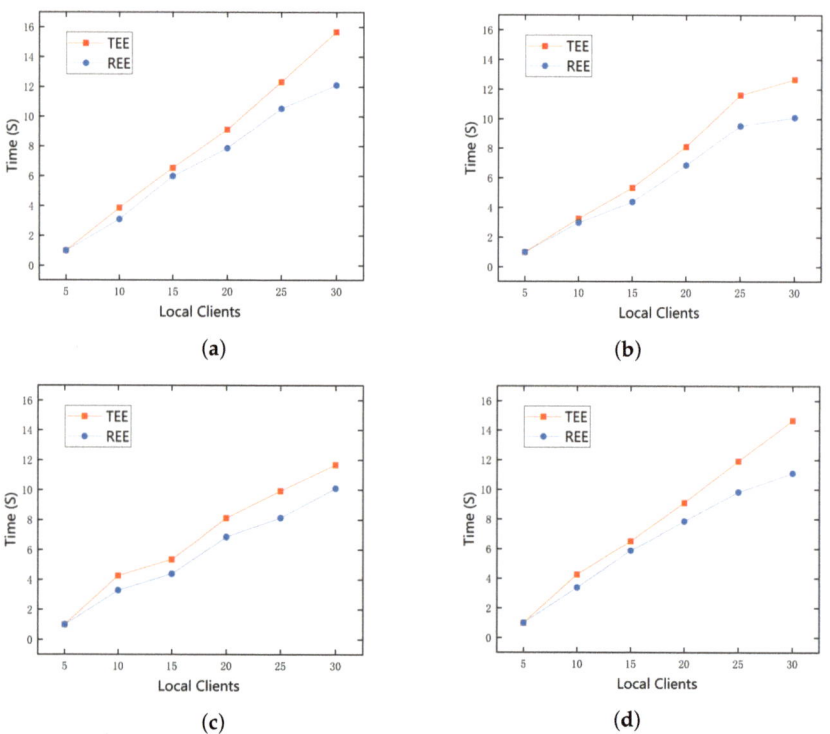

**Figure 6.** Comparison of durations of training processes between the TEE and REE for various deep learning models and the Fashion MNIST dataset. (**a**) ResNet-Fashion MNIST. (**b**) LeNet-MNIST. (**c**) VGG16-MNIST. (**d**) ResNet-MNIST.

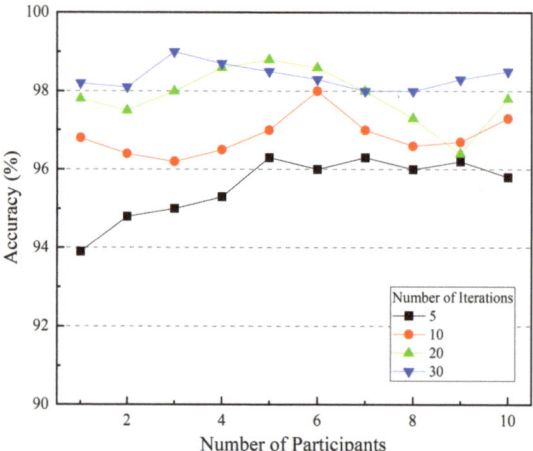

**Figure 7.** Federated learning accuracy.

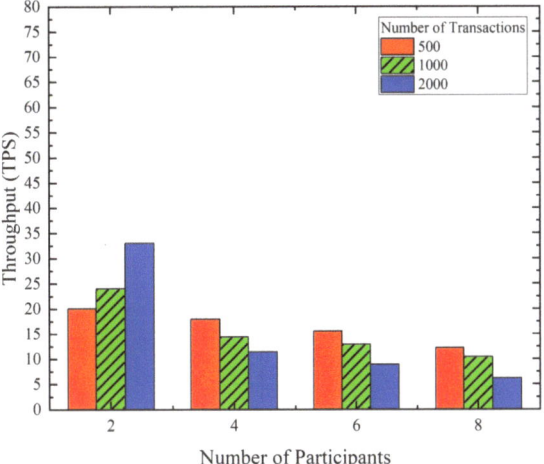

**Figure 8.** Throughput.

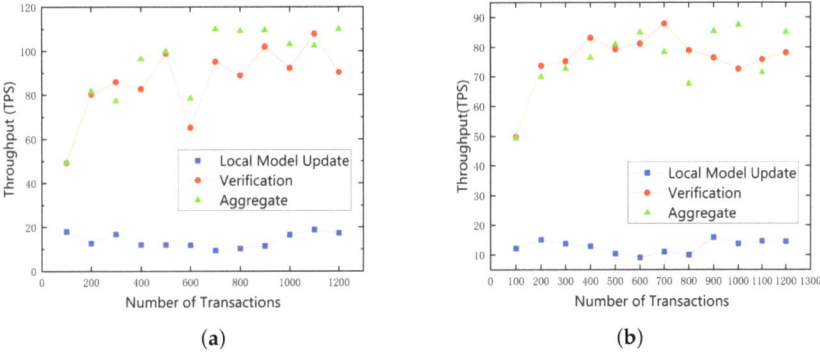

**Figure 9.** The comparison of throughput between 4 nodes and 6 nodes.

We also tested the transaction latency of the system, as well as the evaluation of the system throughput. We still constructed scenarios with 500, 1000, and 2000 transactions and conducted experiments on the average transaction latency of the system with different numbers of participants. Figure 10 shows that as the number of participants increases, the average transaction time delay shows a positive trend. In the case of eight participants, the average time delay for 500 transactions can reach about 40 s. The number of participants remains unchanged, and the increase in transaction volume is also the reason for the increase in average time delay. The reason is that as the number of participants and transactions increase, the system blockchain will increase the overhead of the consensus algorithm and the network communication load, resulting in a decrease in system performance and a delay in transaction completion time. For the evaluation of time delay, we also conducted tests for four and six participants in the same experimental scenarios as the throughput. Figure 11a is a graph of the relationship between transaction volume and throughput for four participants, and Figure 11b is for six participants. As shown in the figure, whether it is four or six participants, the local weight upload stage has a higher time delay than the verification and aggregation stages, which is opposite to the throughput situation. The reason is also that the system reaches a performance bottleneck, resulting in a decrease in throughput and an increase in time delay. Such results provide a reference direction for the subsequent optimization of this system.

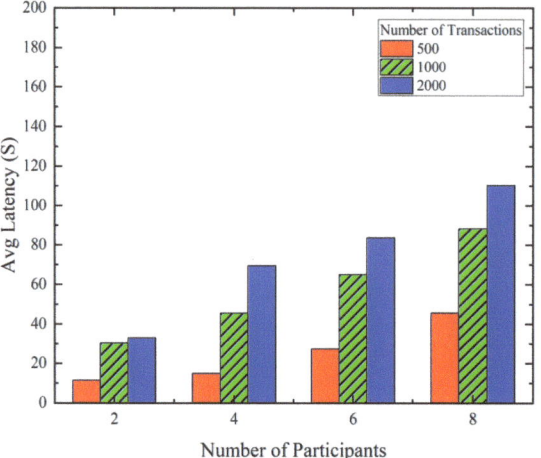

**Figure 10.** Average Latency.

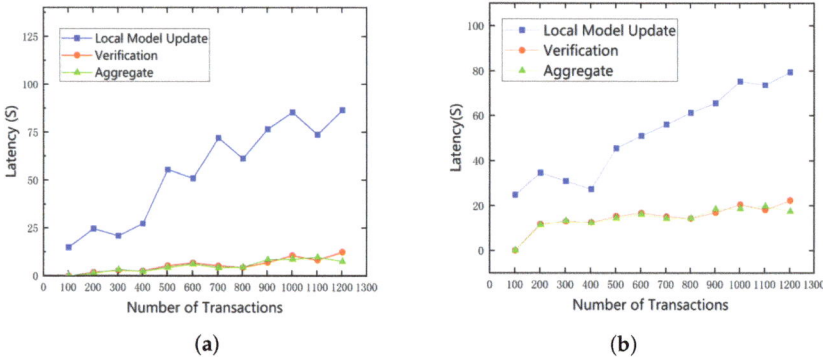

**Figure 11.** The comparison of latency between 4 nodes and 6 nodes.

## 6. Conclusions

In this paper, we propose a TEE and consortium-blockchain-based federated learning framework for the IoT of the supply chain. The main objective of this framework is to ensure the tamper resistance of data in federated learning, protect the data security in the whole federated learning process, and achieve the security and effectiveness of the aggregation results. The local model runs in the TEE. The framework uses an Intel SGX-based TEE to ensure the secure execution of the local model and the trusted output of the local data and then uses consortium blockchain technology to realize the secure transmission of the local data, and finally obtains the aggregated parameter results. In this framework, each blockchain node is equipped with a verification node, which verifies whether the data source is consistent with the set participants and ensures the trustworthiness of data usage. Finally, through blockchain technology, the aggregated global model parameters are added to the blockchain and returned to all local models. We set different numbers of participants and different datasets to test the framework. The experimental results show that the local data-processing time of our proposed framework is almost the same as that of the original federated learning model. In addition, our framework has high throughput performance for normal use by multiple participants.

However, our proposed framework also has some limitations that need to be addressed in future work. First, our system relies on TEE and blockchain technology, which may increase the system's complexity and cost, as well as the hardware and network requirements. We plan to explore how to reduce the system overhead and resource consumption while maintaining security and efficiency. Second, our system uses Intel SGX as a specific implementation of TEE, but Intel SGX also has some known security vulnerabilities, such as Foreshadow and Plundervolt, which may affect the reliability and robustness of our system. We plan to investigate how to deploy our system on different TEE platforms and how to prevent or detect these potential attacks.

**Author Contributions:** Conceptualization, L.Z. and S.H.; methodology, L.Z.; software, S.H.; validation, L.Z., S.H. and M.H.; formal analysis, S.H. and C.M.; investigation, X.Z., C.M. and M.H.; resources, L.Z. and S.H.; writing—original draft preparation, L.Z. and S.H.; writing—review and editing, L.Z. and S.H.; visualization, L.Z., S.H. and M.H.; supervision, L.Z. All authors have read and agreed to the published version of the manuscript.

**Funding:** This work is supported by MOST-FDCT Projects (0058/2019/AMJ, 2019YFE0110300) (Research and Application of Cooperative Multi-Agent Platform for Zhuhai-Macao Manufacturing Service).

**Data Availability Statement:** The data can not be shared due to the project's privacy policy.

**Conflicts of Interest:** The authors declare no conflict of interest.

# References

1. Ben-Daya, M.; Hassini, E.; Bahroun, Z. Internet of Things and Supply Chain Management: A Literature Review. *Int. J. Prod. Res.* **2019**, *57*, 4719–4742. [CrossRef]
2. Qu, T.; Lei, S.; Wang, Z.; Nie, D.; Chen, X.; Huang, G.Q. IoT-Based Real-Time Production Logistics Synchronization System under Smart Cloud Manufacturing. *Int. J. Adv. Manuf. Technol.* **2016**, *84*, 147–164. [CrossRef]
3. Tao, F.; Zuo, Y.; Xu, L.D.; Zhang, L. IoT-Based Intelligent Perception and Access of Manufacturing Resource toward Cloud Manufacturing. *IEEE Trans. Ind. Inform.* **2014**, *10*, 1547–1557.
4. Wen, Q.; Gao, Y.; Chen, Z.; Wu, D. A Blockchain-Based Data Sharing Scheme in the Supply Chain by IIoT. In Proceedings of the 2019 IEEE International Conference on Industrial Cyber Physical Systems (ICPS), Taipei, Taiwan, 6–9 May 2019; pp. 695–700.
5. Yang, Q.; Liu, Y.; Chen, T.; Tong, Y. Federated Machine Learning: Concept and Applications. *ACM Trans. Intell. Syst. Technol.* **2019**, *10*, 12. [CrossRef]
6. Li, A.; Zhang, L.; Tan, J.; Qin, Y.; Wang, J.; Li, X.-Y. Sample-level Data Selection for Federated Learning. In Proceedings of the IEEE INFOCOM 2021—IEEE Conference on Computer Communications, Vancouver, BC, Canada, 10–13 May 2021; pp. 1–10. [CrossRef]
7. Demertzis, K.; Iliadis, L.; Pimenidis, E.; Tziritas, N.; Koziri, M.; Kikiras, P.; Tonkin, M. Federated Blockchained Supply Chain Management: A CyberSecurity and Privacy Framework. In Artificial Intelligence Applications and Innovations. 2021. Available online: http://hdl.handle.net/11615/60214 (accessed on 30 October 2022).
8. Zheng, G.; Kong, L.; Brintrup, A. Federated Machine Learning for Privacy Preserving, Collective Supply Chain Risk Prediction. *Int. J. Prod. Res.* **2023**, 1–18. [CrossRef]
9. Liu, Y.; Yu, W.; Ai, Z.; Xu, G.; Zhao, L.; Tian, Z. A Blockchain-Empowered Federated Learning in Healthcare-Based Cyber Physical Systems. *IEEE Trans. Netw. Sci. Eng.* **2022**. [CrossRef]
10. Wu, J.M.T.; Teng, Q.; Huda, S.; Chen, Y.-C.; Chen, C.-M. A Privacy Frequent Itemsets Mining Framework for Collaboration in IoT Using Federated Learning. *ACM Trans. Sens. Netw.* **2023**, *19*, 27. [CrossRef]
11. Lu, Y.; Huang, X.; Dai, Y.; Maharjan, S.; Zhang, Y. Blockchain and Federated Learning for Privacy-Preserved Data Sharing in Industrial IoT. *IEEE Trans. Ind. Inform.* **2020**, *16*, 4177–4186. [CrossRef]
12. Qammar, A.; Karim, A.; Ning, H.; Ding, J. Securing Federated Learning with Blockchain: A Systematic Literature Review. *Artif. Intell. Rev.* **2023**, *56*, 3951–3985. [CrossRef]
13. Korkmaz, C.; Kocas, H.E.; Uysal, A.; Masry, A.; Ozkasap, O.; Akgun, B. Chain FL: Decentralized Federated Machine Learning via Blockchain. In Proceedings of the 2020 Second International Conference on Blockchain Computing and Applications (BCCA), Antalya, Turkey, 24–26 November 2020; pp. 140–146. [CrossRef]
14. Intel Corporation. *Intel Software Guard Extensions Programming Reference*; Intel Corporation: Santa Clara, CA, USA, 2014.
15. Zhang, Y.; Wang, Y.; Liu, J.; Shi, W. SGX-FPGA: Trusted Execution Environment for CPU-FPGA Heterogeneous Architecture. In Proceedings of the 2021 58th ACM/IEEE Design Automation Conference (DAC), San Francisco, CA, USA, 5–9 December 2021; pp. 1–6.
16. Götzfried, J.; Eckert, M.; Schinzel, S.; Müller, T. Cache attacks on intel sgx. In Proceedings of the 10th European Workshop on Systems Security, Paris, France, 23–24 April 2017; p. 2.
17. Brasser, F.; Müller, U.; Dmitrienko, A.; Kostiainen, K.; Capkun, S.; Sadeghi, A.R. Software grand exposure:SGX cache attacks are practical. In Proceedings of the 11th USENIX Workshop on Offensive Technologies (WOOT17), Vancouver, BC, Canada, 14–15 August 2017; p. 15.

18. Van Bulck, J.; Minkin, M.; Weisse, O.; Genkin, D.; Kasikci, B.; Piessens, F.; Silberstein, M.; Wenisch, T.F.; Yarom, Y.; Strackx, R. Foreshadow: Extracting the keys to the intel sgx kingdom with transient out-of-order execution. In Proceedings of the 27th USENIX Security Symposium (USENIX Security 18), Baltimore, MD, USA, 15–17 August 2018; pp. 991–1008.
19. VanNostrand, P.M.; Kyriazis, I.; Cheng, M.; Guo, T.; Walls, R.J. Confidential Deep Learning: Executing Proprietary Models on Untrusted Devices. In Proceedings of the 2020 IEEE International Conference on Pervasive Computing and Communications Workshops (PerCom Workshops), Austin, TX, USA, 23–27 March 2020; pp. 1–62.
20. Mothukuri, V.; Parizi, R.M.; Pouriyeh, S.; Huang, Y.; Dehghantanha, A.; Srivastava, G. A survey on security and privacy of federated learning. *Future Gener. Comput. Syst.* **2021**, *115*, 619–640. [CrossRef]
21. Zhang, Y.; Zeng, D.; Luo, J.; Xu, Z.; King, I. A Survey of Trustworthy Federated Learning with Perspectives on Security, Robustness, and Privacy. *arXiv* **2023**, arXiv2302.10637.
22. Abadi, M.; Chu, A.; Goodfellow, I.; McMahan, H.B.; Mironov, I.; Talwar, K.; Zhang, L. Deep Learning with Differential Privacy. In Proceedings of the 2016 ACM SIGSAC Conference on Computer and Communications Security (CCS'16), Vienna, Austria, 24–28 October 2016; pp. 308–318.
23. Zhang, C.; Xie, Y.; Bai, H.; Yu, B.; Li, W.; Gao, Y. A survey on federated learning. *Knowl.-Based Syst.* **2021**, *216*, 106775. [CrossRef]
24. McMahan, B.; Moore, E.; Ramage, D.; Hampson, S.; y Arcas, B.A. Communication-efficient learning of deep networks from decentralized data. In Proceedings of the 20th International Conference on Artificial Intelligence and Statistics, PMLR, Fort Lauderdale, FL, USA, 20–22 April 2017; pp. 1273–1282.
25. Lim, W.Y.B.; Luong, N.C.; Hoang, D.T.; Jiao, Y.; Liang, Y.-C.; Yang, Q.; Niyato, D.; Miao, C. Federated learning in mobile edge networks: A comprehensive survey. *IEEE Commun. Surv. Tutor.* **2020**, *22*, 2031–2063. [CrossRef]
26. Li, X.; Jiang, P.; Chen, T.; Luo, X.; Wen, Q. A survey on the security of blockchain systems. *Future Gener. Comput. Syst.* **2020**, *107*, 841–853. [CrossRef]
27. Zheng, Z.; Xie, S.; Dai, H.-N.; Chen, X.; Wang, H. Blockchain challenges and opportunities: A survey. *Int. J. Web Grid Serv.* **2018**, *14*, 352–375. [CrossRef]
28. Dai, H.-N.; Zheng, Z.; Zhang, Y. Blockchain for Internet of Things: A survey. *IEEE Internet Things J.* **2019**, *6*, 8076–8094. [CrossRef]
29. Maesa, D.D.F.; Mori, P. Blockchain 3.0 applications survey. *J. Parallel Distrib. Comput.* **2020**, *138*, 99–114. [CrossRef]
30. Wang, Y.; Zhang, Y.; Li, Z.; Liu, Y. Integrating blockchain technology into the energy sector—From theory of blockchain to research and application of energy blockchain. *Comput. Sci. Rev.* **2020**, *37*, 100275. [CrossRef]
31. Mirabelli, G.; De Benedetto, L.; Dassisti, M. Blockchain-based solutions for agri-food supply chains: A survey. *Int. J. Simul. Process Model.* **2021**, *17*, 1–15. [CrossRef]
32. Hasselgren, A.; Kralevska, K.; Gligoroski, D.; Pedersen, S.A.; Faxvaag, A. Blockchain in healthcare and health sciences—A scoping review. *Int. J. Med. Inform.* **2020**, *134*, 104040. [CrossRef]
33. Kassen, M. Blockchain and e-government innovation: Automation of public information processes. *Inf. Syst.* **2022**, *103*, 101862. [CrossRef]
34. Dib, O.; Brousmiche, K.-L.; Durand, A.; Thea, E.; Hamida, E.B. Consortium blockchains: Overview, applications and challenges. *Int. J. Adv. Telecommun.* **2018**, *11*, 51–64.
35. Li, Z.; Kang, J.; Yu, R.; Ye, D.; Deng, Q.; Zhang, Y. Consortium blockchain for secure energy trading in industrial internet of things. *IEEE Trans. Ind. Inform.* **2017**, *14*, 3690–3700. [CrossRef]
36. Bonawitz, K.; Eichner, H.; Grieskamp, W.; Huba, D.; Ingerman, A.; Ivanov, V.; Kiddon, C.; Konecny, J.; Mazzocchi, S.; McMahan, H.B.; et al. Towards federated learning at scale: System design. *Proc. Mach. Learn. Syst.* **2019**, *1*, 374–388.
37. Chen, Y.; Luo, F.; Li, T.; Xiang, T.; Liu, Z.; Li, J. A training-integrity privacy-preserving federated learning scheme with trusted execution environment. *Inf. Sci.* **2020**, *522*, 69–79. [CrossRef]
38. Li, Y.; Chen, C.; Liu, N.; Huang, H.; Zheng, Z.; Yan, Q. A blockchain-based decentralized federated learning framework with committee consensus. *IEEE Netw.* **2020**, *35*, 234–241. [CrossRef]

**Disclaimer/Publisher's Note:** The statements, opinions and data contained in all publications are solely those of the individual author(s) and contributor(s) and not of MDPI and/or the editor(s). MDPI and/or the editor(s) disclaim responsibility for any injury to people or property resulting from any ideas, methods, instructions or products referred to in the content.

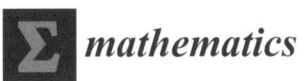

Article

# Healthcare Cost Prediction Based on Hybrid Machine Learning Algorithms

**Shujie Zou [1], Chiawei Chu [1,*], Ning Shen [2] and Jia Ren [3]**

1. Faculty of Data Science, City University of Macau, Macau 999078, China; d21092100231@cityu.mo
2. Department of Innovation, Technology and Entrepreneurship, United Arab Emirates University, Al Ain P.O. Box 15551, United Arab Emirates; ningshen@uaeu.ac.ae
3. School of Information and Communication Engineering, Hainan University, Haikou 570100, China; renjia@hainanu.edu.cn
* Correspondence: cwchu@cityu.mo

**Abstract:** Healthcare cost is an issue of concern right now. While many complex machine learning algorithms have been proposed to analyze healthcare cost and address the shortcomings of linear regression and reliance on expert analyses, these algorithms do not take into account whether each characteristic variable contained in the healthcare data has a positive effect on predicting healthcare cost. This paper uses hybrid machine learning algorithms to predict healthcare cost. First, network structure learning algorithms (a score-based algorithm, constraint-based algorithm, and hybrid algorithm) for a Conditional Gaussian Bayesian Network (CGBN) are used to learn the isolated characteristic variables in healthcare data without changing the data properties (i.e., discrete or continuous). Then, the isolated characteristic variables are removed from the original data and the remaining data used to train regression algorithms. Two public healthcare datasets are used to test the performance of the proposed hybrid machine learning algorithm model. Experiments show that when compared to popular single machine learning algorithms (Long Short Term Memory, Random Forest, etc.) the proposed scheme can obtain similar or higher prediction accuracy with a reduced amount of data.

**Keywords:** healthcare costs; CGBN; regression algorithm; hybrid algorithm

**MSC:** 68T09

## 1. Introduction

With the birth of various advanced medical technologies, the safety of human life has been greatly guaranteed; however, this brings with it larger medical expenses, which represent a great challenge for many patients [1]. Data collected by the Centers for Medicare and Medicaid Services shows that the U.S. spent a larger share of its gross domestic product on healthcare in 2018, increasing by 4.6% from the previous year [2]. Nonetheless, even very large healthcare expenditures may not provide appropriate and affordable healthcare for patients [3]. If the healthcare expenditures can be foreseen in advance, more precise services and treatments can be provided to patients. Thus, predicting healthcare costs can provide protection for patients while assisting healthcare organizations, e.g., drug manufacturers.

Currently, the study of healthcare costs is receiving attention from many researchers. For example, Kharat [4] used descriptive statistics to study the trend of chronic kidney disease in diabetic and non-diabetic patients from 2002 to 2016 and combined it with the associated quality of life to derive the healthcare expenditure of the patients. Yassine [5] used a cross-sectional study to analyze the healthcare expenditures of Moroccan basic health insurers from 2009 to 2014. Zhang studied data on the medical expenditures of lung cancer patients in thirteen provinces in China from 2002 to 2011, deducing that medical and

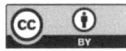

chemotherapy fees were the main factors that increased patients' healthcare cost [6]. Ma [7] collected data on the healthcare expenditures of selected middle-aged and elderly people in Beijing and analyzed the collected data using chi-square tests, t-tests, multivariate analysis, and linear regressions. Gong collected data on the healthcare expenditures of hemophiliacs from China's national insurance database from 2014 to 2016, compared the healthcare cost of employees and residents using the Kolmogorov–Smirnov test, and finally speculated on the factors affecting the healthcare expenditures of hemophiliacs using quantile regression [8]. Yang [9] collected data on medical expenditures of strabismus patients in the First Affiliated Hospital of Harbin Medical University, China and analyzed anesthesia as a major factor influencing medical expenditure of strabismus patients. Wang used Markov and two-part models to analyze healthcare expenditure for the elderly in China from 2011 to 2015 and make predictions about healthcare expenditures for the elderly in China from 2020 to 2060 [10]. Han [11] collected data from the 2018 Peking University Chinese Household Panel Study, used a Heckman sample selection model to analyze the data, and speculated on the extent to which the internet influences personal healthcare expenditures.

The above literature shows good results obtained in the study of healthcare expenditure; however, research in this area requires a large amount of data and extensive expert experience, and the algorithms used encounter difficulty when learning the information contained in the data [2]. With the rapid development of computer technology, researchers have begun to use complex machine learning algorithms to analyze healthcare expenditures. For example, Morid [12] used multiple supervised learning algorithms to learn from a large amount of healthcare cost data and make cost predictions, concluding that artificial neural networks can realize superior performance in the prediction of healthcare costs. Kaushik analyzed time-series healthcare cost data using LSTM (Long Short-Term Memory), CNN (Convolutional Neural Network), and Ensemble Learning to predict the average weekly spending of patients on two pain medications [13–15]. Yang [16] used machine learning algorithms to predict future healthcare expenditures and analyze the temporal correlation of patients' healthcare expenditures, concluding that more historical data leads to better predictive performance on the part of machine learning algorithms. Kuo [17] used machine learning algorithms such as Support Vector Machine, Logistic Regression, Decision Tree, and Random Forest to analyze the healthcare expenditure data of spinal fusion patients in Taiwan from 2021 to 2023 and predict the healthcare expenditures of patients, with Random Forest showing optimal predictive performance. Zeng [18] built a multi-layer self-attention model to learn the relationship between medical codes and medical visits in order to predict future medical expenditures and diseases. The above studies have obtained better results in predicting healthcare cost; however, most of them focus on time-series healthcare expenditure data and require a large amount of data and expertly selected characteristic variables. Meanwhile, many researchers are using advanced single algorithms and expert experience to obtain high prediction accuracy with little consideration of the need to reduce data dimensionality. Irrelevant characteristic variables may represent a kind of "noise" in the dataset that can affect the prediction accuracy of the prediction model. This paper studies non-temporal and small amounts of data that contain partial information (age, gender, previous disease history, etc.) about each individual. More importantly, it focuses on identifying irrelevant characteristic variables in healthcare cost data as a way to reduce the amount of data and the amount of time required by the regression model to analyze the data while improving the prediction accuracy of regression models, an approach that has received little attention from researchers.

## 2. Related Work

Currently, researchers are using CGBN to study healthcare expenditures. For example, Wang [19] used CGBN to analyze data on the healthcare expenditures of lung cancer patients in Taiwan and predict healthcare expenditures based on different disease levels of lung cancer patients. In addition, researchers have used CGBN in other fields of research; for example, Hu [20] used CGBN to process seismic data with a mixture of discrete and continuous variables, then applied CGBN to the prediction of earthquakes in Canterbury from 2010 to 2011; the experimental results showed that the prediction performance of CGBN was better than that of algorithms such as neural networks and support vector machine. Liu in [21] used CGBN to mine gene loci for carotenoid components of maize, finding that CGBN exhibited better performance than other algorithms in the experiment. In this paper, CGBN is used to learn isolated feature variables (variables that do not affect the target variable) from healthcare expenditure data, then regression algorithms are used to learn the data with the isolated variables removed. CGBN plays a key role in filtering data (reducing the amount of data) in the research presented in this paper.

## 3. Prediction Model

In this paper, CGBN is combined with regression algorithms to form hybrid machine learning models used to predict healthcare cost. First, the multiple structural learning algorithms of CGBN are used to learn the information in the dataset in order to build multiple network structures. Then, the number of occurrences of each isolated node in all network structures is counted and the feature variables corresponding to the isolated nodes with the highest number of occurrences are removed from the original dataset. Finally, the regression algorithms are used to learn the processed data and make predictions. The workflow block diagram of the proposed prediction model is shown in Figure 1. The modules in the dotted box in Figure 1 are the steps in which the hybrid machine learning model analyses and processes the data. The processing of the Analysis Module in Figure 1 is shown in Figure 2. The dots in the left three boxes of Figure 2 represent isolated nodes learned by network structure algorithms. Next, the structure learning algorithms used to construct the CGBN are presented.

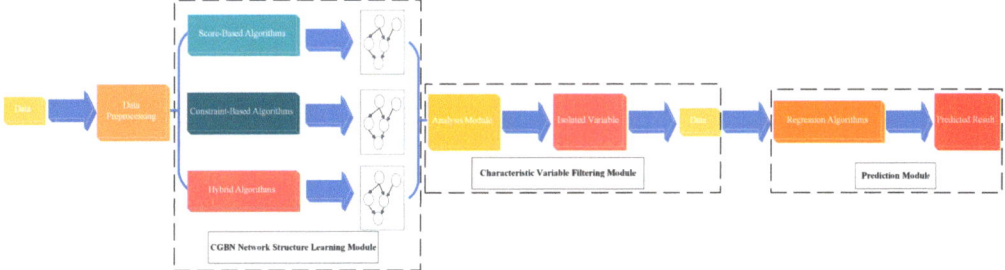

**Figure 1.** Block diagram of the workflow of the hybrid algorithm model.

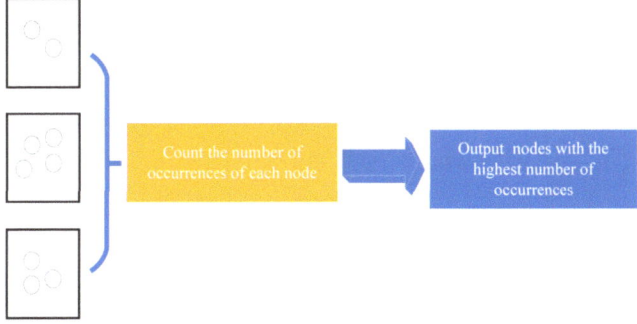

**Figure 2.** Block diagram of the workflow of the analysis module.

## 3.1. Network Structure Learning Algorithm

The attributes of the feature variables (continuous or discrete) are not changed when constructing the CGBN, which does not result in the loss of information in the dataset. In addition, the network structure of the CGBN has the following rules:

1. The nodes corresponding to discrete variables can only have nodes constructed by discrete variables as their parents.
2. The nodes corresponding to continuous variables can have either nodes constructed by discrete variables or nodes constructed by continuous variables as their parents.

Based on the properties of CGBN, in this paper we select two commonly used algorithms from each network structure algorithm to learn the network structure. Next, all network structure learning algorithms used in this paper are introduced in turn.

### 3.1.1. Score-Based Algorithms

In this paper, two score-based algorithms (the Hill Climbing and Tabu algorithms) for learning network structures are used. The BIC (Bayesian Information Criterion) algorithm for evaluating the structure of the network constructed by the Hill Climbing algorithm and the Tabu algorithm is

$$Score(G, D) = \sum_{i=1}^{k_D} (\log P(v_i|pa(v_i)) - \frac{d_{v_i}}{2} \log N) + \sum_{j=1}^{k_C} (\log f(v_j|pa(v_j)) - \frac{d_{v_j}}{2} \log N) \quad (1)$$

where $D$ is the dataset, $G$ is the directed acyclic graph, $N$ is the number of data, $P(\cdot)$ is the conditional probability, $f(\cdot)$ is the probability density function, $d_{v_i}$ and $d_{v_j}$ are the number of network node parameters, $k_D$ is the number of discrete network nodes, $k_C$ is the number of continuous network nodes, $pa(v_i)$ and $pa(v_j)$ are the parents of $v_i$ and $v_j$, respectively, and $v_i$ and $v_j$ are network nodes, where $v_i, v_j \in V = \{v_1, v_2, \ldots, v_n\}$, $k_D + k_C = n$ (with $n$ being the total number of nodes or the number of feature variables), and $V$ is the set of network nodes. The first term on the right side of the equation represents the formula for calculating the scores of the nodes corresponding to discrete variables, while the second term represents the formula for calculating the scores of the nodes corresponding to continuous variables. It is worth noting that when there are nodes of discrete variables in the parent nodes of continuous variables, the expression for the second term on the right side of the equation can be further expressed as follows:

$$\sum_{j=1}^{k_C} (\log f(v_j|pa(v_j)) - \frac{d_{v_j}}{2} \log N) = \sum_{j=1}^{k_C} (\sum_{c \in v_d} \log f(v_j|v_d = c, pa(v_{j \neq d})) - \frac{d_{v_j,c}}{2} \log N) \quad (2)$$

where $v_d$ (discrete variable) represents the parent of node $v_j$, $c$ is the value of node $v_d$, and $d_{v_j,c}$ is the number of network node parameters. Next, the fundamentals of the Hill Climbing algorithm and Tabu algorithm are introduced.

The basic principle of both the Tabu and Hill Climbing (HC) algorithms is to start the search from the network structure (usually an empty graph), then add, delete, or reverse arcs on the network structure until $Score(G, D)$ cannot be improved any more. The Tabu algorithm overcomes the shortcomings of the HC algorithm to a certain extent, and has a better ability to learn the network structure [22].

### 3.1.2. Constraint-Based Algorithms

Two constraint-based network structure learning algorithms (the PC algorithm and Grow–Shrink algorithm) are used as well. The basic principle of the PC and the Grow–Shrink (GS) algorithms is to construct a Bayesian network structure using conditional independent testing. The GS algorithm differs from the PC algorithm in that the GS algorithm learns the Markov blanket of each node. The conditional independence test is based on the principle that, given any two nodes $v_p, v_q \in V(p \neq q)$, finding the subset

$V_S \subset V(v_p, v_q \notin V_S)$ enables the nodes $v_p, v_q$ to be independent given a subset $V_S$ or an arc that exists between the nodes $v_p, v_q$ if no subset $V_S$ exists. Because CGBNs are established in this paper, mutual information is used to test the conditional independence between nodes.

### 3.1.3. Hybrid Algorithms

Two hybrid algorithms (the Max–Min Hill-Climbing (MMHC) and Restricted Maximization (rsmax2) algorithms) are used to learn the network structure of CGBN. These hybrid algorithms combine the benefits of constraint algorithms and score algorithms to learn the network structure of the CGBN. The MMHC algorithm combines Max–Min Parents and Children (the MMPC constraint algorithm) and HC score algorithm. First, the MMPC algorithm learns the candidate parent nodes for each node $v_m \in V$ to form the set $C_m$, then searches for the network structure that maximises the BIC score under the constraints of the set of parent nodes $C_m$. In this paper, the combination of rsmax2 is set to be the same as that of MMHC, with the difference that the rsmax2 algorithm can repeat the network structure learning process of the MMHC algorithm until convergence.

With all of the network structure learning algorithms for CGBN used in this paper described above, we next turn to the regression algorithms.

## 3.2. Regression Algorithms

### 3.2.1. Linear Regression (LR)

The multiple linear regression algorithm used in the paper is a simple and practical machine learning algorithm that plays an important role in regression research. LR algorithms continue to occupy an important place in practical research. Taking the $i$-th instance as an example, the expression for the LR is

$$\overline{y_{l,i}} = w_1 x_{i,1} + w_2 x_{i,2} + \cdots + w_n x_{i,n} + w_0, \tag{3}$$

where $w_{i \neq 0}$ is the partial regression coefficient, $w_0$ is the constant term, $\overline{y_{l,i}}$ is the predicted value, $x_{i,n}$ is the value of the $n$-th feature variable for the $i$-th instance, and $n$ is the number of feature variables.

### 3.2.2. Support Vector Regression (SVR)

Support Vector Machine algorithms are classical machine learning algorithm that use appropriate kernel functions (linear kernel function, Gaussian kernel function, sigmoid kernel function, polynomial kernel function, etc.) and parameters for the analysis of classification or regression. SVR is a part of Support Vector Machine algorithms, and can be used for the prediction of continuous data. SVR builds a hyperplane that tries to keep all sample points from the hyperplane as small as possible. Taking the $i$-th instance as an example, the objective function for finding the hyperplane can be described as follows:

$$\min_{b,W} \frac{||W||^2}{2} + B \sum_{i=1}^{n} (\overline{\xi_i} + \xi_i) \tag{4}$$

$$\overline{\xi_i} = \begin{cases} y_i - \overline{y_{s,i}} - \varepsilon, & y_i > \overline{y_{s,i}} + \varepsilon \\ 0, & \text{other} \end{cases} \tag{5}$$

$$\xi_i = \begin{cases} \overline{y_{s,i}} - \varepsilon - y_i, & y_i < \overline{y_{s,i}} - \varepsilon \\ 0, & \text{other} \end{cases} \tag{6}$$

$$s.t. \begin{cases} y_i - \overline{y_{s,i}} \leq \varepsilon + \overline{\xi_i} \\ \overline{y_{s,i}} - y_i \leq \varepsilon + \xi_i \\ \xi_i, \overline{\xi_i} \geq 0 \end{cases} \tag{7}$$

$$\overline{y_{s,i}} = w_{s,1} x_{i,1} + w_{s,2} x_{i,2} + \cdots + w_{s,n} x_{i,n} + b \tag{8}$$

where $W = (w_{s,1}, w_{s,2}, \ldots, w_{s,n})$ is the vector of coefficients, $\overline{y_{s,i}}$ is the predicted value of the $i$-th instance, $y_i$ is the true value of the $i$-th instance. $\xi_i, \overline{\xi_i}$ are the slack variables, $B$ is the regularisation constant, $\varepsilon$ is the tolerance deviation, and $b$ is a constant term. The correlation algorithm is used to solve the parameters of the above objective function to obtain the hyperplane of the SVR.

### 3.2.3. Backpropagation Neural Networks (BPnet)

Based on the superior performance of neural networks and improvements in computing power, neural networks can approximate the complex nonlinear relationships between variables. Therefore, neural networks provide better results in regression analysis. The simplest neural network architecture consists of three layers: an input layer, a hidden layer, and an output layer. In healthcare cost prediction, BPnet first learns the feature information of patients in the training dataset, then assigns appropriate weights to each feature variable and establishes the relationship between the feature variables and healthcare cost. Based on this, information about the characteristics of the patients in the test dataset can be input into the neural network to predict patients' healthcare costs.

### 3.2.4. Random Forest (RF)

RF consists of multiple decision trees, and belongs to he class of ensemble learning in machine learning. Because RF has better anti-interference ability, many researchers use RF to perform regression analysis research. The basic principle of RF for regression analysis is that the subset of data and the subset of features are randomly selected from the healthcare cost data to build each decision tree of the RF. The test set is input to the trained RF, which averages all the decision tree outputs to output a prediction.

### 3.2.5. Long Short-Term Memory (LSTM)

LSTM is a neural network with good ability to handle sequential data. It is an optimization of the RNN (Recursion Neural Network) model, and has the quality features of RNN. The LSTM structure contains input gates, forgetting gates, and output gates that determine the loss or preservation of information in the data to achieve forgetting and remembering, which overcomes the drawbacks of the single memory overlay approach of RNNs. LSTM currently plays an important role in many research areas, and many researchers have achieved good results using LSTM to predict healthcare costs.

## 4. Dataset

The datasets studied in the paper are all mixed datasets containing both discrete and continuous variables. In order to show the superior performance of the predictive model, two datasets are used to test the predictive ability of the hybrid model. Both datasets collected in this paper are from Kaggle. The first dataset is from a health insurance company and gas 986 instances, each containing ten feature variables and one healthcare cost variable. A specific description of the first dataset is shown in Table 1. The second dataset has a total of 1338 instances, each containing six feature variables and one healthcare cost variable. A specific description of the second dataset is shown in Table 2. There are no missing values in either dataset. Before analyzing the data, characters in the dataset are replaced with numerical values (e.g., 1 for male and 0 for female).

Table 1. Description of the first dataset. × represents that the variable does not have the relevant attribute.

| Variable | Description | Attribute | Min | Max | Mean | Standard Deviation |
|---|---|---|---|---|---|---|
| Age | Age of the patient | Continuous | 18 | 66 | 41.75 | 13.96337 |
| Diabetes | Whether the patient has diabetes | Discrete | × | × | × | × |
| Blood Pressure Problems | Whether the patient has blood pressure disease | Discrete | × | × | × | × |
| Any Transplants | Whether the patient has undergone transplant surgery | Discrete | × | × | × | × |
| Any Chronic Diseases | Whether the patient has any chronic diseases | Discrete | × | × | × | × |
| Height | Patient height | Continuous | 145 | 188 | 168.2 | 10.09815 |
| Weight | Patient weight | Continuous | 51 | 132 | 76.95 | 14.2651 |
| Known Allergiess | Whether the patient has any allergies | Discrete | × | × | × | × |
| History of Cancer in Family | Whether there is any history of cancer in the patient's family | Discrete | × | × | × | × |
| Number of Major Surgeries | The number of major surgeries the patient has undergone | Discrete | × | × | × | × |
| Charges | Healthcare cost | Continuous | 15,000 | 40,000 | 24,337 | 6248.184 |

Table 2. Description of the second dataset. × represents that the variable does not have the relevant attribute.

| Variable | Description | Attribute | Min | Max | Mean | Standard Deviation |
|---|---|---|---|---|---|---|
| Age | Age of the patient | Continuous | 18 | 64 | 39.21 | 14.04996 |
| Sex | Gender of the patient | Discrete | × | × | × | × |
| BMI | Body Mass Index of patient | Continuous | 15.96 | 53.13 | 30.66 | 6.098187 |
| Children | The number of children covered under the medical insurance | Discrete | × | × | × | × |
| Smoker | Whether the patient is a smoker or not | Discrete | × | × | × | × |
| Region | The geographic region of the patient | Discrete | × | × | × | × |
| Charges | Healthcare cost | Continuous | 1122 | 63,770 | 13,270 | 12,110.01 |

## 5. Evaluation Method

To accurately and effectively test the predictive performance of the proposed model, MRE (Mean Relative Error), MSE (Mean Square Error), RMSE (Root Mean Square Error), MAE (Mean Absolute Error), and SMAPE (Symmetric Mean Absolute Percentage Error) are used to test the model performance, all of which play important roles in regression analysis in many fields. Below, the expressions for these evaluation methods are provided in turn:

$$MRE = \frac{\sum_{i=1}^{L} \frac{|\overline{y_i} - y_i|}{y_i}}{L} \tag{9}$$

$$MSE = \frac{\sum_{i=1}^{L} (\overline{y_i} - y_i)^2}{L} \tag{10}$$

$$MAE = \frac{\sum_{i=1}^{L} |\overline{y_i} - y_i|}{L} \tag{11}$$

$$RMSE = \sqrt{\frac{\sum_{i=1}^{L} (\overline{y_i} - y_i)^2}{L}} \tag{12}$$

$$SMAPE = \frac{\sum_{i=1}^{L} \frac{|\overline{y_i} - y_i|}{(\overline{y_i} + y_i)/2}}{L} \tag{13}$$

where $L$ is the number of instances in the test set, $\overline{y_i}$ represents the predicted value, and $y_i$ represents the true value.

## 6. Experimental Analysis

Rstudio was used to build the hybrid models used to predict healthcare cost; 80% of the number of instances of the healthcare data were used for the training set and 20% for the test set. The network structure algorithm for CGBN came from Rstudio's bnlearn package, and the LSTM was built using Rstudio's keras package. The dataset with ten feature variables and one target variable is defined as dataset A and the dataset with six feature variables and one target variable as dataset B. For simplicity of description, the hybrid models built by CGBN with the various regression algorithms are abbreviated as CGBN + RF, CGBN + SVR, CGBN + BPnet, CGBN + LR, and CGBN + LSTM.

### 6.1. Dataset A

The three classes of CGBN structure learning algorithm were first used to learn dataset A. Then, the multiple network structures learned from the CGBN network structure algorithm were analyzed to obtain isolated nodes. After analysis, there was one isolated node with the highest number of occurrences in multiple network structures. The results obtained by the hybrid algorithms after deleting the isolated node corresponding to the feature variables in dataset A are shown in Figure 3. The single models (e.g. RF, SVR, etc.) analyzed the original dataset with no reduction in feature variables. Figure 3 shows the prediction graphs for CGBN + RF, CGBN + SVR, CGBN + BPnet, CGBN + LR, and CGBN + LSTM. Each graph contains the results predicted by the hybrid model, the results predicted by the single model, and the true values in Figure 3. As can be seen from Figure 3, the trend of the prediction curves of the hybrid and single models in Figure 3a,c are very close to the trend of the true curves, which indicates that CGBN + RF, RF, CGBN + BPnet, and BPnet have a better prediction ability on dataset A. The prediction curve of CGBN + LR in Figure 3d almost overlaps with the prediction curve of LR, which indicates that the prediction ability of CGBN + LR is the same as that of LR in the case of reduced data. Moreover, Figure 3b,e exhibit better predictive power than Figure 3d. Overall, the prediction curves of the hybrid models with reduced data volume are similar to those of the single models, which reflects the reasonableness of the hybrid models.

In order to better show the performance advantages of the proposed model, MRE, MSE, RMSE, MAE, and SMAPE were used to evaluate the prediction results of both the hybrid and single models. The error analysis between the prediction results and the true values of the hybrid models and single models is shown in Table 3. As can be seen in Table 3, the error analyses of the various evaluation methods is not necessarily consistent for the hybrid models and single models. For example, the MRE of CGBN + RF is lower than that of RF, while the MRSE of CGBN + RF is slightly higher than that of RF. In general, the MRE better reflects the predictive power of the models in healthcare cost forecasting. As can be seen from Table 3, CGBN + RF has the lowest MRE, followed by CGBN + BPnet, which is in line with the trend of the predicted curves in Figure 3a,b. The MRE of CGBN + LR is essentially the same as that of LR, which is in line with the trend of the predicted curves in Figure 3d. More importantly, Table 3 shows that the MREs and SMAPEs of the hybrid models are lower than the MREs and SMAPEs of the corresponding single models in all cases where the amount of data is reduced, which fully reflects the superior predictive performance of the hybrid models. MSE, RMSE, and MAE can be inconsistent in their evaluation of the hybrid models and single models; however, each evaluation algorithm calculates similar error values for the hybrid and single models, which further reflects the validity of the hybrid models.

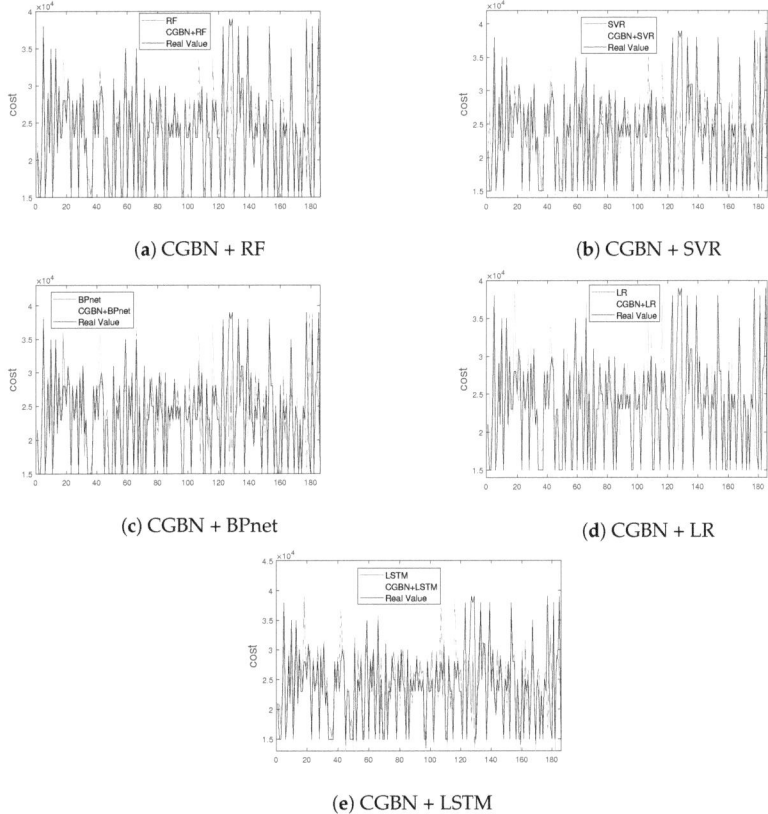

**Figure 3.** Predictive results for hybrid and single models; the horizontal axis represents the number of instances and the vertical axis represents the healthcare cost.

**Table 3.** Evaluation results for hybrid and single models.

| Model \ Method | MRE | MAE | MSE | RMSE | SMAPE |
|---|---|---|---|---|---|
| CGBN + RF | 0.071 | $1.79 \times 10^3$ | $1.49 \times 10^7$ | $3.86 \times 10^3$ | 0.072 |
| CGBN + SVR | 0.113 | $2.65 \times 10^3$ | $2.15 \times 10^7$ | $4.64 \times 10^3$ | 0.110 |
| CGBN + BPnet | 0.074 | $2.018 \times 10^3$ | $1.98 \times 10^7$ | $4.45 \times 10^3$ | 0.075 |
| CGBN + LR | 0.129 | $3.0865 \times 10^3$ | $2.28 \times 10^7$ | $4.77 \times 10^3$ | 0.127 |
| CGBN + LSTM | 0.118 | $2.83 \times 10^3$ | $2.11 \times 10^7$ | $4.59 \times 10^3$ | 0.119 |
| RF | 0.078 | $1.92 \times 10^3$ | $1.45 \times 10^7$ | $3.80 \times 10^3$ | 0.077 |
| SVR | 0.116 | $2.70 \times 10^3$ | $2.16 \times 10^7$ | $4.65 \times 10^3$ | 0.112 |
| BPnet | 0.077 | $2.047 \times 10^3$ | $1.82 \times 10^7$ | $4.26 \times 10^3$ | 0.078 |
| LR | 0.130 | $3.0869 \times 10^3$ | $2.28 \times 10^7$ | $4.77 \times 10^3$ | 0.127 |
| LSTM | 0.123 | $2.87 \times 10^3$ | $2.08 \times 10^7$ | $4.56 \times 10^3$ | 0.119 |

## 6.2. Dataset B

In order to test the generality of the hybrid models, dataset B was analyzed using the hybrid models. Similarly to dataset A, the three classes of CGBN structure learning algorithms were used to learn dataset B, then the multiple network structures learned from the CGBN network structure algorithm were analyzed to obtain isolated nodes. After analysis, there were two isolated nodes with the highest number of occurrences in multiple network structures. The prediction results obtained by the hybrid models after deleting the feature variables in dataset B corresponding to the isolated nodes are shown in Figure 4. The single models analyzed the original dataset with no reduction in feature variables. As can be seen from Figure 4, the trend of the prediction curves of the hybrid and single models in Figure 4b,e are very close to the trend of the true curves, which suggests that CGBN + SVR, SVR, CGBN + LSTM, and LSTM have better prediction ability on dataset B. Compared to the prediction curves shown in the other figures, the trends of the prediction curves of the hybrid and single models in Figure 4d deviate from the trend of the true curves more, indicating that the prediction performances of CGBN + LR and LR on dataset B are poor. Similar to the case of Figure 3, the prediction curves of the hybrid models with reduced data volumes are demonstrated in Figure 4 to be similar to that of the single models, further demonstrating the superior performance of the hybrid models.

Again, MRE, MSE, RMSE, MAE, and SMAPE were used to evaluate the prediction results of hybrid models and single models in order to highlight the prediction performance of each model. The error analysis between the prediction results and the true values of the hybrid models and single models is shown in Table 4. As can be seen from Table 4, the MRE of CGBN + SVR is the lowest among the hybrid models and the MRE of LSTM is the lowest among the single models, which is in line with the trend of the curves in Figure 4b,e. The MRE of CGBN + LR is the highest among the hybrid models, while the MRE of LR is the highest among the single models, which indicates that LR cannot analyze dataset B as well as the other regression algorithms. Although the prediction performance of CGBN + LSTM is lower than LSTM, the predictive performance of the other hybrid models is similar to or better than that of the corresponding single models. Overall, the hybrid models can obtain better prediction results with reduced data volume.

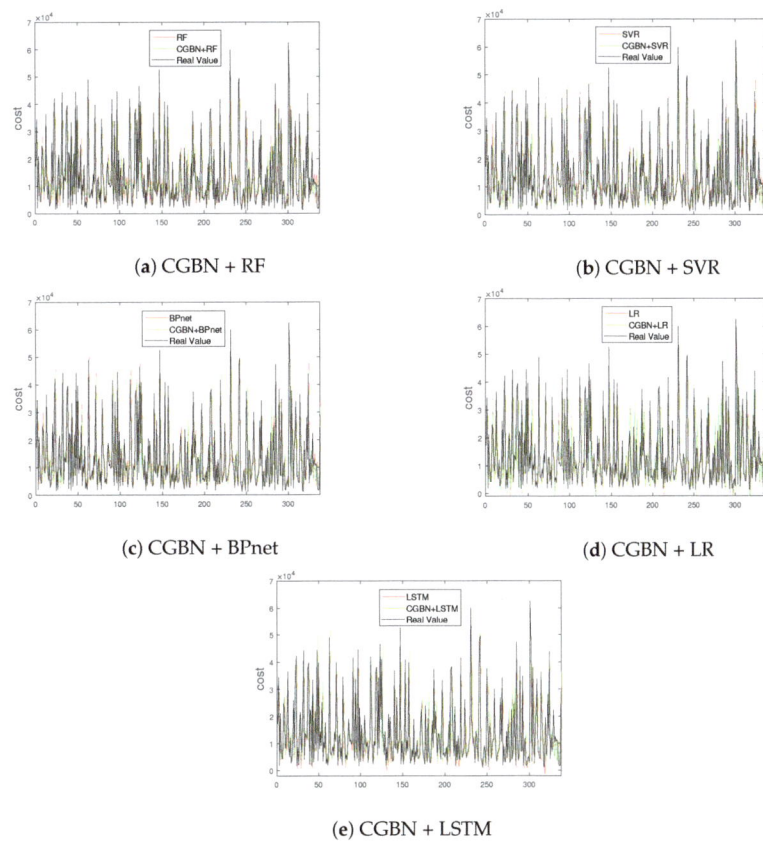

**Figure 4.** Predictive results for hybrid and single models. The horizontal axis represents the number of instances and the vertical axis represents the healthcare cost.

**Table 4.** Evaluation results for hybrid and single models.

| Model \ Method | MRE | MAE | MSE | RMSE | SMAPE |
|---|---|---|---|---|---|
| CGBN + RF | 0.27 | $3.91 \times 10^3$ | $3.57 \times 10^7$ | $5.97 \times 10^3$ | 0.27 |
| CGBN + SVR | 0.21 | $2.60 \times 10^3$ | $2.79 \times 10^7$ | $5.28 \times 10^3$ | 0.22 |
| CGBN + BPnet | 0.24 | $2.86 \times 10^3$ | $2.62 \times 10^7$ | $5.12 \times 10^3$ | 0.25 |
| CGBN + LR | 0.32 | $4.52 \times 10^3$ | $4.34 \times 10^7$ | $6.58 \times 10^3$ | 0.34 |
| CGBN + LSTM | 0.25 | $3.05 \times 10^3$ | $2.81 \times 10^7$ | $5.30 \times 10^3$ | 0.26 |
| RF | 0.24 | $3.28 \times 10^3$ | $2.93 \times 10^7$ | $5.41 \times 10^3$ | 0.25 |
| SVR | 0.25 | $2.91 \times 10^3$ | $2.77 \times 10^7$ | $5.26 \times 10^3$ | 0.26 |
| BPnet | 0.24 | $3.02 \times 10^3$ | $2.73 \times 10^7$ | $5.23 \times 10^3$ | 0.25 |
| LR | 0.32 | $4.46 \times 10^3$ | $4.29 \times 10^7$ | $6.55 \times 10^3$ | 0.34 |
| LSTM | 0.19 | $2.75 \times 10^3$ | $3.03 \times 10^7$ | $5.51 \times 10^3$ | 0.16 |

Although the addition of the CGBN algorithm increases the complexity of the overall prediction model, only the network structure learning algorithms of CGBN are used in the paper. During the experiment, the proposed model spends little computation and time in processing the data. Meanwhile, the feature variables filtered out by the proposed model can provide a reference for staff and facilitate the collection and processing of data which cannot be done by a single algorithm.

## 7. Conclusions

This paper proposes combining CGBN with various regression algorithms to form hybrid models to predict healthcare costs. First, CGBN network structure learning algorithms reduce the amount of data in the dataset by deleting irrelevant information, then regression algorithms are used to learn the rest of the dataset, and finally regression algorithms make predictions. The predictive performance of the hybrid models was tested separately on two healthcare cost datasets, with the hybrid models obtaining better predictive results than the single models. Therefore, the proposed hybrid models can obtain better prediction performance with reduced data volumes, which can provide a corresponding reference for related workers and reduce the workload of data collection and processing. Although the CGBN structure learning algorithms can accurately identify the irrelevant variables in the dataset, it is difficult for the current CGBN network structure learning algorithms to independently learn the legitimate network structure from medical cost data. In future studies, we intend to optimise the CGBN network structure algorithm in order to enable them to learn legitimate network structures without relying on expert experience. In addition, time-series healthcare cost data will be investigated to further improve the applicability of the hybrid models.

**Author Contributions:** Conceptualization, S.Z. and C.C.; methodology, S.Z.; software, S.Z.; validation, S.Z. and C.C.; formal analysis, S.Z.; investigation, S.Z.; resources, S.Z. and C.C.; data curation, S.Z.; writing—original draft preparation, S.Z.; writing—review and editing, J.R. and N.S.; visualization, S.Z.; supervision, J.R. and N.S.; project administration, C.C.; funding acquisition, C.C. All authors have read and agreed to the published version of the manuscript.

**Funding:** MOST-FDCT Projects: 0058/2019/AMJ Research and Application of Cooperative Multi-Agent Platform for Zhuhai–Macao Manufacturing Service.

**Data Availability Statement:** The dataset A is available at https://www.kaggle.com/datasets/tejashvi14/medical-insurance-premium-prediction (accessed 20 August 2023). The dataset B is available at https://www.kaggle.com/datasets/harshsingh2209/medical-insurance-payout (accessed 20 August 2023).

**Conflicts of Interest:** We declare that we have no financial and personal relationships with other people or organizations that could inappropriately influence our work, and no professional or other personal interests of any nature or kind in any product, service, and/or company that could be construed as influencing the position presented in or the review of the manuscript entitled "Healthcare Cost Prediction Based on Hybrid Machine Learning Algorithms".

## References

1. Kane, J. Health costs: How the US compares with other countries. *PBS Newshour* **2012**, *22*, 1–32.
2. Zeng, X.; Lin, S.; Liu, C. Multi-view deep learning framework for predicting patient expenditure in healthcare. *IEEE Open J. Comput. Soc.* **2021**, *2*, 62–71. [CrossRef]
3. Kaushik, S.; Choudhury, A.; Natarajan, S.; Pickett, L.A.; Dutt, V. Medicine Expenditure Prediction via a Variance-Based Generative Adversarial Network. *IEEE Access* **2020**, *8*, 110947–110958. [CrossRef]
4. Kharat, A.A.; Muzumdar, J.; Hwang, M.; Wu, W. Assessing trends in medical expenditures and measuring the impact of health-related quality of life on medical expenditures for US adults with diabetes associated chronic kidney disease using 2002–2016 medical expenditure panel survey data. *J. Pharm. Health Serv. Res.* **2020**, *11*, 365–373. [CrossRef]
5. Yassine, A.; Hangouche, A.J.; El Malhouf, N.; Maarouf, S.; Taoufik, J. Assessment of the medical expenditure of the basic health insurance in Morocco. *Pan Afr. Med. J.* **2020**, *35*, 115. [CrossRef] [PubMed]
6. Zhang, X.; Shi, J.-F.; Liu, G.-X.; Ren, J.-S.; Guo, L.-W.; Huang, W.-D.; Shi, L.-M.; Ma, Y.; Huang, H.-Y.; Bai, Y.-N.; et al. Medical expenditure for lung cancer in China: A multicenter, hospital-based retrospective survey. *Cost Eff. Resour. Alloc.* **2021**, *19*, 53. [CrossRef] [PubMed]
7. Ma, C.; Jiang, Y.; Li, Y.; Zhang, Y.; Wang, X.; Ma, S.; Wang, Y. Medical expenditure for middle-aged and elderly in Beijing. *BMC Health Serv. Res.* **2019**, *19*, 360. [CrossRef] [PubMed]

8. Gong, G.-w.; Chen, Y.-c.; Fang, P.-q.; Min, R. Medical expenditure for patients with hemophilia in urban China: Data from medical insurance information system from 2013 to 2015. *Orphanet J. Rare Dis.* **2020**, *15*, 137. [CrossRef]
9. Yang, L.; Min, Y.; Jia, Z.; Wang, Y.; Zhang, R.; Sun, B. Medical expenditure for strabismus: A hospital-based retrospective survey. *Cost Eff. Resour. Alloc.* **2022**, *20*, 27. [CrossRef] [PubMed]
10. Wang, L.; Tang, Y.; Roshanmehr, F.; Bai, X.; Taghizadeh-Hesary, F.; Taghizadeh-Hesary, F. The health status transition and medical expenditure evaluation of elderly population in China. *Int. J. Environ. Res. Public Health* **2021**, *18*, 6907. [CrossRef] [PubMed]
11. Han, J.; Zhang, X.; Meng, Y. The impact of internet medical information overflow on residents' medical expenditure based on China's observations. *Int. J. Environ. Res. Public Health* **2020**, *17*, 3539. [CrossRef] [PubMed]
12. Morid, M.A.; Kawamoto, K.; Ault, T.; Dorius, J.; Abdelrahman, S. Supervised learning methods for predicting healthcare costs: Systematic literature review and empirical evaluation. *AMIA Annu. Symp. Proc.* **2018**, *2017*, 1312–1321. [PubMed]
13. Kaushik, S.; Choudhury, A.; Dasgupta, N.; Natarajan, S.; Pickett, L.A.; Dutt, V. Ensemble of multi-headed machine learning architectures for time-series forecasting of healthcare expenditures. In *Applications of Machine Learning*; Springer: Singapore, 2020; pp. 199–216.
14. Kaushik, S.; Choudhury, A.; Dasgupta, N.; Natarajan, S.; Pickett, L.A.; Bisht, D. Evaluating single-and multi-headed neural architectures for time-series forecasting of healthcare expenditures. In *Computational Intelligence Theoretical Advances and Advanced Applications*; De Gruyter Publisher: Berlin, Germany, 2020; pp. 159–176.
15. Kaushik, S.; Choudhury, A.; Sheron, P.K.; Dasgupta, N.; Natarajan, S.; Pickett, L.A.; Dutt, V. AI in healthcare: Time-series forecasting using statistical, neural, and ensemble architectures. *Front. Big Data* **2020**, *3*, 4. [CrossRef] [PubMed]
16. Yang, C.; Delcher, C.; Shenkman, E.; Ranka, S. Machine learning approaches for predicting high cost high need patient expenditures in health care. *Biomed. Eng. Online* **2018**, *17*, 131. [CrossRef] [PubMed]
17. Kuo, C.-Y.; Yu, L.-C.; Chen, H.-C.; Chan, C.-L. Comparison of models for the prediction of medical costs of spinal fusion in Taiwan diagnosis-related groups by machine learning algorithms. *Healthc. Inform. Res.* **2018**, *24*, 29–37. [CrossRef] [PubMed]
18. Zeng, X.; Feng, Y.; Moosavinasab, S.; Lin, D.; Lin, S.; Liu, C. Multilevel self-attention model and its use on medical risk prediction. In *Pacific Symposium on Biocomputing 2020*; World Scientific: Singapore, 2019; pp. 115–126.
19. Wang, K.-J.; Chen, J.-L.; Wang, K.-M. Medical expenditure estimation by Bayesian network for lung cancer patients at different severity stages. *Comput. Biol. Med.* **2019**, *106*, 97–105. [CrossRef] [PubMed]
20. Hu, J.; Wang, J.; Zhang, Z.; Liu, H. Continuous-discrete hybrid Bayesian network models for predicting earthquake-induced liquefaction based on the Vs database. *Comput. Geosci.* **2022**, *169*, 105231. [CrossRef]
21. Liu, J.; Kang, Y.; Liu, K.; Yang, X.; Sun, M.; Hu, J. Maize Carotenoid Gene Locus Mining Based on Conditional Gaussian Bayesian Network. *IEEE Access* **2020**, *8*, 15223–15231. [CrossRef]
22. Scutari, M.; Denis, J.-B. *Bayesian Networks: Examples R*, 2nd ed.; CRC Press: Boca Raton, FL, USA, 2021.

**Disclaimer/Publisher's Note:** The statements, opinions and data contained in all publications are solely those of the individual author(s) and contributor(s) and not of MDPI and/or the editor(s). MDPI and/or the editor(s) disclaim responsibility for any injury to people or property resulting from any ideas, methods, instructions or products referred to in the content.

# Predicting Typhoon Flood in Macau Using Dynamic Gaussian Bayesian Network and Surface Confluence Analysis

Shujie Zou [1], Chiawei Chu [1,*], Weijun Dai [2], Ning Shen [3], Jia Ren [4] and Weiping Ding [5]

1. Faculty of Data Science, City University of Macau, Macau 999078, China; d21092100231@cityu.mo
2. Artificial Intelligence College, Guangdong Polytechnic Institute, Guangzhou 510091, China; wjdai@gdrtvu.edu.cn
3. Department of Innovation, Technology and Entrepreneurship, United Arab Emirates University, Al Ain 15551, United Arab Emirates; ningshen@uaeu.ac.ae
4. School of Information and Communication Engineering, Hainan University, Haikou 570100, China; renjia@hainanu.edu.cn
5. School of Information Science and Technology, Nantong University, Nantong 226000, China; ding.wp@ntu.edu.cn
* Correspondence: cwchu@cityu.mo

**Abstract:** A typhoon passing through or making landfall in a coastal city may result in seawater intrusion and continuous rainfall, which may cause urban flooding. The urban flood disaster caused by a typhoon is a dynamic process that changes over time, and a dynamic Gaussian Bayesian network (DGBN) is used to model the time series events in this paper. The scene data generated by each typhoon are different, which means that each typhoon has different characteristics. This paper establishes multiple DGBNs based on the historical data of Macau flooding caused by multiple typhoons, and similar analysis is made between the scene data related to the current flooding to be predicted and the scene data of historical flooding. The DGBN most similar to the scene characteristics of the current flooding is selected as the predicting network of the current flooding. According to the topography, the influence of the surface confluence is considered, and the Manning formula analysis method is proposed. The Manning formula is combined with the DGBN to obtain the final prediction model, DGBN-m, which takes into account the effects of time series and non-time-series factors. The flooding data provided by the Macau Meteorological Bureau are used to carry out experiments, and it is proved that the proposed model can predict the flooding depth well in a specific area of Macau under the condition of a small amount of data and that the best predicting accuracy can reach 84%. Finally, generalization analysis is performed to further confirm the validity of the proposed model.

**Keywords:** dynamic Gaussian Bayesian network; Manning formula; flood prediction; surface confluence

**MSC:** 68T09

## 1. Introduction

Nowadays, flood disaster is still a major problem faced by many cities. The probability of flood disaster is very high, especially in coastal cities. In coastal cities, when the typhoon comes, it will cause heavy rainfall, seawater backflow and other phenomena. There will be surface confluence in areas with larger terrain fluctuations, which will lead to severe flood disaster in areas with lower terrain. According to statistics, flood disaster in various regions of the world will cause huge economic losses and casualties every year [1]. For example, several provinces in China were hit by floods in 2017, resulting in tens of millions of people being affected, of which Macau was heavily hit. If the trend of flooding can be predicted in advance, some protective measures can be taken in advance to avoid casualties and reduce economic losses.

Flood disaster prediction is a concern of many researchers, and many prediction schemes have been proposed. Among them, machine learning methods have been successfully applied to flood disaster prediction by many researchers, and have achieved good results in terms of computational speed and accuracy [2]. For example, Tehrany et al. [3] combined a support vector machine and decision tree to analyze the correlation between flood risk level and various influencing factors. Satria et al. [4] developed a system to predict flood depth in Manila city using K-nearest neighbors (KNNs) and inverse-distance-weighted interpolation (IDW). Wasiq et al. [5] combined machine learning models and data analysis methods with Internet of Things (IoT) sensor data to predict flood risk levels, but the prediction results were intervals, which can only provide vague reference results. Du et al. [6] used Soil Moisture Active Passive (SMAP) and Landsat monitoring to evaluate and predict flood inundation, and achieved good results, but the model used was complex and difficult to implement. Due to the rapid development of deep learning, some researchers use the advantages of artificial neural networks to describe the linear and nonlinear characteristics of data to establish flood prediction models. For example, Ramil et al. [7] combined a back propagation (BP) neural network with a Kalman filter to model the upstream and downstream data of the water flow to predict the water level downstream of the water flow. Sunita et al. [8] conducted a study of water catchments in the UK using an improved artificial neural network. Imrie et al. [9] built a complex flood early warning model using neural networks and achieved good prediction results, which provided help for flood prevention. Kim et al. [10] used an artificial neural network to predict after-runner storm surges on the coast of Tottori, Japan. The prediction of storm surges can indirectly prevent flooding disasters. Gude et al. [11] combined autoregressive integrated moving average (ARIMA) and a long short-term memory network (LSTM) to build the model for predicting flood depth. Kourgialas et al. [12] built a neural network to predict extreme water flow in a small agricultural watershed in the Mediterranean, demonstrating the predictive advantage of neural networks for such scenarios. In addition, Dai et al. [13,14] used a neural network and ensemble learning methods to predict the flood depth of Macau during a typhoon period, respectively, conducting many experiments and exploring a variety of research paths to obtain effective research and prediction results, and also provided a good research foundation for the work of the paper.

Although the above various machine learning algorithms (neural network, ensemble learning, etc.) have achieved certain results in flood disaster prediction, these algorithms require a large amount of training data to obtain a better prediction ability. Taking Macau flooding as an example, the data provided by the Macau Meteorological Bureau show that, due to equipment conditions, the amount of data generated by the flood disaster in Macau caused by typhoons is relatively small. There are currently only six recorded typhoons, of which the typhoon with the longest duration of flooding (Mangkhut) produced only 759 pieces of data on the flooding depth (data recorded every one minute), and the data volume of other typhoons causing flooding in Macau is below 300. More importantly, the prediction model established by a neural network cannot know the relationship between each flooding factor and the relationship between each flooding factor and the flooding depth (direct or indirect influence), which is the reason for why the neural network is called a black box. In most cases, it is necessary not only to predict the flooding depth but also to know which flooding factors have a direct or indirect impact on the flooding depth so that appropriate and accurate measures can be taken to prevent the flooding disaster. Therefore, a DGBN is adopted as the predicting network of flooding depth in this paper, which has the following advantages in Macau's flooding depth prediction scenario:

- When the amount of data is small, expert experience can be added in the construction of the Bayesian network to guide the direction of algorithm learning. And, the characteristic information of the flooding factor is further enhanced, and the learned network structure will also better fit the characteristics of the data.

- Bayesian networks have multiple network structures (stationary, non-stationary, high-order, low-order) to deal with changing scenarios. According to different scene characteristics, the appropriate network structure is selected to process the data.
- After the Bayesian network is established, the relationship between various flooding factors and the relationship between flooding factors and flooding depth can be clearly known, which will help relevant departments to take effective flood control measures.

The content of this paper is arranged as follows: Section 2 introduces the literature on the use of Bayesian networks for related research; Section 3 introduces the principle and construction process of the DGBN; Section 4 presents the surface confluence analysis, which leads to the Manning formula analysis method; Section 5 designs the prediction model of the DGBN combined with the Manning formula; Section 6 conducts experiments to prove the effectiveness of the proposed scheme based on the flooding data provided by the Macau Meteorological Bureau; Section 7 analyzes and summarizes the full paper.

## 2. Related Work

At present, many researchers used a Bayesian network for predictive analysis and obtained better results. For example, Lu used expert knowledge to establish a Bayesian network to assess the flood risk of the Xianghongdian Reservoir, and used the unique attributes of the Bayesian network to make a flexible two-way inference to obtain the probability distribution of each node, more comprehensively understanding and controlling floods [15]. Sebastian used observations from hundreds of tropical cyclones in the Gulf of Mexico to build a non-parametric Bayesian network to simulate storm surges in coastal watersheds and infer possible floods and some uncertain events during storm surges [16]. Sen constructed two dynamic Bayesian networks to assess resilience after natural disasters in various parts of Barak Valley in northeastern India, describing trends over time and differences in resilience among regions [17]. Chen et al. [18] used the uncertainty between expert knowledge and variables to build a dynamic Bayesian network, and used Monte Carlo simulation to provide input data for the dynamic Bayesian network to assess the real-time flood control dispatch risk of a multi-reservoir system in China. In addition, some researchers use Bayesian networks for research in other fields. David et al. [19] established a high-order DGBN to predict the temperature in an industrial furnace for a long time, and the prediction results show that the long-term prediction ability of the DGBN is better than that of a convolutional recursive neural network. Fateme et al. [20] built a dynamic Bayesian belief network to dynamically assess Australia's energy reserves to provide reference and support for power system suppliers' decision making. Dong et al. [21] used a dynamic Bayesian network to model the characteristics of battery degradation during charging and used the established dynamic Bayesian network to predict the health of the battery. Some researchers also used Bayesian networks for risk assessment in different scenarios [22–26]. For example, Zhang et al. [22] proposed fuzzy probabilistic Bayesian networks for network security assessment in industrial control systems; Ma et al. [23] used the dynamic Bayesian network to make a reasonable quantitative assessment of the risks associated with driving, etc. It can be seen that the dynamic Bayesian network has a powerful inference and prediction function. Although much effort has been dedicated toward prediction typhoon flooding, the noted algorithms suffer from the following limitations and challenges:

i   The data studied are basically from the same scene, which is equivalent to the same features involved in the events studied.
ii  These Bayesian network models are built under a large amount of data without considering a small amount of data.
iii The Bayesian network structure of some of the literature is completely established by experts' experience, which may not capture the uncertainties during the flood.

The data analyzed come from different typhoon scenarios in this paper because the characteristics of each typhoon and the trends and ranges of changes in related weather attributes caused by typhoons are basically not the same or are even very different. More importantly, the various factors that cause floods in Macau are not exactly the same for each typhoon. For example, some flooding events are caused by heavy rainfall, and some flooding events are caused by a combination of rainfall and storm surge. Therefore, it is necessary to consider how to deal with the different scenarios of flood disasters caused by typhoons before establishing the prediction model. For example, Xu et al. [27] proposed to use similar historical flood alarm sequences to predict the upcoming alarm events of the current flood alarm sequence. In this paper, similarity analysis (Euclidean distance) is used to calculate the similarity between the relevant scene features of the flooding that needs to be predicted and the historical scene features. Then, the DGBN is found as the network model of the flood to be predicted, which is established by the historical flood event most similar to the flood to be predicted. Furthermore, the influence of surface confluence is analyzed, and the surface confluence model is combined with the DGBN (the terrain factor is successfully added to the prediction model), which makes the prediction model of this paper have a convincing and better prediction ability.

## 3. Dynamic Gaussian Bayesian Network

Bayesian networks are probabilistic graphical models and are directed acyclic, consisting of nodes and directed arcs [19]. Bayesian networks can deal with discrete and continuous variables, and each node in Bayesian networks has a probability distribution: Gaussian distribution (continuous variable) or conditional probability distribution (discrete variable). The expression for the joint probability distribution of the static Gaussian Bayesian network (SGBN) is

$$P(V) = \prod_{i=1}^{k} f(v_i | pa(v_i)) = \prod_{i=1}^{k} N(\gamma_{0,i} + \sum_{j=1}^{k_i} \gamma_{j,i} pa_j(v_i); \delta_i^2) \tag{1}$$

where $k$ is the number of network nodes, $k_i$ is the number of parent nodes of the $i$-th node, $f(\cdot)$ is the probability density function, $V = (v_1, v_2, \ldots, v_k)$ is the node set, $v_i$ is the $i$-th node, $pa(v_i) = \{pa_1(v_i), pa_2(v_i), \ldots, pa_{k_i}(v_i)\}$ is the parent set of the $i$-th node, $pa_j(v_i)$ is the $j$-th parent node of the node $v_i$, $\delta_i^2$ is the variance of the $i$-th node, $\gamma_{0,i}$ is the intercepts of the $i$-th node and $\gamma_{j,i}$ is the coefficient of the $j$-th parent node of the $i$-th node. Generally speaking, SGBNs become DGBNs after adding the time factor, and the expression of the joint probability distribution of the DGBN is

$$P(V_0, V_1, \ldots, V_T) = f(V_0) \prod_{t=0}^{T-1} f(V_{t+1} | V_0, \ldots, V_t) \tag{2}$$

where $V_t = (v_{1,t}, \ldots, v_{k,t})$ is the node set of the $t$-th time slice, $v_{i,t}$ is the $i$-th node in the $t$-th time slice and $T$ represents the number of time slices. The first-order Markov DGBN represents that the nodes in the current time slice are only affected by the nodes in the current time slice and the previous time slice and have nothing to do with the nodes in the earlier time slice. And, the high-order Markov DGBN represents that the nodes in the current time slice are affected by the nodes in the earlier time slice. For the convenience of description, the expression for the first-order Markov DGBN is given:

$$\begin{aligned} P(V_0, V_1, \ldots, V_T) &= f(V_0) \prod_{t=0}^{T-1} f(V_{t+1} | V_t) \\ &= \prod_{i=1}^{k} N(\gamma_{0,i,0} + \sum_{j=1}^{k_{i,0}} \gamma_{j,i,0} pa_j(v_{i,0}); \delta_{i,0}^2) \\ &\quad \prod_{t=0}^{T-1} \prod_{i=1}^{k} N(\gamma_{0,i,t+1} + \sum_{j=1}^{k_{i,t+1}} \gamma_{j,i,t+1} pa_j(v_{i,t+1}); \delta_{i,t+1}^2) \end{aligned} \tag{3}$$

where $\gamma_{0,i,t}$ represents the intercept of the $i$-th node in the Bayesian network of the $t$-th time slice, $\delta^2_{i,t}$ represents the variance of the $i$-th node in the Bayesian network of the $t$-th time slice, $\gamma_{j,i,t}$ represents the coefficient of the $j$-th parent node of the $i$-th node in the Bayesian network of the $t$-th time slice and $k_{i,t}$ represents the number of parent nodes of the $i$-th node in the Bayesian network of the $t$-th time slice. The Bayesian network of each time slice can be regarded as an SGBN whose nodes may be affected by the nodes of the previous time slice.

### 3.1. Data Preprocessing

Before building the DGBNs, the data need to be preprocessed. Some monitoring sensors may malfunction during flooding, resulting in partial data loss. When a small amount of data are lost, linear interpolation is used to fill in the lost data. When a large amount of data are lost, the corresponding data are chosen to be discarded. In this case, the data that need to be filled have lost a large amount of feature information, and the relevant algorithms have difficulty in recovering the lost information. The expression of the linear interpolation is

$$y_c = y_a + \frac{y_b - y_a}{t_b - t_a}(t_c - t_a) \qquad (4)$$

where $t_a < t_c < t_b$, $y_c$ is the missing value at time $t_c$ and $y_a$ and $y_b$ are the known values at time $t_a$ and $t_b$, respectively.

### 3.2. Network Structure Learning

The DGBN's structure $G_D$ consists of the initial network $G_0$ and the transition network $G_\rightarrow$, $G_D = (G_0, G_\rightarrow)$. Here, the initial network $G_0$ is taken as an example. Firstly, stochastic Bayesian networks are established by using the uniform random acyclic directed graph algorithm. The uniform random acyclic directed graph algorithm is shown in Algorithm 1. The algorithm complexity of Algorithm 1 is lower than $O(|V|^4)$ and the details of Algorithm 1 can be found in [28]. When the Markov chain $MC$ in Algorithm 1 converges to a uniform distribution, $MC$ is defined to generate an acyclic digraph every $i$ iterations. A total of $N$ acyclic digraphs are generated, which can ensure the diversity of the generated random acyclic digraph [29]. Then, the randomly generated $N$ Bayesian networks are used as the starting network of the tabu search algorithm combined with the Bayesian information criterion (BIC) scoring algorithm. The tabu search algorithm is shown in Algorithm 2, where the computational complexity of Algorithm 2 is lower than $O(Np'M^2)$. The expression of the BIC scoring algorithm is

$$Score(G, D) = \sum_{i=1}^{|V|} [\log f(v_i | pa(v_i)) - \frac{|d_i|}{2} \log n] \qquad (5)$$

where $n$ is the number of samples, $f(\cdot)$ is the probability density function, $|V|$ is the number of network nodes, $v_i$ is the $i$-th network node, $pa(v_i)$ is the parent node of node $v_i$, $|d_i|$ is the number of parameters of the node, $G$ is a directed acyclic graph and $D$ is the dataset. It is worth noting that the blacklist variables in Algorithm 2 are combined with expert experience to optimize the algorithm, so that the network structure learned by Algorithm 2 fits the data better. After repeated analysis and comparison, the blacklist set in this paper includes:

i  Other flooding factors and flooding depths are prohibited from becoming the parent node of the typhoon track because the typhoon track is mainly affected by factors such as gravity and subtropical high pressure.

ii  It is forbidden for the flooding depth to become the parent node of the flooding factor because the flooding factor affects the change in the flooding depth.

**Algorithm 1** Uniform Random Acyclic Directed Graph Algorithm

**Input:** network node $V = (v_1, v_2, \ldots, v_k)$; a Markov Chain $MC$ whose state space $ST = \{s_1, \ldots, s_t, \ldots, \}$ is all acyclic directed graphs composed of network nodes $V$, $s_t$ is the state of the Markov chain $MC$ at time $t$.

1: **Initialization:** the initial state of $MC$ is an empty graph.
2: set the state transition function $f(s_t)$ of the Markov chain:
3:     uniformly randomly set ordered pairs $(v_i, v_j)$, $v_i, v_j \in V$, $v_i \neq v_j$.
4:     if there is an arc $e$ between the ordered pair $(v_i, v_j)$ in $s_t$, then $s_{t+1} = s_t \backslash e$, which means that the arc $e$ is removed from the state $s_t$.
5:     if there is no arc $e$ between the ordered pair $(v_i, v_j)$ in $s_t$, then $s_{t+1}$ is equal to adding arc $e$ in $s_t$, and check whether $s_{t+1}$ is acyclic, if $s_{t+1}$ is a cyclic graph, then $s_{t+1} = s_t$.
6: **for** $t = 1$ to $p$ **do**
7:     uniform random selection of number $i$ from $1:k$ to get $v_i$.
8:     uniform random selection of number $j$ from $1:k\backslash i$ to get $v_j$.
9:     $s_{t+1} = f(s_t)$
10: **end for**
11: after $p$ iterations, the Markov chain $MC$ converges to a uniform distribution.

After learning from Algorithm 2, $N$ Bayesian networks are obtained. Two thresholds, $\alpha$ and $\beta$ ($0 < \alpha < 1, 0 < \beta < 1$), are set to represent the connection strength and arc direction strength of the arc between any two vertices $(v_i, v_j)$, respectively. Then, we compute the ratio $\alpha'$ of occurrence of each arc and the ratio $\beta'$ of occurrence of its direction separately in $N$ Bayesian networks. If the conditions of $\alpha' \geq \alpha$, $\beta' \geq \beta$ are satisfied at the same time, the corresponding arc with direction is recorded, and the recorded arcs are defined as the set $Ar = (a_1, \ldots, a_\epsilon), \epsilon \geq 1$. Finally, an initial Bayesian network $G_0$ is established by the set $Ar$. Similarly, the network structure of the transfer network $G_\rightarrow$ and other time slices is jointly established by Algorithms 1 and 2.

It is worth noting that the network structure of each time slice and the transition network $G_\rightarrow$ are allowed to change, which means that the number of parent nodes of each node may change in the Bayesian network of each time slice, as shown in Figure 1. Figure 1 shows the schematic of the simple DGBN with three time slices, where there are three network nodes in each time slice. The DGBN established in this way is realistic, and some flooding factors do not always have an effect on flooding depth. For example, early flooding depths may be affected by rainfall, while later flooding depths may be affected by storm surges.

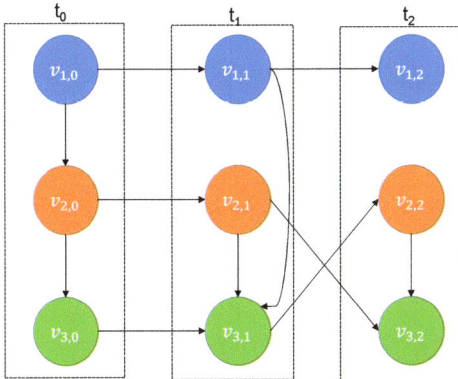

**Figure 1.** Schematic diagram of the one-order unsteady DGBN. Each dotted box represents a time slice, solid circles represent network nodes, the different colored nodes represent different variables, initial network $G_0 = \{v_{1,0}, v_{2,0}, v_{3,0}\}$, the network structure of the three time slices $(t_0, t_1, t_2)$ is different and the structure of the two transfer networks $G_\rightarrow = \{G_{t_0 \rightarrow t_1}; G_{t_1 \rightarrow t_2}\}$ is also different.

**Algorithm 2** Tabu Search Algorithm

**Input:** the starting Bayesian network $G = (G_1, \ldots, G_N)$, dataset $D$, blacklist $blacklist = (e'_1, \ldots, e'_i, \ldots)$.
1: **Initialization:** tabu list $tabulist = \emptyset$, tabu length $tabulong = TL$, the number of iterations $p'$, neighborhood solution network $G_O = (G_{O,1}, \ldots, G_{O,N})$, optimal scoring network $G_B = (G_{B,1}, \ldots, G_{B,N})$, $G_B = G_O = G$, empty list $list = zeros(1, M)$.
2: **Definition:** the neighborhood solution network $G_O$ is equal to the operation of adding, subtracting, and reversing the direction of the arc to the current network $G_B$, and the set of operated arcs $eo = (e_1, \ldots, e_M)$.
3: **for** $i = 1$ to $N$ **do**
4:   **for** $j = 1$ to $p'$ **do**
5:     **for** $k = 1$ to $M$ **do**
6:       $list(1, k) = BIC(G_{O,i}, e_k, D)$
7:     **end for**
8:     **while** $length(list) != 0$ **do**
9:       $[a, b] = find(list == max(list))$
10:       **if** $e_b \in blacklist$ **then**
11:         remove $b$ from $list$
12:         continue
13:       **end if**
14:       **if** $e_b \in tabulist$ **then**
15:         **if** $max(list) > BIC(G_{B,i}, D)$ **then**
16:           remove $e_b$ from $tabulist$
17:           $G_{B,i} = (G_{O,i}, e_b)$
18:           $G_{O,i} = G_{B,i}$
19:           add $e_b$ to the tail of $tabulist$
20:           break
21:         **else**
22:           remove $b$ from $list$
23:           continue
24:         **end if**
25:       **else**
26:         $G_{B,i} = (G_{O,i}, e_b)$
27:         $G_{O,i} = G_{B,i}$
28:         add $e_b$ to the tail of $tabulist$
29:         **if** $length(tabulist) > TL$ **then**
30:           remove the first element in the $tabulist$
31:         **end if**
32:         break
33:       **end if**
34:     **end while**
35:   **end for**
36: **end for**
**Output:** $G_B$

### 3.3. Network Parameter Learning

If the variable is discretized, the flooding depth will be discretized into multiple intervals. However, the variation range of the flooding depth caused by each typhoon is different. When the current predicted flooding depth exceeds or is lower than the historical flooding depth interval, the discrete Bayesian network cannot predict. Therefore, the use of continuous data to build Bayesian networks (Gaussian Bayesian networks) facilitates predictive reasoning. The maximum likelihood parameter estimation is used to learn

DGBN parameters to characterize the degree of influence between nodes. Taking a single node $v_{i,t}$ as an example, the expression for maximum likelihood parameter estimation is

$$L(\theta|D, G_D) = P(D, G_D|\theta) = \prod_{j=1}^{n} f(v_{j,i,t}|\theta) = \prod_{j=1}^{n} N(\gamma_{0,i,t} + \sum_{j'=1}^{k_i} \gamma_{j',i,t} pa_{j'}(v_{i,t}); \delta_{i,t}^2) \quad (6)$$

$$l(\theta|D, G_D) = \ln L(\theta|D, G_D) = \sum_{j=1}^{n} \ln N(\gamma_{0,i,t} + \sum_{j'=1}^{k_i} \gamma_{j',i,t} pa_{j'}(v_{i,t}); \delta_{i,t}^2) \quad (7)$$

$$\hat{\theta} = \arg\max_{\theta} l(\theta|D, G_D) \quad (8)$$

where $\theta = (\gamma_{0,i,t}, \gamma_{j',i,t}, \delta_{i,t}^2)$, $v_{j,i,t}$ represents the $j$-th sample point of node $v_{i,t}$, $n$ is the sample size, $D$ is the dataset, $G_D$ is DGBN network structure, $\gamma_{j',i,t}$ represents the coefficient of the $j'$-th parent node of the $i$-th node in the Bayesian network of the $t$-th time slice, $\gamma_{0,i,t}$ represents the intercept of the $i$-th node in the Bayesian network of the $t$-th time slice, $\delta_{i,t}^2$ represents the variance of the $i$-th node in the Bayesian network of the $t$-th time slice, $\hat{\theta}$ represents the maximum likelihood estimator.

*3.4. Network Reasoning*

In this paper, the approximate reasoning method (likelihood weighting algorithm) is used to perform predictive reasoning. The likelihood weighted algorithm has a better predictive reasoning ability than the logical sampling algorithm. Only the sampling process of the likelihood weighting algorithm is used here, as shown in Algorithm 3. According to the sampled data, the mean value of the sample is calculated to approximate the value of the query node conditioned on the evidence node.

---

**Algorithm 3** Likelihood Weighting Algorithm

**Input:** DGBN $G_D$, evidence node set $E = (v_{1,0} = ev_1, \ldots, v_{i,t} = ev_i), i \leq k-1, 0 \leq t \leq T$, query node $Q$
**Sampling:**
1. Use the value of the evidence node to instantiate the corresponding node in the Bayesian network, and sample all non-evidence nodes according to the topology and network parameters of the $G_D$ network to obtain $N'$ samples.
2. The sample output of node $Q$ will be queried to obtain a sample set $(q_1, \ldots, q_{N'})$.

$\overline{Q} = \frac{\sum_{i=1}^{N'} q_i}{N'}$

**Output:** $\overline{Q}$

---

This section briefly introduces network construction, network parameter learning and network inference for DGBNs. In order to understand the DGBN construction and reasoning process, the overall flow chart is given, as shown in Figure 2. The left side of Figure 2 is the construction process of the initial network and the right side is the construction process of the transfer network. The top of Figure 2 is the data preprocessing part and the tail is the process of DGBN parameter learning and predictive inference. Data adjustment represents lagging the data and dividing the lagged data equally according to the number of time slices. Next, we analyze the phenomenon of surface confluence caused by topography.

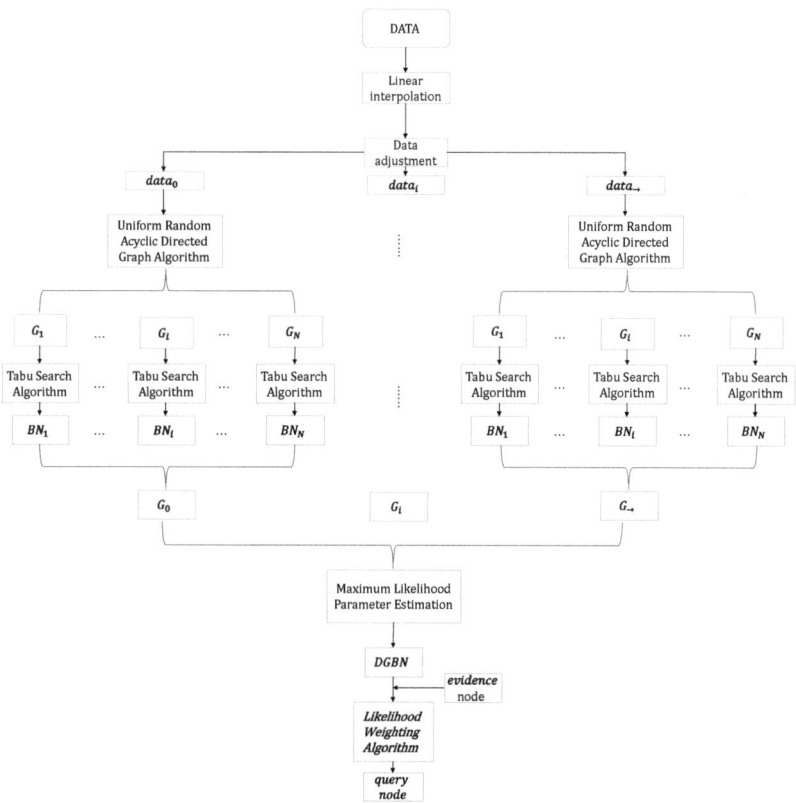

**Figure 2.** Construction and inference of DGBN. $data_0$ represents the data required to establish the initial network $G_0$, $data_{\rightarrow}$ represents the data required to establish the transfer network $G_{\rightarrow}$, $data_i$ represents the data required to establish the $i$-th time slice network $G_i$, $BN_i$ represents Bayesian network structure learned from tabu search algorithm, evidence node represents the value of the characteristic variable (excluding flooding depth) of the flooding to be predicted.

## 4. Surface Confluence Analysis

The stagnant water in the high-terrain areas will flow to the low-terrain areas in the event of flooding disasters, resulting in a further increase in flooding depth in the low-terrain areas. What we predict is the depth of flooding in a specific area of Macau, and the topographic factor has no time attribute in the flooding in Macau. Thus, the topographic factor is not added when constructing the DGBN. In the past, when the typhoon passed or landed in Macau, flooding would occur at the Inner Harbor Station. The flooding data recorded at the Inner Harbor Station are relatively complete and valuable for research. According to the map provided by the Macau Meteorological Bureau, a number of water level monitoring points in different directions and near the Inner Harbor Station are selected. The Manning formula is used to analyze the surface confluence phenomenon at the Inner Harbor Station. The Manning formula is often used to calculate the open channel flow, which is more reasonable to calculate from high terrain to low terrain. Taking the $i$-th high terrain as an example, the expression of the Manning formula is

$$W_i = \frac{AR^{2/3}S_i^{1/2}}{\varphi} \tag{9}$$

where $W_i$ (m$^3$/s) is the flow rate from the $i$-th high terrain to Inner Harbor Station. $A$ is the conversion coefficient, the international standard is 1 m, $R$ (m) is the hydraulic radius and $S_i$ is the slope. $\varphi$ is the Manning coefficient, which is the ground roughness. And, the flooding depth caused by multiple high terrains to low terrains is approximately calculated in the future period, which is defined as $H_G = (H_{G,1}, \ldots, H_{G,n'})$, where $n'$ is the number of water level monitoring points in different directions on the high terrain, and

$$H_{G,i} = 60 \frac{W_i}{w} m \tag{10}$$

where $H_{G,i}$ is the flooding depth caused by the $i$-th high terrain to Inner Harbor Station, $w$ (m$^2$) is the coverage area of Inner Harbor Station and $m$ (min) is the length of the future period. Because the data provided by the Macau Meteorological Bureau are collected every minute, the above formula needs to be multiplied by a constant 60 when converting minutes into seconds.

## 5. Prediction Model Construction

In the previous two sections, the DGBN and the surface confluence model are constructed. Combining the DGBN with the surface confluence model yields the prediction model, referred to as DGBN-m.

According to the flooding data provided by the Macau Meteorological Bureau, we select $F$ flooding events at the Inner Harbor Station with relatively complete data, and define $TY = (ty_1, \ldots, ty_F)$ as the set of selected flood events in the Inner Harbor Station. According to the data contained in $TY$, $F$ DGBNs are built, which are defined as $model = \{DGBN_1, \ldots, DGBN_F\}$. After a similar analysis is performed between the scene data of the flooding event $ty_{pre}$ of the Inner Harbor Station to be predicted and the scene data of the $F$ flooding events, the $DGBN_i$ model with the most similar characteristics to $ty_{pre}$ is selected from $model$. The scene data for similar analysis are collected before flooding occurs. The Euclidean distance is used for similarity analysis between flooding events, and the expression is

$$dist(B_{ty_{pre}}, C_{ty_i}) = \frac{\sum_{j=1}^{n''} \sqrt{\sum_{i=1}^{k-1}(b_{i,j} - c_{i,j})^2}}{n''} \tag{11}$$

$$DGBN_i \propto \min\{dist(B_{ty_{pre}}, C_{TY})\} \tag{12}$$

where $B_{ty_{pre}} = (b_{1,1}, \ldots, b_{k-1,n''})$ and $C_{ty_i} = (c_{1,1}, \ldots, c_{k-1,n''})$ are the flooding factor sample (excluding flooding depth) of the current flooding to be predicted and the $i$-th flooding, respectively, $C_{TY} = (C_{ty_1}, \ldots, C_{ty_F})$ is the set of flooding factor samples of $F$ flooding events, $b_{i,j}$ and $c_{i,j}$ are the $j$-th samples of the $i$-th flooding factor and $n''$ is the number of data of the flooding factor before flooding occurred. We define the flooding depth predicted by the $DGBN_i$ as $H_B$.

Generally speaking, when the ponding in the high terrain exceeds a certain depth, the water flow to the low terrain will be generated. Therefore, a threshold $\tau$ is set to decide whether to generate surface confluence. Define the set of flooding depth as $H_H = (H_{h,1}, \ldots, H_{h,n'})$ at different azimuth high topographies, where $H_{h,i}$ is the flooding depth of the $i$-th high topography. Based on the above analysis, the following prediction expression is obtained:

$$H_{NG} = \begin{cases} H_B, & H_H \leq \tau \\ H_B + \sum_{i=1}^{n'_\tau} H_{G,i}, & \exists H_{h,i} \geq \tau, 1 \leq n'_\tau \leq n' \end{cases} \tag{13}$$

where $H_{NG}$ is the predicted flooding depth of the Inner Harbor Station and $n'_\tau$ is the number of water level monitoring points whose stagnant water exceeds the threshold $\tau$. The final prediction model DGBN-m of this paper is shown in Figure 3. The prediction model in Figure 3 consists of three modules: the DGBN module, similarity module and surface confluence module. Based on the above analysis and the construction of the DGBN-m, the performance of the proposed scheme will be tested against the real data provided by the Macau Meteorological Bureau in the next section.

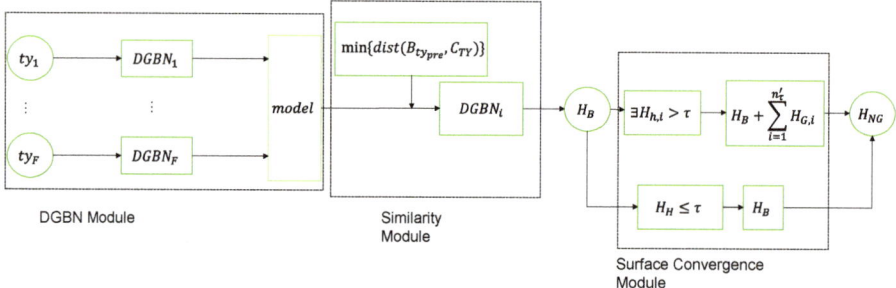

**Figure 3.** Prediction model DGBN-m. DGBN Module represents the set of DGBNs built from historical flooding disasters, Similarity Module represents the process of selecting the appropriate DGBN from the *model* and performing the initial prediction and Surface Confluence Module represents the process of combining Manning formula with DGBN to predict the flooding depth.

## 6. Experimental Analysis

### 6.1. Dataset Selection

According to the data provided by the Macau Meteorological Bureau, three flood events with complete data are selected to establish three DGBNs. The three typhoons associated with the three flooding events are Mangkhut, Nida and Bebinca. These three typhoons have relatively complete flooding data, and the amount of data is relatively large. And, typhoon Hato is selected as the predicted flooding (test set). The flood disaster caused by typhoon Hato to Macau is the most serious in historical records, causing a flooding depth that exceeds 3 m (higher than that of other flooding events). The Macau Meteorological Bureau only recorded data on the rise in flooding depth caused by typhoon Hato but not on the fall in flooding depth because the water level detector was damaged when the flooding depth reached the maximum. Based on the above analysis, the data of typhoon Hato are not suitable for building the DGBN but they are suitable for use as the test set.

### 6.2. Flooding Factor Selection

The flooding caused by typhoons in Macau is a complicated process. There are many factors that cause flooding in Macau (such as heavy rainfall, storm surge, etc.). Therefore, many factors need to be considered when selecting the flooding factor. The test cases are the flooding events at the Inner Harbor Station in Macau. Based on the above analysis, we select eight factors: the location of the typhoon center (longitude and latitude), the wind speed of the typhoon center, city wind speed (values measured by the Tai Tam Shan Meteorological Observatory in Macau), the rainfall of Macau, the tide (Macau tide and Jiuzhou Port tide) and the flooding depth. These eight factors are used to build the DGBN, referred to as DGBN8. The prediction model is referred to as DGBN8-m. The specific description of the eight factors is shown in Table 1.

**Table 1.** Abbreviations and units of 8 flooding factors.

| | Record Data for 8 Factors Every Minute | | | | | | | |
|---|---|---|---|---|---|---|---|---|
| Name of Factor | Latitude | Longitude | Typhoon Wind Speed | City Wind Speed | Rainfall in Macau | Macau Tide | Jiuzhou Port Tide | Flooding Depth |
| Signs and units of factors | La (°N) | Lo (°E) | WD (m/s) | CWD (m/s) | Rain (mm/m) | MC (m) | JZ (m) | D (m) |

According to the map of water level monitoring points provided by the Macau Meteorological Bureau, three water level monitoring points are selected in different directions of the Inner Harbor Station, namely Inner Harbor North Station, Kang Kung Temple Station and Xiahuan Street Station.

## 6.3. Parameter Settings

Set the number of nodes to $k = 8$ in the Bayesian network per time slice, the connection strength of the arc to $\alpha = 0.85$, the direction strength of the arc to $\beta = 0.5$, hydraulic radius to $R = 4/17$ m, Inner Harbor Station coverage area to $w = 4000$ m$^2$, Manning coefficient to $\varphi = 0.014$, the number of DGBNs to $F = 3$, the number of high-terrain water level monitoring sites to $n' = 3$ and threshold to $\tau = 0.3$.

## 6.4. Performance Analysis

Firstly, similarity analysis is made between the data of the flooding factor of typhoon Hato and the data of the flooding factor of Mangkhut, Nida and Bebinca, as shown in Figure 4. It can be seen from Figure 4 that the attributes of typhoon Hato and typhoon Mangkhut are closest to each other and that the difference is about 5. However, the attributes of typhoon Hato and the other two typhoons are far apart, and the difference is about 25 and 27, respectively. Therefore, the DGBN established by typhoon Mangkhut is selected as the network model of typhoon Hato.

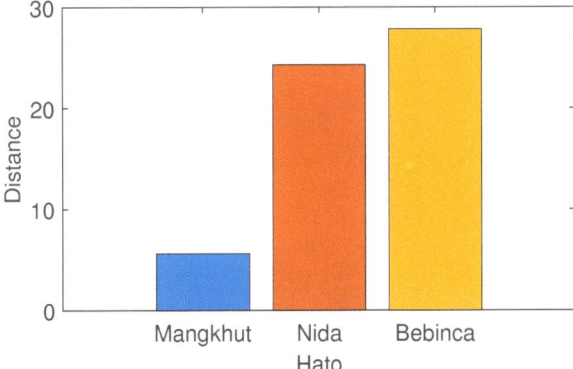

**Figure 4.** Similarity analysis of Typhoon Hato and Typhoon Mangkhut, Nida and Bebinca.

The flooding depth prediction after 15 min is conducted for the flooding of Macau Inner Harbour Station caused by typhoon Hato, as shown in Figure 5. The abscissa represents the time axis, and the ordinate represents the flooding depth in Figure 5. DGBN8 with two time slices is used for predictive analysis, and the interval between time slices is 15 min. Figure 5 shows the curves of the actual flooding depth, the flooding depth predicted by the DGBN8 model and the flooding depth predicted by the DGBN8-m model. It can be seen from the picture that the predicted curves of DGBN8 and DGBN8-m are coincident before 130 min, which means that the surface confluence has not yet occurred. After 130 min, the predicted curves of DGBN8 and DGBN8-m begin to separate, where the predicted curve of DGBN8-m gradually approaches the real flooding depth curve and the predicted curve of DGBN8 gradually deviates from the real curve. Overall, the prediction curves in Figure 5 can reflect the effectiveness of DGBN8-m proposed in the paper.

Relative error (RE), mean square error (MSE), root mean square error (RMSE) and mean absolute error (MAE) are used to analyze the error in predicting the flooding depth after 15 min for the DGBN8 and DGBN8-m models, as shown in Table 2. It can be seen from Table 2 that the error values of DGBN8-m calculated by various error algorithms are all smaller than the error value of DGBN8. In general, RE is more indicative of the reliability of the predictive model. Therefore, the RE is used to calculate the prediction accuracy of the prediction model. The prediction accuracy of DGBN8-m is 84%, and the prediction accuracy of DGBN8 is 77%, which fully demonstrates the prediction ability of the DGBN8-m model.

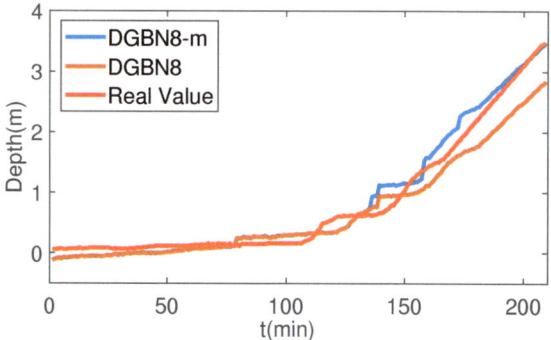

**Figure 5.** Prediction of flooding depth after 15 min. The abscissa represents the time and the vertical axis represents the flooding depth.

**Table 2.** Prediction error analysis of DGBN8 and DGBN8-m.

| Model \ Algorithm | RE | MSE | RMSE | MAE |
|---|---|---|---|---|
| DGBN8-m | 0.16 | 0.026 | 0.16 | 0.13 |
| DGBN8 | 0.23 | 0.066 | 0.25 | 0.19 |

However, it can be seen from Figure 5 that the predicted values of DGBN8 and DGBN8-m are less than 0 (negative value) before about 50 min, which is contrary to the real phenomenon. To solve this problem, the network structure and network parameters of DGBN8 are carefully studied, and we find that the flooding factor $CWD$ can cause the network structure to show unreasonable connections (for example, urban wind speed affects typhoon wind speed). Therefore, we choose to discard the flooding factor $CWD$ and establish the seven-variable DGBN to form the new prediction model, referred to as DGBN7-m.

DGBN7-m and DGBN7 models are used to predict the flooding depth after 15 min at Macau Inner Harbor Station under the typhoon Hato scenario, as shown in Figure 6. Similar to the prediction model in Figure 5, a DGBN with two time slices is used for prediction analysis, and the interval between time slices is 15 min. The change trends of the curves of DGBN7-m and DGBN7 models in Figure 6 are basically the same as those in Figure 5. The biggest difference between Figures 5 and 6 is that the predicted values of DGBN7-m and DGBN7 are both positive and close to the real values in the early prediction, which can better reflect the changing trend of flooding depth.

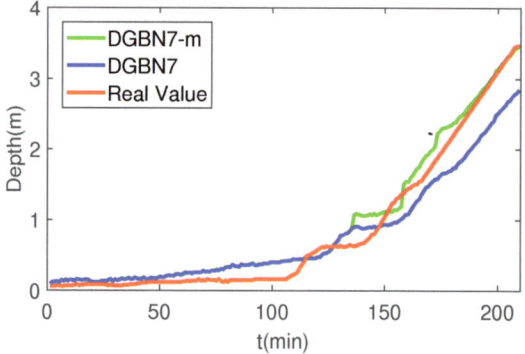

**Figure 6.** Prediction of flooding depth after 15 min. The abscissa represents the time and the vertical axis represents the flooding depth.

In order to more accurately reflect the prediction performance of the new prediction model DGBN7-m, RE, MSE, RMSE and MAE are also used to analyze the error of DGBN7 and DGBN7-m models in predicting the flooding depth after 15 min, as shown in Table 3. It can be seen that the error values of DGBN7-m calculated by various error algorithms are the same as those of DGBN8-m. The RE is used to calculate the prediction accuracy of the model, and the prediction accuracy of DGBN7-m and DGBN7 is 84% and 75%, respectively. The prediction accuracy of DGBN7 is not much different from that of DGBN8. Further, the number of parameters of DGBN7 and DGBN8 is analyzed, where the number of parameters of the DGBN7 network is 92 and the number of parameters of the DGBN8 network is 106, which shows that the DGBN7-m model runs faster and requires fewer computational resources than the DGBN8-m model under the same prediction accuracy. Therefore, the DGBN7-m model will be used for subsequent experimental analyses.

**Table 3.** Predicting error analysis of DGBN7 and DGBN7-m.

| Algorithm<br>Model | RE | MSE | RMSE | MAE |
| --- | --- | --- | --- | --- |
| DGBN7-m | 0.16 | 0.026 | 0.16 | 0.13 |
| DGBN7 | 0.25 | 0.076 | 0.27 | 0.21 |

To further demonstrate the performance of the prediction model DGBN7-m, the flooding depth after 30 min is predicted for the flooding at Macau Inner Harbor Station caused by Typhoon Hato. The DGBN7 of two time slices (the interval between time slices is 30 min), the three-time-slice one-order DGBN7 (the interval between time slices is 15 min) and three-time-slice two-order DGBN7 (the interval between time slices is 15 min) are established, respectively, to predict the flooding depth after 30 min, as shown in Figure 7. The above three prediction models are abbreviated as 2TDGBN7-m, 3T1ODGBN7-m and 3T2ODGBN7-m, respectively. From Figure 7, we can see that all three types of DGBN7-m can approximately predict the changing trend of the flooding depth. Figure 7 shows that 3T2ODGBN7-m has the best prediction performance before about 130 min; 3T1ODGBN7-m has the best prediction performance after about 130 min; 2TDGBN7-m only exhibits a better prediction performance in the later period and its prediction performance is not optimal in the whole prediction period. Although the prediction performance of 3T2ODGBN7-m is slightly better than that of 3T1ODGBN7-m in the early stage, the prediction curves of the two models are close. In the later prediction, the prediction performance of 3T2ODGBN7-m is much worse than that of 3T1ODGBN7-m, and the prediction trend of 3T2ODGBN7-m has deviated from the change trend of the real value.

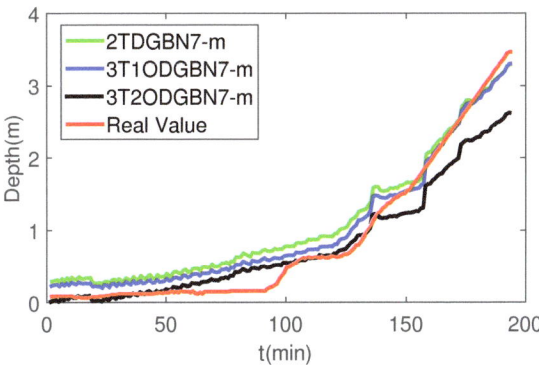

**Figure 7.** Prediction of flooding depth after 30 min. The abscissa represents the time and the vertical axis represents the flooding depth.

Similarly, RE, MSER, RMSE and MAE are used to analyze the prediction errors of 2TDGBN7-m, 3T1ODGBN7-m and 3T2ODGBN7-m, as shown in Table 4. It can be seen from Table 4 that the prediction errors of the 3T1ODGBN7-m model calculated by various error algorithms are smaller than those of the 2TDGBN7-m model and 3T1ODGBN7-m model. Through RE analysis, we can further obtain that the prediction accuracy of the 3T1ODGBN7-m model is 80%, the prediction accuracy of the 2TDGBN7-m model is 71% and the prediction accuracy of the 3T2ODGBN7-m model is 78%. Compared with the prediction accuracy of the prediction model that predicts the flooding depth after 15 min, the prediction accuracy of the 3T1ODGBN7-m model for predicting the flooding depth after 30 min decreased by only 4%.

**Table 4.** Prediction error analysis for 2TDGBN7-m, 3T1ODGBN7-m and 3T2ODGBN7-m.

| Algorithm<br>Model | RE | MSE | RMSE | MAE |
| --- | --- | --- | --- | --- |
| 2TDGBN7-m | 0.29 | 0.082 | 0.28 | 0.25 |
| 3T1ODGBN7-m | 0.20 | 0.042 | 0.20 | 0.17 |
| 3T2ODGBN7-m | 0.22 | 0.088 | 0.29 | 0.20 |

6.4.1. Robustness Analysis

When the flood disaster occurs, various detectors often fail. Once a device such as the detector fails, data loss will occur. When faced with a large number of missing data and some characteristic variables being completely missing, the corresponding complementary algorithm is useless. But, we still hope that the predictive model can have a certain predictive ability in this case. In this section, the robustness of the DGBN7-m will be tested in the case of a complete loss of data for some flood factors, as shown in Figure 8. Figure 8 represents the flooding depth after 30 min predicted by 3T1ODGBN7-m in the case where each flood factor is lost once (the data of the corresponding flood factor are completely lost). The prediction curves in Figure 8 (except the true value curve) represent the results predicted by the 3T1ODGBN7-m model after the corresponding variable is lost. It can be seen from the picture that the change trend of all predicted curves (except the prediction curve corresponding to variable $D$) is basically similar to the change trend of the real curve, in which the prediction curves corresponding to variables $JZ$, $Lo$ and $Rain$ are close to the real value about 120 min ago. After 120 min, the predicted curve of the $JZ$ variable deviates to a greater extent than the predicted curve of the $Lo$ and $Rain$ variables deviates from the true curve. This phenomenon shows that 3T1ODGBN7-m still has a well-predictive ability after the data loss of the $Lo$ or $Rain$ variable, and that 3T1ODGBN7-m can withstand the data loss of the $JZ$ variable in the early period. Furthermore, it can be seen that the prediction curves corresponding to $La$ and $WD$ variables are close to the real curves after 150 min, which indicates that 3T1ODGBN7-m can withstand the data loss of these two variables in the later period. The picture shows that only the prediction curves corresponding to $MC$ and $D$ variables deviate from the true curve to a large extent during the whole prediction period. The above analysis shows that 3T1ODGBN7-m has strong robustness.

To better describe the predictive ability of the 3T1ODGBN7-m model after the flood factor is missing, the RE analysis graph is given, as shown in Figure 9. It can be seen that when the prediction error of 3T1ODGBN7-m is lower than 0.5, the corresponding variables are $La$, $Lo$, $Rain$ and $JZ$; when the prediction error is higher than 0.5, the corresponding variables are $WD$, $MC$ and $D$, which is consistent with the prediction result in Figure 8.

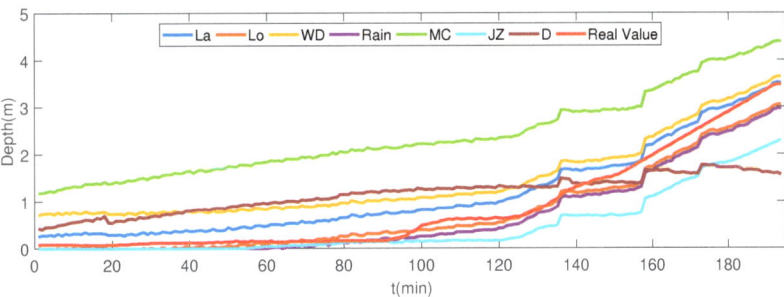

**Figure 8.** Prediction of flooding depth for 3T1ODGBN7-m with missing flood factor. The abscissa represents the time and the vertical axis represents the flooding depth.

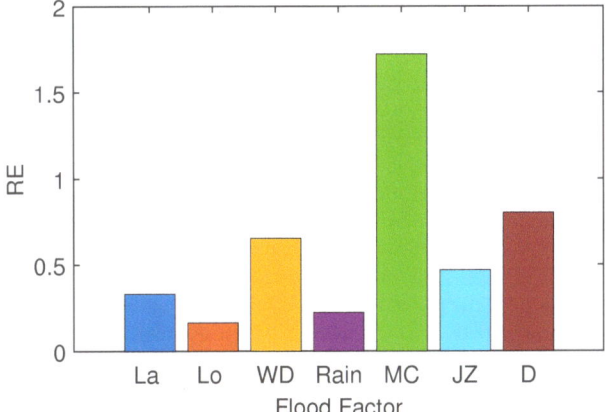

**Figure 9.** Relative error analysis. The abscissa represents that the corresponding variable is lost and the vertical axis represents the error.

### 6.4.2. Algorithm Comparison

Due to the rapid development of deep learning, neural networks have achieved better results in prediction. Therefore, the prediction performance of the back propagation (BP) neural network and linear regression is compared with that of the DGBN7-m model. We build the three-layer BP neural network, input layer, hidden layer and output layer. We set the input layer to have 6 nodes (the number of flood factor), the output layer to have 1 node (flooding depth) and the hidden layer to have 13 neurons (according to Kolmogorov's theorem). The corresponding parameters of the BP neural network are set with a learning rate of 0.01, loss threshold of 0.03 and 10,000 training times. The data of the three typhoons of Mangkhut, Nida and Bebinca are used as the training set of the BP neural network and linear regression, and the data of Typhoon Hato are used as the test set of the BP neural network and linear regression. As shown in Figure 10, the BP neural network and linear regression predict the flooding depth after 15 min at Macau Inner Harbor Station. As can be seen from the picture, the neural network and linear regression cannot accurately predict the changing trend of flooding depth. Through the analysis of RE, the prediction accuracy of the neural network is only 39%, and the prediction accuracy of linear regression is only 22%. The low prediction performance of the BP neural network may be caused by the small amount of data and the difference in flooding scenes, which makes it difficult for the BP neural network to accurately learn the relationship between the flooding factor and the flooding depth. This further reflects the advantages of the prediction model DGBN7-m in scenarios where the amount of data is small and the flooding scenarios are different.

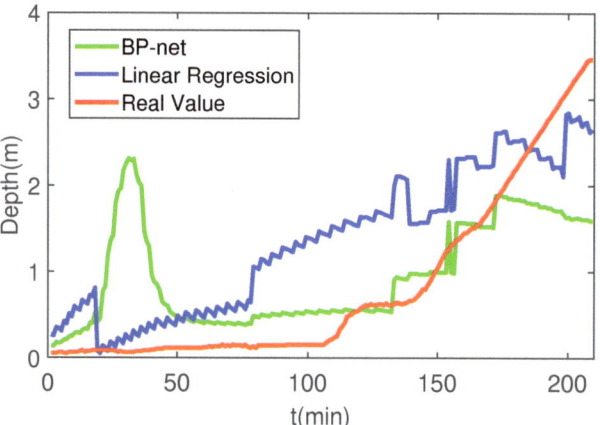

**Figure 10.** BP neural network and linear regression predict the flooding depth after 15 min. The abscissa represents the time and the vertical axis represents the flooding depth.

6.4.3. Generalization Analysis

In order to verify the validity and reliability of the DGBN7-m model, this section tests the generalization of the DGBN7-m model. Another typhoon (Dianmu) that caused the flooding at the Macau Inner Harbor Station is selected as the test set. The data of the flooding factor of typhoon Dianmu and the data of the flooding factor of typhoon Mangkhut, Nida and Bebinca are analyzed for similarity, as shown in Figure 11. We can see from the picture that typhoon Dianmu is most similar to typhoon Bebinca. However, the gap between typhoon Dianmu and typhoon Bebinca is about 15, which is larger than the gap between typhoon Hato and typhoon Mangkhut. In other words, the DGBN7 established by typhoon Bebinca has a low degree of matching with the characteristics of flooding caused by typhoon Dianmu. Given the limited number of typhoons currently recorded by the Macau Meteorological Bureau, the DGBN7 established by typhoon Bebinca is still selected as the prediction network for typhoon Dianmu.

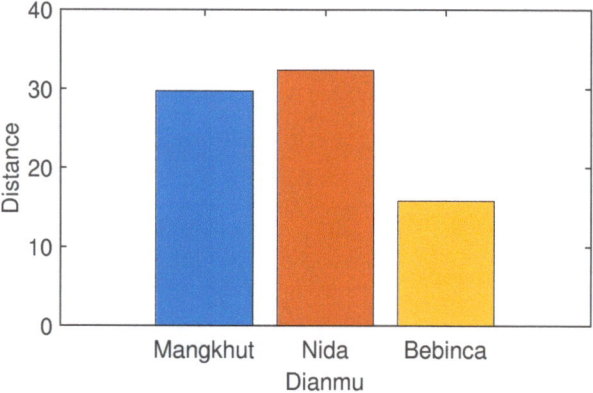

**Figure 11.** Similarity analysis of typhoon Dianmu and typhoon Mangkhut, Nida and Bebinca.

The flooding depth prediction after 15 min is shown in Figure 12. The change trend of the predicted curve of DGBN7-m in the early and late stages is similar to that of the real flooding depth curve. The change trend of the predicted curve of DGBN7-m in the mid-term has a large deviation from the change trend of the real flooding depth curve. According to the error analysis in Table 5, the difference between the flooding depth predicted by

DGBN7-m and the real flooding depth is small. The prediction accuracy of DGBN7-m calculated by the RE can reach 72%. Therefore, the above analysis shows that the DGBN7-m model still has a good prediction performance in the case of large differences, which further confirms that the DGBN7-m model has good generalization.

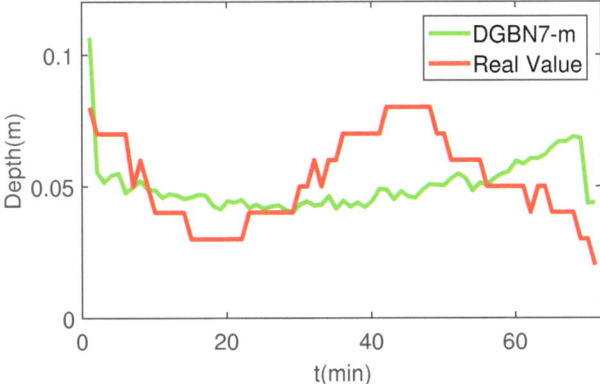

**Figure 12.** Flooding depth prediction after 15 min. The abscissa represents the time and the vertical axis represents the flooding depth.

**Table 5.** Error analysis table of DGBN-m.

| Algorithm<br>Model | RE | MSE | RMSE | MAE |
|---|---|---|---|---|
| DGBN7-m | 0.28 | 0.0003 | 0.018 | 0.015 |

## 7. Conclusions

This paper designs a prediction model for flooding in Macau. A more accurate prediction model, DGBN7-m, is obtained by combining the DGBN with the surface confluence, and achieves better prediction results proved by simulation. The work carried out in this paper can be summarized as follows:

i    In the case of a small amount of data, some expert experience is useful for guiding the learning direction of the algorithm to establish a more reasonable DGBN.
ii   In the case of different flooding scenarios, multiple historical flooding scenarios are used to establish multiple DGBNs, and then a similar analysis is made between the scenarios of flooding to be predicted and the scenarios of multiple historical flooding; finally, the DGBN established by the historical flooding that is most similar to the flooding to be predicted is chosen as the prediction network.
iii  According to the topography of Macau, the influence of surface confluence is studied, and the Manning formula analysis method is put forward. And, the DGBN and Manning formula are combined to obtain the final prediction model, DGBN-m, which has a high prediction ability.

The prediction model that we designed has growth potential: with the accumulation of more scene data of flooding, scene similarity analysis will have more advantages, and the accuracy and effectiveness of DGBN-m model prediction can be further improved. For example, the current flooding can be constructed as the DGBN, which is added to the set of DGBNs to enhance the ability of the prediction model to predict the flood depth of future flooding. Due to the lack of relevant data, this paper does not analyze the effects of infiltration and drainage systems on the flooding areas. In the case of severe typhoons and little changes in the urban drainage system, the impact of infiltration and the drainage system is small in different scenarios. But, the analysis of infiltration and the drainage system can further improve the effectiveness of the prediction model, which can achieve a more accurate and timely prevention of flooding disasters. Therefore, the more difficult infiltration phenomena and the effects of drainage systems will be worked on in the future. In future research, we will study flooding in different terrains and incorporate scenarios of the confluence and diversion of ponding into the prediction model to achieve a more comprehensive prediction of flooding. In addition, we will explore the characteristics of flooding in different coastal cities to find out the same and different factors that allow the predictive model to be built adaptively for different environments.

**Author Contributions:** Conceptualization, S.Z. and C.C.; Methodology, S.Z.; Software, S.Z. and C.C.; Validation, S.Z.; Formal analysis, S.Z.; Investigation, S.Z. and W.D. (Weiping Ding); Resources, W.D. (Weijun Dai); Data curation, S.Z. and W.D. (Weijun Dai); writing—original draft, S.Z.; writing—review and editing, C.C., N.S., J.R. and W.D. (Weiping Ding); Supervision, C.C., N.S., J.R. and W.D. (Weiping Ding); Project administration, C.C.; Funding acquisition, C.C. and W.D. (Weijun Dai). All authors have read and agreed to the published version of the manuscript.

**Funding:** This study was supported by: National Natural Science Foundation of China and Macau Science and Technology Development Joint Project (0066/2019/AFJ): Research on Knowledge-oriented Probabilistic Graphical Model Theory based on Multi-source Data. MOST-FDCT Joint Projects (0058/2019/AMJ, 2019YFE0110300): Research and Application of Cooperative Multi-Agent Platform for Zhuhai-Macau Manufacturing Service. Natural Science Characteristic Innovation Project of Guangdong General Universities (2022KTSCX323). Heyuan Social Development Science and Technology Project (2021/62/138).

**Data Availability Statement:** Macau Meteorological Bureau data are available at https://www.smg.gov.mo/zh/subpage/355/report/typhoon-yearly-report (accessed on 1 May 2023).

**Conflicts of Interest:** We declare that we have no financial and personal relationships with other people or organizations that can inappropriately influence our work and that there is no professional or other personal interest of any nature or kind in any product, service and/or company that could be construed as influencing the position presented in, or the review of, the manuscript entitled, "Predicting Typhoon Flood in Macau by Dynamic Gaussian Bayesian Network and Surface Confluence Analysis".

## References

1. Kellens, W.; Terpstra, T.; De Maeyer, P. Perception and communication of flood risks: A systematic review of empirical research. *Risk Anal. Int. J.* **2013**, *33*, 24–49. [CrossRef] [PubMed]
2. Mosavi, A.; Ozturk, P.; Chau, K.W. Flood prediction using machine learning models: Literature review. *Water* **2018**, *10*, 1536. [CrossRef]
3. Tehrany, M.S.; Jones, S.; Shabani, F. Identifying the essential flood conditioning factors for flood prone area mapping using machine learning techniques. *Catena* **2019**, *175*, 174–192. [CrossRef]
4. Paradilaga, S.N.; Sulistyoningsih, M.; Lestari, R.K.; Laksitaningtyas, A.P. Flood Prediction Using Inverse Distance Weighted Interpolation of K-Nearest Neighbor Points. In Proceedings of the 2021 IEEE International Geoscience and Remote Sensing Symposium IGARSS, Brussels, Belgium, 11–16 July 2021; pp. 4616–4619.
5. Khan, W.; Hussain, A.J.; Alaskar, H.; Baker, T.; Ghali, F.; Dhiya, A.; Al-Shamma'a, A. Prediction of Flood Severity Level via Processing IoT Sensor Data Using a Data Science Approach. *IEEE Internet Things Mag.* **2020**, *3*, 10–15. [CrossRef]
6. Du, J.; Kimball, J.S.; Sheffield, J.; Pan, M.; Fisher, C.K.; Beck, H.E.; Wood, E.F. Satellite flood inundation assessment and forecast using SMAP and landsat. *IEEE J. Sel. Top. Appl. Earth Obs. Remote Sens.* **2021**, *14*, 6707–6715. [CrossRef] [PubMed]
7. Adnan, R.; Ruslan, F.A.; Zain, Z.M. Flood water level modelling and prediction using artificial neural network: Case study of Sungai Batu Pahat in Johor. In Proceedings of the 2012 IEEE Control and System Graduate Research Colloquium, Shah Alam, Malaysia, 16–17 July 2012; pp. 22–25.
8. Sinha, S.; Mandal, N. Design and analysis of an intelligent flow transmitter using artificial neural network. *IEEE Sens. Lett.* **2017**, *1*, 1–4. [CrossRef]
9. Imrie, C.E.; Durucan, S.; Korre, A. River flow prediction using artificial neural networks: Generalisation beyond the calibration range. *J. Hydrol.* **2000**, *233*, 138–153. [CrossRef]
10. Kim, S.; Matsumi, Y.; Pan, S.; Mase, H. A real-time forecast model using artificial neural network for after-runner storm surges on the Tottori coast, Japan. *Ocean Eng.* **2016**, *122*, 44–53. [CrossRef]
11. Gude, V.; Corns, S.; Long, S. Flood prediction and uncertainty estimation using deep learning. *Water* **2020**, *12*, 884. [CrossRef]
12. Kourgialas, N.N.; Dokou, Z.; Karatzas, G.P. Statistical analysis and ANN modeling for predicting hydrological extremes under climate change scenarios: The example of a small Mediterranean agro-watershed. *J. Environ. Manag.* **2015**, *154*, 86–101. [CrossRef]

13. Dai, W.; Cai, Z. Predicting coastal urban floods using artificial neural network: The case study of Macau, China. *Appl. Water Sci.* **2021**, *11*, 161. [CrossRef]
14. Dai, W.; Tang, Y.; Zhang, Z.; Cai, Z. Ensemble Learning Technology for Coastal Flood Forecasting in Internet-of-Things-Enabled Smart City. *Int. J. Comput. Intell. Syst.* **2021**, *14*, 166. [CrossRef]
15. Lu, Q.; Zhong, P.A.; Xu, B.; Zhu, F.; Ma, Y.; Wang, H.; Xu, S. Risk analysis for reservoir flood control operation considering two-dimensional uncertainties based on Bayesian network. *J. Hydrol.* **2020**, *589*, 125353. [CrossRef]
16. Sebastian, A.; Dupuits, E.J.C.; Morales-Nápoles, O. Applying a Bayesian network based on Gaussian copulas to model the hydraulic boundary conditions for hurricane flood risk analysis in a coastal watershed. *Coast. Eng.* **2017**, *125*, 42–50. [CrossRef]
17. Sen, M.K.; Dutta, S.; Kabir, G. Modelling and quantification of time-varying flood resilience for housing infrastructure using dynamic Bayesian Network. *J. Clean. Prod.* **2022**, *361*, 132266. [CrossRef]
18. Chen, J.; Zhong, P.A.; An R.; Zhu, F.; Xu, B. Risk analysis for real-time flood control operation of a multi-reservoir system using a dynamic Bayesian network. *Environ. Model. Softw.* **2019**, *111*, 409–420. [CrossRef]
19. Quesada, D.; Valverde, G.; Larrañaga, P.; Bielza, C. Long-term forecasting of multivariate time series in industrial furnaces with dynamic Gaussian Bayesian networks. *Eng. Appl. Artif. Intell.* **2021**, *103*, 104301. [CrossRef]
20. Fahiman, F.; Disano, S.; Erfani, S.M.; Mancarella, P.; Leckie, C. Data-driven dynamic probabilistic reserve sizing based on dynamic Bayesian belief networks. *IEEE Trans. Power Syst.* **2018**, *34*, 2281–2291. [CrossRef]
21. Dong, G.; Han, W.; Wang, Y. Dynamic Bayesian Network-Based Lithium-Ion Battery Health Prognosis for Electric Vehicles. *IEEE Trans. Ind. Electron.* **2020**, *68*, 10949–10958. [CrossRef]
22. Zhang, Q.; Zhou, C.; Tian, Y.C.; Xiong, N.; Qin, Y.; Hu, B. A fuzzy probability Bayesian network approach for dynamic cybersecurity risk assessment in industrial control systems. *IEEE Trans. Ind. Inform.* **2017**, *14*, 2497–2506. [CrossRef]
23. Ma, Y.; Qi, S.; Fan, L.; Lu, W.; Chan, C.Y.; Zhang, Y. Dynamic Bayesian network approach to evaluate vehicle driving risk based on on-road experiment driving data. *IEEE Access* **2019**, *7*, 135050–135062. [CrossRef]
24. Keprate, A.; Ratnayake, R.C. Assessment of Reliability and Remaining Fatigue Life of Topside Piping Using Dynamic Bayesian Network. In Proceedings of the 2019 IEEE International Conference on Industrial Engineering and Engineering Management (IEEM), Macao, China, 15–18 December 2019; pp. 1114–1118.
25. Wang, J.; Han, M.; Wei, S. Discrete Dynamic Bayesian Network Threat Assessment Method Based on Cloud Parameter Learning. In Proceedings of the 2019 IEEE International Conference on Signal, Information and Data Processing (ICSIDP), Chongqing, China, 11–13 December 2019; pp. 1–6.
26. Fan, L.-M.; Jia, L.-L.; Ren, Y.; Wang, K.-S.; Yang, D.-Z. Risk Analysis of Discrete Dynamic Event Tree Based on Dynamic Bayesian Network. In Proceedings of the 2019 International Conference on Quality, Reliability, Risk, Maintenance, and Safety Engineering (QR2MSE), Zhangjiajie, China, 6–9 August 2019; pp. 141–147.
27. Xu, Y.; Wang, J.; Yu, Y. Alarm event prediction from historical alarm flood sequences based on Bayesian estimators. *Proc. IEEE Trans. Autom. Sci. Eng.* **2019**, *17*, 1070–1075. [CrossRef]
28. Melançon, G.; Dutour, I.; Bousquet-Mélou, M. Random generation of directed acyclic graphs. *Electron. Notes Discret. Math.* **2001**, *10*, 202–207. [CrossRef]
29. Scutari, M.; Denis, J.-B. *Bayesian Networks: Examples R*, 2nd ed.; CRC Press: Boca Raton, FL, USA, 2021.

**Disclaimer/Publisher's Note:** The statements, opinions and data contained in all publications are solely those of the individual author(s) and contributor(s) and not of MDPI and/or the editor(s). MDPI and/or the editor(s) disclaim responsibility for any injury to people or property resulting from any ideas, methods, instructions or products referred to in the content.

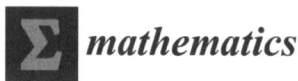

Article

# CLG: Contrastive Label Generation with Knowledge for Few-Shot Learning

Han Ma, Baoyu Fan, Benjamin K. Ng * and Chan-Tong Lam

Faculty of Applied Sciences, Macao Polytechnic University, Macao 999078, China; han.ma@mpu.edu.mo (H.M.); baoyu.fan@mpu.edu.mo (B.F.); ctlam@mpu.edu.mo (C.-T.L.)
* Correspondence: bng@mpu.edu.mo

**Abstract:** Training large-scale models needs big data. However, the few-shot problem is difficult to resolve due to inadequate training data. It is valuable to use only a few training samples to perform the task, such as using big data for application scenarios due to cost and resource problems. So, to tackle this problem, we present a simple and efficient method, contrastive label generation with knowledge for few-shot learning (CLG). Specifically, we: (1) Propose contrastive label generation to align the label with data input and enhance feature representations; (2) Propose a label knowledge filter to avoid noise during injection of the explicit knowledge into the data and label; (3) Employ label logits mask to simplify the task; (4) Employ multi-task fusion loss to learn different perspectives from the training set. The experiments demonstrate that CLG achieves an accuracy of 59.237%, which is more than about 3% in comparison with the best baseline. It shows that CLG obtains better features and gives the model more information about the input sentences to improve the classification ability.

**Keywords:** few-shot learning; contrastive learning; knowledge graph; natural language processing; transfer learning

**MSC:** 68T50

Citation: Ma, H.; Fan, B.; Ng, B.K.; Lam, C.-T. CLG: Contrastive Label Generation with Knowledge for Few-Shot Learning. *Mathematics* **2024**, *12*, 472. https://doi.org/10.3390/math12030472

Academic Editor: Faheim Sufi

Received: 5 January 2024
Revised: 24 January 2024
Accepted: 30 January 2024
Published: 1 February 2024

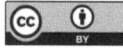

Copyright: © 2024 by the authors. Licensee MDPI, Basel, Switzerland. This article is an open access article distributed under the terms and conditions of the Creative Commons Attribution (CC BY) license (https://creativecommons.org/licenses/by/4.0/).

## 1. Introduction

Big data have become a considerable treasure due to their scale effect with the rapid development of storage technology in the past few years. The model achieves a huge improvement based on the big data in natural language processing (NLP) (BERT [1], RoBERTa [2], ALBERT [3], XLNet [4], BART [5], GPT-1 [6], GPT-2 [7], GPT-3 [8], T5 [9], ERNIE 1.0 [10], ERNIE 2.0 [11], and ERNIE 3.0 [12]) and computer vision (ViT [13], DALL-E [14], DALL-E 2 [15]), and Flamingo [16]). However, a few training samples cannot provide enough information as big data to train a model. Therefore, the performance of this problem is not satisfactory.

Based on [17], we would expect to find a function in the few-shot problem; when we input $x$, then the function can return $y$. $x$ and $y$ are the corresponding data and label. In this case, the model parameters shall ideally reach the optimal point. Training a model to reach the optimal point is similar to looking for treasure. When someone reaches the optimal point, he or she can obtain the treasure. However, in the process of searching for treasure, there are two traps: one is approximation error, and the other is estimation error. The model architecture determines the search space. When the search space does not contain the optimal point, the nearest point to the optimal point in the space is the best point that can be reached. The distance between the optimal point and the best point is the approximation error. When the amount of data is insufficient, the distance between the best point and the actual point is the estimation error. The estimation error is more prominent in the few-shot problem. That is the reason few-shot learning may produce inferior results.

In this work, we advance contrastive label generation with knowledge for few-shot learning (CLG), as shown in Figure 1. We inject the text and label with the context prompt and knowledge triplets to enhance their semantic information. Then, we input them into the CLG model. We shrink the output logits candidate space to simplify the task. Finally, we train the model with three objects.

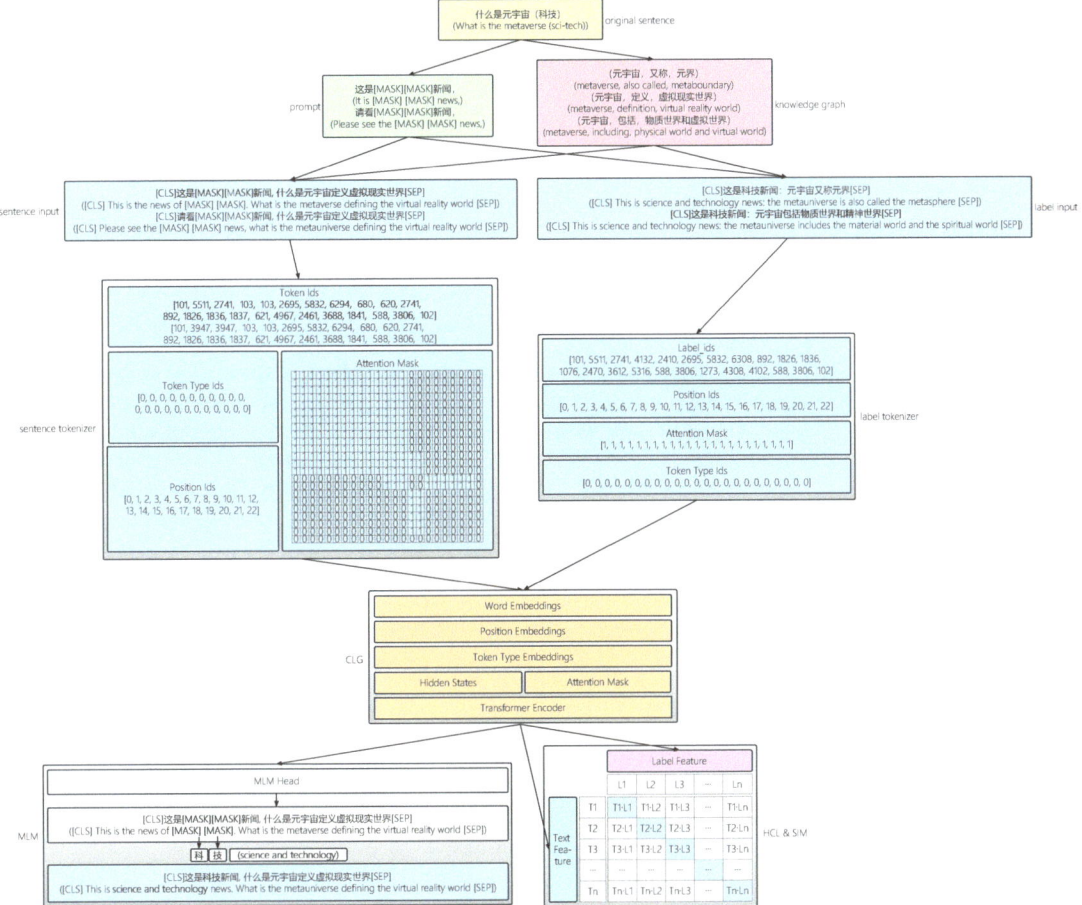

**Figure 1.** Overview of the structure of CLG. The text and label are augmented by the prompt and knowledge and then input into the model. In the model, there are three embedding layers to map the text and label to the vector space. Then, the encoder is used to extract the features. In the end, the features of the text and label are used to perform the downstream tasks.

The external knowledge base contains some content unrelated to the training data. In order to avoid the noise of external knowledge, we propose the label knowledge filter, which can skip the unrelated entity and relation to avoid the knowledge noise.

In the contrastive prompt and knowledge context, the text has been much enhanced, which creates a gap between the enhanced text with the unenhanced label. Therefore, the similarities will be far less. To solve this problem, we propose the label alignment method, which aligns the label with the text by introducing the prompt and knowledge.

Masked Language Modeling (MLM) searches the answers in the whole vocabulary list. There are many noise candidates in the search space. To solve this problem, we propose the MLM mask strategy, which can mask the noise candidates to narrow the search space into the label candidates.

We adopt multi-task fusion loss, HCL (Contrastive Learning with Hard negative samples), SIM (SIMilarity), and MLM. In order to obtain the common benefits of the three objective functions, all of the objective functions are weighted and summed to obtain the final loss.

The contributions of this work can be summarized as:

- Contrastive label generation (CLG). We propose contrastive label generation to align labels with the data. The input text has undergone semantic enhancement when associated with the label, but the label did not perform these operations, resulting in a lack of semantic information in the label. Therefore, we align the labels with the data and perform the same processing on the labels to reduce the difficulty of the model learning task;
- Label knowledge filter. We propose a label knowledge filter to avoid injecting noise into the text during the injection of knowledge. The traditional injection method matches the entities in the sentence with the head entities of the knowledge graph and injects the matched relations and tail entities after the center head entity. This kind of matching introduces knowledge that is not related to the sentence, so we eliminate the irrelevant noise by constructing a label knowledge filter to improve the effectiveness of the knowledge injection;
- Label logits mask. We employ the label logits mask to simplify the task. When the model outputs the logits, its candidate space is 8021 in the entire domain, while our task only needs to predict the first word of each label, which is a total of 15 words. Therefore, the first word in all of the labels is different. Hence, we constrain the output space to the task-related word range by masking the probability of other irrelevant candidate spaces so that the model can focus on outputting task-related words and improve its focus and performance;
- Multi-task fusion loss. We adopt the multi-task fusion loss. Different tasks could help the model to learn the different perspectives of the training set. Based on this, we adopt three different objects to help the model learn different perspectives of the training set to improve the final test task performance.

Extensive analysis verifies that CLG improves accuracy for the few-shot classification task.

This paper is organized as follows. Section 2 presents the literature review of data augmentation, model augmentation, and algorithm augmentation. Section 3 introduces the problem setup to clarify the problem to be resolved and presents the specific methodology of CLG concerning data, model, and algorithm. Section 4 features the experimental results and the conclusion about CLG. Section 5 includes the conclusion about CLG.

## 2. Related Work

Data augmentation uses some strategies to create more data. It is divided into homologous data augmentation and heterologous data augmentation. Homologous data augmentation is a method that creates data from the same source as the data set. It mainly increases new data from the training set, weakly labeled set, and unlabeled set in the same source. For the training set, it can translate [18–20], flip [20,21], shear [20], scale [19,22], reflect [23,24], crop [22,25], rotate [26], and so on to enrich the training set. For the weakly labeled or unlabeled set, there are some noisy or rare labeled data. Firstly, we can use these data to train a model and then use this model to obtain the pseudolabels for the weakly or unlabeled data. It only gives the label to the data with high confidence until the accuracy does not increase. Refs. [27,28] automatically annotate unlabeled data with pseudolabels to improve the accuracy and robustness of the model. Ref. [29] decodes the unlabeled data feature vectors via a large language model to generate the pseudolabels. The tail data of the long-tailed problem are also similar to those of the few-shot problem. Ref. [30] proposes a data-balanced review to keep the model learning all classifications. This method certifies the effect of multi-stage knowledge transfer to improve the classification accuracy of a few training samples of the tail. Heterologous data augmentation uses similar domain data sets to train the model. The more similar the used domain data sets are, the better the result.

Prompt creates a prompting function that results in the most effective performance on the downstream task. Based on [31], there are four paradigms of modern NLP technology development. Paradigm I is fully supervised learning without a non-neural network. It mainly extracts features of data by hand-crafting. Paradigm II is fully supervised learning with a neural network. It mainly designs the architecture of models to obtain better results. Paradigm III is pre-training and fine-tuning. It mainly designs the objective function to fit the downstream task. Paradigm IV is pre-training, prompt, and prediction. It mainly uses the prompt as context to close the distance between downstream tasks and pre-training tasks. These paradigms are shown in the development of NLP. According to [31], the prompt in the pre-trained language model is seen as the parameter. So, there are two methods using the prompt in few-shot learning. On the one hand, the prompt is dynamic in fine-tuning. For instance, in prefix-tuning [32] and warp [33], they freeze all of the pre-trained language model parameters while only updating the prompt parameters. AutoPrompt [34] dynamically obtains the optimal prompt template through model training. This method can alleviate the problems of difficult construction of the manual templates and unstable effects. The dynamic prompt is common and easy to carry out. It can keep the knowledge in the model of the pre-trained task. However, its performance is limited in terms of data scale because more data usually lead to better results. On the other hand, the prompt is static in fine-tuning, such as PET-TC [35], PET-Gen [36], and LM-BFF [37]. The static prompt only trains model parameters and sees the prompt as a part of the input. It can update the parameters of the large language model with the downstream task without introducing new parameters, but it needs to design the prompt template, and its robustness is not strong. The prompt is a useful method to extend the training set and convert the downstream task form to fit the pre-training task.

Explainability is important to certify the answer reasonably. Ref. [38] proposes an unsupervised approach to generate explanations for Machine Reading Comprehension (MRC) tasks. Ref. [39] proposes a modularized pre-training model framework to enable the model to train two sub-modules independently. It also proposes a knowledge retriever and a knowledge retrieval task (KRT) to train the ability of the model to retrieve correct knowledge entities from the knowledge base (KB) to improve the ability to generate dialogue. The KG provides external information to improve the explainability of the model. There are two main methods of applying a KG: explicit knowledge representation and implicit knowledge representation. Explicit knowledge representation injects the KG triplet text into sentences. KnowBERT [40] proposes the embedding of multiple knowledge bases into large-scale models to enhance the representation. SentiLR [41] adds emotional polarity to each word in the sentence and designs a new pre-trained task, which can establish the relationship between sentence-level emotional tags and word-level emotional words. KEPLER [42] proposes a unified model for knowledge embedding and language representation. It uses a large model to jointly learn knowledge embedding (KE) and MLM objective functions to align the actual knowledge and language representation into the same semantic space. CoLAKE [43] proposes word–knowledge graphs, which are undirected and heterogeneous. These graphs can realize the representation of language and knowledge and then improve the performance of the model in downstream tasks through pre-trained tasks. K-BERT [44] uses three embedding layers to represent the input sentences. The token embedding obtains the token information. The soft-position embedding obtains the relative position information. The segment embedding obtains the sentence pair information. K-BERT constructs the sentence tree, including the sentence and KG triplet. The triplet injects into the positions that are after the matched head entity, which enriches the information of the input to obtain better results. PK-BERT [45] attempts to resolve the few-shot problem. Firstly, it adds a prompt before the original sentence. Secondly, it injects the KG triplet (head, relation, tail) after sentences. Thirdly, in the attention matrix, the sentence tokens can see each other, but the head token can only see its relation token. The relation token can see both its head and its tail token. The tail token can only see its relation token. Finally, PK-BERT constructs the relative position ID to provide the token index information for the word and KG triplet in a sentence. The results show that PK-BERT can dig into the potential of the model, provide the knowledge, and guide the model to better complete the downstream tasks. Implicit knowledge representation embeds the KG triplets into vector space and then injects them into sentence vectors. ERNIE (THU) [46] uses TransE, which is a method of mapping the knowledge to a vector in the feature space to express and learn the KG. It first obtains the features of the token and entity, respectively; then codes and fuses them; and, finally, separates the features. This method can make the features of the token and entity contain each other's information to achieve the goal of text and knowledge fusion. For MLM tasks, ERNIE (Baidu) 1.0 [10] uses three different fine-grained mask strategies, namely, the random word-level mask strategy, entity-level mask strategy, and phrase-level mask strategy, so that the model can understand the language from different levels. ERNIE (Baidu) 2.0 [11] uses continual multi-task learning and introduces a series of tasks to let the model pay attention to words, sentences, and semantics, which can make models more knowledgeable. In addition to the advantages of the first generation and the second generation, ERNIE (Baidu) 3.0 [12] adds the universal knowledge–text prediction task to enable model learning, knowledge memory, and reasoning ability. In Ref. [47], the authors propose leveraging negative enhanced knowledge, using augmented knowledge pieces as hard negatives to improve knowledge representations.

To deal with the few-shot problem, Ref. [48] uses triplet information for data augmentation in relationship extraction, Ref. [49] uses clustering algorithms to construct pseudo-labeled data to alleviate the problem of insufficient sample size, and Ref. [50] obtains more comprehensive and accurate interaction information from other prototype networks to train the prototype network.

## 3. Methodology

In this section, we first introduce the problem setting and the challenges in few-shot classification. We address the challenges by proposing contrastive label generation, a knowledge graph with a block list, a logits–labels mask, multiple-task training, and some other methods.

*3.1. Problem Setting*

For a few-shot single-classification task, there are some sentences, $S$, corresponding to labels, $L$, in a small data set $D$ as shown in Equations (1)–(3), where the sentences list $S$ includes $N$ sentences, the label list $L$ includes $C$ labels, and the data set $D$ includes $I$ pairs of a sentence and a label $(S, L)$. For the few-shot setting, the value of $I$ is only 240 in our experiments.

$$S = \{S_1, \ldots, S_N\} \qquad (1)$$
$$L = \{L_1, \ldots, L_C\} \qquad (2)$$
$$D = \{(S_1, L_1), \ldots, (S_I, L_I)\} \qquad (3)$$

For a pair of one sentence $S_I$ and one label $L_I$ as shown in Equations (4) and (5), where $n$ sentence tokens, $t$, and $m$ label tokens, $l$, are included.

$$S_I = \{t_1, \ldots, t_n\} \tag{4}$$
$$L_I = \{l_1, \ldots, l_m\} \tag{5}$$

To solve this problem, we propose the method $CLG$ that can generate label tokens to solve the classification task as shown in Equation (6), where $m$ are sentence tokens and $x$ and $i$ are label tokens.

$$\{y_1, \ldots, y_i\} = CLG(\{x_1, \ldots, x_m\}) \tag{6}$$

*3.2. Contrastive Label Generation*

The traditional classification task converts the labels as the indexes from 0 to the classification number $C$, which loses the semantic meanings of the labels and limits the output space of the language model. So, we first adopt the original label phrases instead of indexes as the labels to keep the semantic information of the labels and then construct the context sentences for the labels to improve the label semantic information. In addition, we set the masked language modeling object to predict the label words, which activates the language ability of the model, aligns the downstream task with the pre-training task for transfer performance, and enlarges the output space of the task for other similar tasks. However, this makes the search space for the output larger than the classification number. To solve this problem, we adopt a logits mask, which masks all token probability, except for the label tokens, to shorten the search space.

To solve these two problems and improve the performance of the model, we propose contrastive label generation (CLG), as shown in Figure 1, which activates the language ability of the model, enlarges the output space of the model, and improves the label representation. Specifically, to make the model learn the semantic meanings of the labels and align the downstream task with the pre-training task, which is the language modeling (LM), we propose label generation to let the model output the language tokens of the label instead of the index of the classification. To improve the label feature representation, we consider that the task has its candidate classification list; it would be easy to perform a classification task via the elimination method. So, we present the contrastive label to make both the label tokens obtain better representations in the feature space and compare the candidates to make the task easy to perform.

CLG makes the model output the language tokens of the label instead of the index of the classification and makes the model learn the semantic meanings of the labels and enhance the output space of the model.

The classification task is similar to answering the choice question. When we make choices, we always have some alternative answers. It could be easier to answer the question when we consider the difference between choices. So, in this case, we compare the similarity of each input sentence with the labels and select the most similar label as the prediction answer.

Inspired by CLIP [51], we use the text and label pairs to calculate the similarity. In the training phase, the form is almost the same as the common pre-training phase as shown in Table 1. $t_i$ means the index of the text. $l_i$ means the index of the label. Each line has a number 1, indicating the correct label for the text. The only difference in the common pre-training phase is the use of sentences with two different prompts; however, in the training phase, labels with prompt prefixes are used.

**Table 1.** Training inputs matrix. The key to contrastive learning is to construct positive samples and negative samples. In this task, positive samples are correct text–label pairs that represent the value 1, and negative samples are incorrect text–label pairs that represent the value 0.

|       | $l_1$ | $l_2$ | $l_3$ | $l_4$ | $l_5$ | $l_6$ | $l_7$ | $l_8$ | $l_9$ | $l_{10}$ | $l_{11}$ | $l_{12}$ | $l_{13}$ | $l_{14}$ | $l_{15}$ |
|---|---|---|---|---|---|---|---|---|---|---|---|---|---|---|---|
| $t_1$ | 0 | 0 | 0 | 0 | 1 | 0 | 0 | 0 | 0 | 0 | 0 | 0 | 0 | 0 | 0 |
| $t_2$ | 0 | 0 | 0 | 0 | 0 | 0 | 0 | 0 | 0 | 0 | 0 | 1 | 0 | 0 | 0 |
| $t_3$ | 0 | 0 | 0 | 0 | 0 | 0 | 0 | 0 | 1 | 0 | 0 | 0 | 0 | 0 | 0 |
| $t_4$ | 0 | 1 | 0 | 0 | 0 | 0 | 0 | 0 | 0 | 0 | 0 | 0 | 0 | 0 | 0 |
| $t_5$ | 0 | 0 | 0 | 0 | 0 | 0 | 0 | 0 | 0 | 0 | 0 | 0 | 0 | 1 | 0 |
| $t_6$ | 0 | 0 | 0 | 0 | 0 | 0 | 1 | 0 | 0 | 0 | 0 | 0 | 0 | 0 | 0 |
| $t_7$ | 0 | 0 | 0 | 1 | 0 | 0 | 0 | 0 | 0 | 0 | 0 | 0 | 0 | 0 | 0 |
| $t_8$ | 0 | 0 | 0 | 0 | 0 | 0 | 0 | 0 | 0 | 0 | 1 | 0 | 0 | 0 | 0 |

### 3.3. Logits Mask and Label Mask

MLM is a head that is used to output raw hidden states. It uses a special token [MASK] to let the model predict the word that is masked. This method can shorten the distance between the downstream task and the pre-trained task to improve the effect of transfer learning.

When carrying out the MLM task, the original method randomly masks some single words, but there are many phrases in sentences. Masking only one word cannot provide the whole meaning. So, the Whole Word Masking (WWM) strategy is proposed to solve this question. If one word in a phrase has been masked, then it also masks the whole phrase.

The search space of the MLM object is the vocabulary size, which, in our experiment, is 8021, but the label words are much fewer than the vocabulary words. So, a natural idea is to shorten the search space. In our task, there are 15 phrases of the labels in the data set. In the pre-training stage, without the MLM logits mask, the task needs to search in the whole vocabulary space. However, we found that the first words of all labels are different. Therefore, it only needs to predict the first word, and then the subsequent words of the labels can be auto-completed. Hence, with the MLM logits mask, the task only needs to search the 15 words that are the first words of the 15 label phrases. So, this method can effectively shorten the search space and complete the task more easily.

MLM labels mask is also used to avoid unrelated words in the vocabulary. This can shrink the choices space of the task. It can be viewed as solving multiple choice questions by elimination. For example, when we perform a generative task, the standard method will choose some words from the whole vocabulary list. The labels mask will also select some words from part of the vocabulary list that only includes the first words of the 15 label phrases. This could greatly reduce the number of alternative words and simplify the task.

MLM mask indexes are the token ID 103 of the special token [MASK]. It can avoid unuseful information and let the model focus on the importance of the task.

### 3.4. Knowledge-Enhanced Label

The KG can provide semantic information for the model. It is a huge semantic network with many head entities, relation edges, and tail entities about people, things, and objects. The KG contains explicit knowledge, which is comprised the relations between entities and the attributes of entities. This can provide the knowledge for sentences. Therefore, it is logical, reasonable, and interpretable. The effectiveness is knowledge-driven and depends on the quantity and quality of the KG.

The KG usually represents the head entities, relation edges, and tail entities as triplets [h,r,t]. It can identify the phrases of sentences in the KG, and then inject the related relations and tails of the phrases into the sentence. The KG may not exactly match the domain of the data set, so the KG block list is used to avoid injecting the knowledge noise into the input sentence. If there are many triplets injected into the sentences, the algorithm will randomly sample the candidates to make sure that it will not obtain too much knowledge to influence the semantic information of the original sentences. Inspired by K-BERT [44] and CoLAKE [43], we use the KG and divide the sentence include two parts. One is the word graph; the other is the KG. The word graph is a fully connected word semantic network. In such a network, each word can be visible to others. They can be calculated by the model to map the word token to the embedding vector and then obtain the semantic representation. The KG is a knowledge semantic network composed of nodes and edges. The nodes mean the entities, and the edges mean the relations between the entities. If a phrase in its sentence can match a head entity in the KG, then the corresponding relation and tail entity of the head entity will be injected into the sentence. After that, the model will map the word tokens in the KG to the vectors in the feature representation space. In contrastive learning, we inject the KG triplets into the labels and add the prompt prefix before the labels to align with the text. Then, we input them into the model to obtain the feature vectors of the labels.

*3.5. Data Preprocessing*

Due to the few-shot problem setup, we can only use a few training samples to train the model. The task is about news title classification. The training set includes 240 news titles and the corresponding 15 classifications. So, effectively using it is a challenge. Given that the challenge is the data scale, the natural idea is to obtain more data to train. Considering the gap between the downstream and the pre-training task, we use the prompt to convert the downstream task form into the pre-training task form. This allows the model to better understand the task and improve the performance. Based on the prompt, the sentences differ in prefixes but convey the same semantics. So, they all have the same label. It is an easy but effective method for achieving data augmentation as shown in the following Equation (7).

$$D_{fsl} = \sum_{i=1}^{I} \sum_{j=1}^{J} \sum_{n=1}^{N} (p_i s_j t_n) \qquad (7)$$

The $D_{fsl}$ means the few-shot learning data set, $P_i$ means the $i$-th prompt, $S_j$ means the $j$-th symbol, $T_n$ means the $n$-th sentence, $I$ is the total number of prompts, $J$ is the total number of symbols, and $N$ is the total amount of training data. This way can create $I * J * N$ data for training, which can significantly enrich the training set.

*3.6. Prompt Prefix*

The prompt consists of templates and symbols, which can shorten the search space of the answers and prompt their retrieval. Since the downstream task may not be the same as the pre-trained task, the prompt can convert downstream data into pre-trained data, which helps to improve the effect of transfer learning. It can stimulate the potential power of the large language models and shorten the distance between the downstream objective and the pre-trained objective, as shown in the following example.

It is [MASK][MASK] news.

Inspired by the GPT series [10–12], we use the prompt as the prefix template to augment data. Specifically, we use different prefix templates before sentences. Each prefix template can create a set of input sentences. Through this method, we can obtain more data to train the model.

The prompt gives models more insights to let models generate output that better align with the task scenario. We manually craft and compare some prompts to obtain the results.

As shown in Table 2, the token IDs are the results of the tokenizer tokenizing the Token Word. Some special tokens need to be explained. Token [CLS] means the head of the sentence. It can represent the whole sentence. Token [MASK] means the word that is masked. It masks the sentence label that the model needs for prediction. Token [SEP] means the end of the sentence.

Table 2. Input sentence. The input words are tokenized to the token IDs.

| Type | Inputs |
|---|---|
| Token Word | ZH: [CLS]这是[MASK][MASK]新闻，什么是元宇宙定义虚拟现实世界[SEP]<br>(EN: [CLS]It is [MASK][MASK] news, What is metaverse define virtual reality world [SEP]) |
| Token IDs | [101, 5511, 2741, 103, 103, 2695, 5832, 119, 680, 620, 2741, 892, 1826, 1836, 1837, 621, 4967, 2461, 3688, 1841, 588, 3806, 102] |

When labels are determined, the main difference between templates is how to reasonably build prefix templates for two-character Chinese labels through natural language. Finally, we manage to pick some prompt templates that positively impact our results.

### 3.7. Multi-Task Fusion Loss

HCL loss [52] is concerned with contrastive learning with hard negative samples. It calculates the similarity of the samples to determine the label of the data. This can close the distance between positive samples and, at the same time, push away the distance between the negative samples.

$$\mathcal{L}_h = -\sum_{i=1}^{N} log \frac{e^{[f(x_i)f(y_i^+)^T]/\tau}}{e^{[f(x_i)f(y_i^+)^T]/\tau} + \sum_{j=1}^{M} e^{[f(x_i)f(y_j^-)^T]/\tau}} \quad (8)$$

In Equation (8), $x$ means the input sentence, $y^+$ means the positive label of the input sentence, $y^-$ means the negative label of the input sentence, $i$ means the $i$-th of the batch, $j$ means the $j$-th of the negative sentences, the function $f()$ maps the text to the vector, $\tau$ means the dynamic temperature, $N$ means the batch size, and $M$ means the number of negative classes.

The SIM loss calculates the similarity between the text feature vectors and the label feature vectors. It uses cross-entropy to calculate loss and updates the model weights.

$$\mathcal{L}_{s1} = -\sum_{i=1}^{N} log \frac{e^{[f(x_i)f(y_i^+)^T]/\tau}}{\sum_{j=0}^{M} e^{[f(x_i)f(y_j)^T]/\tau}} \quad (9)$$

$$\mathcal{L}_{s2} = -\sum_{i=1}^{N} log \frac{e^{[f(y_i^+)f(x_i)^T]/\tau}}{\sum_{j=0}^{M} e^{[f(y_j)f(x_i)^T]/\tau}} \quad (10)$$

$$\mathcal{L}_s = (\mathcal{L}_{s1} + \mathcal{L}_{s2})/2.0 \quad (11)$$

In Equations (9)–(11), $y$ means the sentence label, and the other symbols are the same as above.

The MLM loss function converts the downstream task into the pre-trained task, which can improve the effectiveness of the performance of transfer learning.

$$\mathcal{L}_m = -\sum_{i=1}^{N} log \frac{e^{f(x_i)_{[MASK]} \cdot g(y_i)}}{\sum_{j=0}^{M} e^{f(x_i)_{[MASK]} \cdot g(y_j)}} \quad (12)$$

In Equation (12), the function $g()$ maps the label to the vector, $[MASK]$ means the index of the mask in the sentence, and the other symbols are the same as above.

$$\mathcal{L} = w_h * \mathcal{L}_h + w_s * \mathcal{L}_s + w_m * \mathcal{L}_m \qquad (13)$$

The total loss calculates the weighted sum of the above three loss functions. In Equation (13), $\mathcal{L}_h$, $\mathcal{L}_s$, and $\mathcal{L}_m$ are the losses of the HCL, SIM, and MLM. The $w_h$, $w_s$, and $w_m$, which are set manually, are the weights of the HCL, SIM, and MLM objective functions.

*3.8. Training Algorithm*

The algorithm is the strategy used to search for the best parameters in the search space. Algorithm augmentation can provide a better direction for reaching the optimal point in each iteration.

The warmup is a method that lets the learning rate begin from a small value in the initial stage and grow to normal after the warmup period. It needs to set the warmup epochs. In the warmup epochs period, the parameters of the model will move more slowly. In this case, the gradient descent direction is at a small step length in the warmup stage, and it is more likely to avoid falling into the local optimal solution.

The learning scheduler is used to operate and process the learning rate. It can calculate the loss of the evaluation set. When the loss cannot decrease, the learning rate scheduler will decrease the learning rate to try more directions for updating.

Inspired by physical experiments, the algorithm simulates the process of observing the cooling of solids and gradually reduces the internal energy through annealing, so that the internal state reaches the ground state from the stable state. The simulated annealing (SA) algorithm is a method that can weaken the difference in each gradient at the initial training stage so that the model has more exploration directions and the overfitting of model training and model parameters falling into the local optimal solution are avoided. The simulated annealing algorithm keeps the temperature slowly down at some rate. It is possible to jump out from the local optimum solution.

The early stop is another trick that can end the training in advance under certain conditions. Such conditions are generally key indicators of the experiment, such as preparation rate, recall rate, F1, and loss. The first three are that the larger the numerical value, the better the model effect. Therefore, in this case, the condition for leaving early is that when the numerical value is still less than or equal to the highest value in the past within a certain number of times, the training ends. Correspondingly, the smaller the loss value, the better the effect of the model. Therefore, in this case, the condition for the early stop is that when the value is still greater than or equal to the lowest value in the past within a certain number of times, the training ends. Here, a certain number of times is a hyper-parameter, which can be given manually.

*3.9. Pseudocode*

The pseudocode for the implementation of CLG is shown in the Algorithm 1, and it can be summarized as follows. First, load the text and label from the data set. Second, add the prompt and inject the KG into the text and label. Third, tokenize the text and label from natural language to token ID. Fourth, input the tokens to embeddings and encoder layers and obtain the feature vectors of text and label. Fifth, calculate the similarity of the feature vectors of the text and label. Sixth, predict the token IDs of the position $[MASK]$ in sentences by the MLM head. Finally, calculate the final loss.

**Algorithm 1** CLG Pseudocode

1: $text, label \leftarrow load\_data(dataset)$
2: **for** $t, l$ in $zip(text, label)$ **do**
3:    $t\_p \leftarrow add\_prompt(t)$
4:    $l\_p \leftarrow add\_prompt(l)$
5:    $t\_pk \leftarrow inject\_kg(t\_p)$
6:    $l\_pk \leftarrow inject\_kg(l\_p)$
7: **end for**
8: **for** $t\_input, l\_input$ in $zip(t\_pk, l\_pk)$ **do**
9:    $text\_feature \leftarrow get\_feature(t\_input)$
10:    $label\_feature \leftarrow get\_feature(l\_input)$
11:    $hcl\_logits \leftarrow text\_feature\_vector@label\_feature\_vector.T/hcl\_temperature$
12:    $sim\_logits \leftarrow text\_feature\_vector@label\_feature\_vector.T/sim\_temperature$
13:    $mlm\_logits \leftarrow mlm\_head(text\_sequence\_output)$
14:    $index\_label \leftarrow$ index of the label_ids in each batch
15:    $onehot\_label \leftarrow index\_label$ in each batch
16:    $pos\_logits \leftarrow hcl\_logits * onehot\_label$
17:    $neg\_logits \leftarrow hcl\_logits * (1 - onehot\_label)$
18:    $hcl\_loss \leftarrow -log(pos\_logits/(pos\_logits + neg\_logits)).mean()$
19:    $text\_loss \leftarrow cross\_entropy(sim\_logits, onehot\_label).mean()$
20:    $label\_loss \leftarrow cross\_entropy(sim\_logits.T, onehot\_label.T).mean()$
21:    $sim\_loss \leftarrow (text\_loss + label\_loss)/2.0$
22:    $mlm\_loss \leftarrow cross\_entropy(mlm\_logits, label\_ids)$
23:    $loss \leftarrow w_{hcl} * hcl\_loss + w_{sim} * sim\_loss + w_{mlm} * mlm\_loss$ # $w_{hcl}, w_{sim}, w_{mlm}$ are the weights of the losses
24: **end for**

## 4. Experiment

### 4.1. Data Set

The TNEWS data set is a Chinese short text classification data set about news titles. It is divided into 15 categories, including technology, entertainment, automobiles, tourism, finance, education, international, real estate, e-sports, military, stories, culture, sports, agriculture, and stocks. The whole data set contains 73,360 pieces of data, and each piece of data contains a label, label description, sentence, keywords, and ID.

In FewCLUE [53], only a few training samples are used to achieve the classification task. There are 240 pieces of data in the training set, 240 pieces of data in the evaluation set, and 20,000 pieces of data in the test set.

In this work, we use the same data set as FewCLUE [53]. So, there are 15 labels, and each label has 16 pieces of sentences in the training set (15-way–16-shot), which are used for the few-shot learning. The training set size is 240, which is for the few-shot setting. The validation set size is 1200, which is for the feedback of the training phase and saves the model weights when the accuracy is better. The test set size is 2010, which is used to show the task performance of the model.

### 4.2. Inputs

Our experiments are on 15 categories of the text classification task. Note that the experiment does not use full data. In the training phase, each category has only 16 pieces of data, which is the few-shot setting.

#### 4.2.1. Input Token IDs

This method converts the input token words to token IDs by the tokenizer. The input includes the prompt that transfers the current task to the pre-training task for training models, and the KG triplet enhances the sentence information. We choose the prompt with the best accuracy as the label prompt, as shown in Table 3.

Table 3. Label prompts experiment. The bold number is the best accuracy in the experiment. In this task, we select the best prompt as the label prompt to perform the continued experiments.

| No. | Label Prompt | Acc. (%) |
|---|---|---|
| 1 | zh: 这是[MASK][MASK]新闻<br>en: This is [MASK] news | 19.167 |
| 2 | zh: 看看[MASK][MASK]新闻<br>en: See [MASK] News | 21.563 |
| 3 | zh: [MASK][MASK]新闻即将播放<br>en: [MASK] News coming soon | 21.458 |
| 4 | zh: [MASK][MASK]新闻来啦<br>en: Here comes the [MASK] news | **25.677** |
| 5 | zh: 这条新闻的类别是[MASK][MASK]<br>en: The category of this news is [MASK] | 14.896 |
| 6 | zh: 这条新闻是[MASK][MASK]类别的<br>en: This news is in the category of [MASK] | 25.625 |
| 7 | zh: 我认为这是[MASK][MASK]新闻<br>en: I think this is [MASK] news | 23.854 |
| 8 | zh: 这是[MASK][MASK]新闻吧<br>en: Is this [MASK] news | 22.604 |
| 9 | zh: 这是[MASK][MASK]新闻吗<br>en: Is this [MASK] news | 19.74 |
| 10 | zh: 这是什么新闻？[MASK][MASK]新闻<br>en: What news is this? [MASK] News | 23.229 |

There are 10 prompts and 10 symbols with their accuracies, as shown in Tables 4 and 5. In this experiment, we select, respectively, the top 5 prompts and the top 2 symbols of the group to expand the training set by 10 times.

Table 4. Text prompts experiment. The bold number is the best accuracy in the experiment. In this task, we select the top 5 prompts as the text prompts to perform the continued experiments.

| No. | Text Prompt | Acc. (%) |
|---|---|---|
| 1 | zh: 这是[MASK][MASK]新闻<br>en: This is [MASK] news | 23.698 |
| 2 | zh: 看看[MASK][MASK]新闻<br>en: See [MASK] News | **27.604** |
| 3 | zh: [MASK][MASK]新闻即将播放<br>en: [MASK] News coming soon | **28.333** |
| 4 | zh: [MASK][MASK]新闻来啦<br>en: Here comes the [MASK] news | **26.198** |
| 5 | zh: 这条新闻的类别是[MASK][MASK]<br>en: The category of this news is [MASK] | **31.25** |
| 6 | zh: 这条新闻是[MASK][MASK]类别的<br>en: This news is in the category of [MASK] | **29.74** |
| 7 | zh: 我认为这是[MASK][MASK]新闻<br>en: I think this is [MASK] news | 24.74 |
| 8 | zh: 这是[MASK][MASK]新闻吧<br>en: Is this [MASK] news | 18.854 |
| 9 | zh: 这是[MASK][MASK]新闻吗<br>en: Is this [MASK] news | 24.948 |
| 10 | zh: 这是什么新闻？[MASK][MASK]新闻<br>en: What news is this? [MASK] News | 25.521 |

**Table 5.** Text symbols experiment. The bold number is the best accuracy in the experiment. In this task, we select the top 2 symbols as the text symbols to perform the continued experiments.

| No. | Prompt | Acc. (%) |
| --- | --- | --- |
| 1 | ， | 25.052 |
| 2 | 。 | **27.24** |
| 3 | ? | 22.187 |
| 4 | : | 25.938 |
| 5 | ; | 24.427 |
| 6 | 、 | 25.729 |
| 7 | ! | **30.26** |
| 8 | - | 25.365 |
| 9 | —— | 25.417 |
| 10 | —> | 27.031 |

#### 4.2.2. Knowledge Graph

CN-DBpedia [54] is a large-scale general-domain structured encyclopedia KG that includes 5,168,865 pairs of head entities, relation edges, and tail entities.

Due to fewer pieces of information in the short text of the classification task, we use KG triplets to enhance the sentence head entity. This gives the model more information about the sentences and improves the explainability. For example, there is a sentence and a KG triplet, as shown in Table 6. For token type IDs, it is a sentence usually with two types of tokens, [0: the first sentence, 1: the second sentence]. Type 0 represents the original sentence tokens, including the head entity tokens. Type 1 represents the relation edge tokens and tail entity tokens in the KG triplet. In our task, we construct only one sentence that includes the original sentence and KG triplets to perform the continuous experiments. So, the final sequence is an all-zero sequence.

For position IDs, it is numbered in the order of the tokens in the sentence, but we need to note that it first tokenizes the original sentence from 0 to the length of the sentence minus 1. Then, it adopts the relative position code to tokenize KG triplets. Specifically, we add the KG positions, which are the indexes after the end word of the head entities, and the relation edge indexes are the next index at the end of the token of the head entities. The tail entity indexes are the next index of the end of the token of the relation edges. Finally, we combine all of them as the position IDs' input.

For the label, as the same text, we also add the prompt and inject KG relations and tails into the label words to construct label sentences. The label sentences have the label token IDs, label attention mask, and label type IDs.

We convert the input text from words to IDs. Those are unfriendly to humans but friendly to models, which means we can allow the model to understand what we want to say in natural language.

#### 4.2.3. Attention Mask

The input IDs consist of original sentences, entities, and relations of the KG. To avoid the knowledge token's interference in the sentence meaning, the relation edges can only be seen by their corresponding head and tail entities, and the tail entities can only be seen by the corresponding relation edges. The relation edges and tail entities cannot be seen by other original sentence tokens and other head entities.

The attention mask is also called the attention matrix, which can determine whether the tokens in a sentence can be seen by each other. The standard is that all tokens in the original sentence can see each other. If the first entity is identified in the original sentence, the relational edge and tail entity in the KG triplet will be injected into the end of the sentence as the second sentence and input into the model together. Based on [44], the relational edges and tail entities injected into the sentence are independent of the tokens of the non-head entities in the original sentences, so we use the attention mask attention matrix to achieve it. When two tokens see each other, their intersection position in the two-dimensional table is 1. On the contrary, when two tokens do not see each other, their intersection position in the two-dimensional table is 0, as shown in Table 7.

**Table 6.** The inputs converted from words to IDs.

| Inputs | Data |
|---|---|
| Text | 什么是元宇宙<br>(What is metaverse) |
| Label | 科技<br>(sci-tech) |
| prompt | 这是[MASK][MASK]新闻<br>(It is [MASK] news) |
| symbol | (,) |
| KG | （元宇宙，又称，元界）（元宇宙，定义，虚拟现实世界）<br>(metaverse, define, virtual reality world) |
| Text Token | [CLS]这是[MASK][MASK]新闻，什么是元宇宙定义虚拟现实世界[SEP]<br>([CLS] It is [MASK] news, what is metaverse define virtual reality world [SEP]) |
| Text Token IDs | [101, 5511, 2741, 103, 103, 2695, 5832, 6294, 680, 620, 2741, 892,<br>1826, 1836, 1837, 621, 4967, 2461, 3688, 1841, 588, 3806, 102] |
| Text Type IDs | [0, 0, 0, 0, 0, 0, 0, 0, 0, 0, 0, 0, 0, 0, 0, 0, 0, 0, 0, 0, 0, 0, 0] |
| Text Position IDs | [0, 1, 2, 3, 4, 5, 6, 7, 8, 9, 10, 11, 12, 13, 14, 15, 16, 17, 18, 19, 20, 21, 22] |
| Label Token | [CLS]这是科技新闻：元宇宙或称元界[SEP]<br>([CLS] This is technology news: metaverse is also called meta world [SEP]) |
| Label Token IDs | [101, 5511, 2741, 4132, 2410, 2695, 5832, 6308,<br>892, 1826, 1836, 2360, 4143, 892, 3806, 102] |
| Label Token Type IDs | [0, 0, 0, 0, 0, 0, 0, 0, 0, 0, 0, 0, 0, 0, 0, 0] |
| Label Position Ids | [0, 1, 2, 3, 4, 5, 6, 7, 8, 9, 10, 11, 12, 13, 14, 15] |

### 4.3. Training Strategy

There are some strategies for models to update the parameters effectively.

The warmup can increase the learning rate from a certain small value to the set value so that the model can explore more gradient update directions at the initial training stage and prevent the model from falling into local optimization. The learning rate scheduler decreases the learning rate until certain epochs, where a designated metric, such as loss not decreasing or accuracy not increasing, indicates a halt in improvement. A simulated annealing gradient can decrease the learning rate. We use simulated annealing to let the model explore more gradient update directions in the initial training stage to prevent the model from falling into local optimization. When the performance of models cannot improve or match certain conditions, then the models will stop learning. Dropout can be used as a feature augmentation method for training the model. In the training process, the weight of each neuron in the model has a certain probability $p$ to set it to zero, so that the neuron cannot have an impact on the neural network. This method can reduce the dependence between neurons in the network; that is, it does not rely too much on some local features, thus enhancing the generalization ability of the model.

### 4.4. Benchmark

In the FewCLUE [53] benchmark test, the data set was randomly disrupted, and the entire data set was divided into smaller data sets, including the training set, evaluation set, and test set. The training set consists of 15 categories and 16 samples of each category, also known as 15-way–16-shot.

The model is trained by using the corpus, which is the same source as the task data. So, using such a model can help it understand the data and improve its performance The inference ability is better than the models with other sources of the data set. In the model, the most important parts are the embeddings and encoder. The embedding layers are used to map the token IDs to the vectors, and the encoder layer is used to extract the features.

**Table 7.** The attention mask matrix shows that the relation tokens can only be seen by their own head entity tokens and tail entity tokens. The value 1 means the two words can be seen by each other and the value 0 means the words can not be seen by each other. The tail entity tokens can only be seen by the relation tokens. The two hashes ## indicate that it is a suffix following some other words.

| Attention Mask | [CLS] | 这 (It) | 是 (is) | [MASK] | [MASK] | 新 (news) | ##闻 | , | 什 (What) | ##么 | 是 (is) | 元 (metaverse) | ##宇 | ##宙 | 定 (definition) | 义 (definition) | 虚 (virtual) | ##拟 | 现 (reality) | ##实 | 世 (world) | ##界 | [SEP] |
|---|---|---|---|---|---|---|---|---|---|---|---|---|---|---|---|---|---|---|---|---|---|---|---|
| [CLS] | 1 | 1 | 1 | 1 | 1 | 1 | 1 | 1 | 1 | 1 | 1 | 1 | 1 | 1 | 0 | 0 | 0 | 0 | 0 | 0 | 0 | 0 | 1 |
| 这 (It) | 1 | 1 | 1 | 1 | 1 | 1 | 1 | 1 | 1 | 1 | 1 | 1 | 1 | 1 | 0 | 0 | 0 | 0 | 0 | 0 | 0 | 0 | 1 |
| 是 (is) | 1 | 1 | 1 | 1 | 1 | 1 | 1 | 1 | 1 | 1 | 1 | 1 | 1 | 1 | 0 | 0 | 0 | 0 | 0 | 0 | 0 | 0 | 1 |
| [MASK] | 1 | 1 | 1 | 1 | 1 | 1 | 1 | 1 | 1 | 1 | 1 | 1 | 1 | 1 | 0 | 0 | 0 | 0 | 0 | 0 | 0 | 0 | 1 |
| [MASK] | 1 | 1 | 1 | 1 | 1 | 1 | 1 | 1 | 1 | 1 | 1 | 1 | 1 | 1 | 0 | 0 | 0 | 0 | 0 | 0 | 0 | 0 | 1 |
| 新 (news) | 1 | 1 | 1 | 1 | 1 | 1 | 1 | 1 | 1 | 1 | 1 | 1 | 1 | 1 | 0 | 0 | 0 | 0 | 0 | 0 | 0 | 0 | 1 |
| ##闻 | 1 | 1 | 1 | 1 | 1 | 1 | 1 | 1 | 1 | 1 | 1 | 1 | 1 | 1 | 0 | 0 | 0 | 0 | 0 | 0 | 0 | 0 | 1 |
| , | 1 | 1 | 1 | 1 | 1 | 1 | 1 | 1 | 1 | 1 | 1 | 1 | 1 | 1 | 0 | 0 | 0 | 0 | 0 | 0 | 0 | 0 | 1 |
| 什 (What) | 1 | 1 | 1 | 1 | 1 | 1 | 1 | 1 | 1 | 1 | 1 | 1 | 1 | 1 | 0 | 0 | 0 | 0 | 0 | 0 | 0 | 0 | 1 |
| ##么 | 1 | 1 | 1 | 1 | 1 | 1 | 1 | 1 | 1 | 1 | 1 | 1 | 1 | 1 | 0 | 0 | 0 | 0 | 0 | 0 | 0 | 0 | 1 |
| 是 (is) | 1 | 1 | 1 | 1 | 1 | 1 | 1 | 1 | 1 | 1 | 1 | 1 | 1 | 1 | 0 | 0 | 0 | 0 | 0 | 0 | 0 | 0 | 1 |
| 元 (metaverse) | 1 | 1 | 1 | 1 | 1 | 1 | 1 | 1 | 1 | 1 | 1 | 1 | 1 | 1 | 1 | 1 | 0 | 0 | 0 | 0 | 0 | 0 | 1 |
| ##宇 | 1 | 1 | 1 | 1 | 1 | 1 | 1 | 1 | 1 | 1 | 1 | 1 | 1 | 1 | 1 | 1 | 0 | 0 | 0 | 0 | 0 | 0 | 1 |
| ##宙 | 1 | 1 | 1 | 1 | 1 | 1 | 1 | 1 | 1 | 1 | 1 | 1 | 1 | 1 | 1 | 1 | 0 | 0 | 0 | 0 | 0 | 0 | 1 |
| 定 (definition) | 0 | 0 | 0 | 0 | 0 | 0 | 0 | 0 | 0 | 0 | 0 | 1 | 1 | 1 | 0 | 0 | 1 | 1 | 1 | 1 | 1 | 1 | 1 |
| 义 (definition) | 0 | 0 | 0 | 0 | 0 | 0 | 0 | 0 | 0 | 0 | 0 | 1 | 1 | 1 | 0 | 0 | 1 | 1 | 1 | 1 | 1 | 1 | 1 |
| 虚 (virtual) | 0 | 0 | 0 | 0 | 0 | 0 | 0 | 0 | 0 | 0 | 0 | 0 | 0 | 0 | 1 | 1 | 0 | 0 | 0 | 0 | 0 | 0 | 1 |
| ##拟 | 0 | 0 | 0 | 0 | 0 | 0 | 0 | 0 | 0 | 0 | 0 | 0 | 0 | 0 | 1 | 1 | 0 | 0 | 0 | 0 | 0 | 0 | 1 |
| 现 (reality) | 0 | 0 | 0 | 0 | 0 | 0 | 0 | 0 | 0 | 0 | 0 | 0 | 0 | 0 | 1 | 1 | 0 | 0 | 0 | 0 | 0 | 0 | 1 |
| ##实 | 0 | 0 | 0 | 0 | 0 | 0 | 0 | 0 | 0 | 0 | 0 | 0 | 0 | 0 | 1 | 1 | 0 | 0 | 0 | 0 | 0 | 0 | 1 |
| 世 (world) | 0 | 0 | 0 | 0 | 0 | 0 | 0 | 0 | 0 | 0 | 0 | 0 | 0 | 0 | 1 | 1 | 0 | 0 | 0 | 0 | 0 | 0 | 1 |
| ##界 | 0 | 0 | 0 | 0 | 0 | 0 | 0 | 0 | 0 | 0 | 0 | 0 | 0 | 0 | 1 | 1 | 0 | 0 | 0 | 0 | 0 | 0 | 1 |
| [SEP] | 1 | 1 | 1 | 1 | 1 | 1 | 1 | 1 | 1 | 1 | 1 | 1 | 1 | 1 | 1 | 1 | 1 | 1 | 1 | 1 | 1 | 1 | 1 |

### 4.5. Baseline Line

BERT [1] is the first large-scale model that is pre-trained in big data. BERT has a good ability for generalization and can reuse the parameters of models to obtain a better result in the downstream task. RoBERTa [2] is a model that uses bigger data, more parameters, and some other tricks to pre-train a model based on BERT. GPT [8] is a big model that first uses the generative task to pre-train the model and obtains a better result in few-shot learning and zero-shot learning. Fine-tune is a method that first pre-trains in a big data set and then trains in a small data set to transfer the knowledge from big data to small data by model parameters. Few-shot uses a few training samples to train the model. Zero-shot uses no training data and just directly makes inferences. PET [55] uses prompt and MLM head to convert the task from a classification to generative task. Then, the downstream task form is similar to the pre-training task, which can improve the effect of transfer learning and the performance of the model. LM-BFF [37] automatically creates the prompt prefix. In the training phase, it constructs demonstrations to perform few-shot learning. P-tuning [56] transforms the problem of constructing the prompt into a continuous parameter optimization problem. The non-natural language is used to construct the prompt, which makes the space of the hypothesis of the prompt larger and more likely to find the best prompt. This method is simple and effective, giving GPT the ability of natural language understanding. EFL [57] transforms the downstream task into an implication task and a binary classification problem. It constructs sentence pairs and labels to judge whether the sentence pair is the implication. This method reduces the difficulty of the task. At the same time, the method transforms the downstream task into the pre-training task, which improves the effect of transfer learning. ERNIE 1.0 [10] is pre-trained by masking the knowledge entity, which gives the model more knowledge of words and phrases. In these results, our method CLG reaches the top of the list. It uses a smaller model but obtains better accuracy than other methods. especially when using ERNIE methods. This proves the effectiveness of our method.

### 4.6. Evaluation Metric

The confusion matrix is an important and common metric for measuring the classification performance of the models. The confusion matrix divides the results into four situations, as shown in Table 8.

Table 8. Calculate the evaluation metric through the confusion matrix.

| Confusion Matrix | | Ground Truth | |
|---|---|---|---|
| | | True | False |
| Prediction | Positive | TP | FP |
| | Negative | FN | TN |

They are True Positive (*TP*), False Positive (*FP*), False Negative (*FN*), and True Negative (*TN*) in the confusion matrix. The accuracy is shown in Equation (14). Similar to other studies, accuracy is the metric of our experiments.

$$Accuracy = \frac{(TP + TN)}{(TP + TN + FP + FN)} \quad (14)$$

*4.7. Results and Discussion*

There are some methods performing the same task that can compared to CLG, as shown in Table 9. For intuitive comparison, we put all of the readiness rates in one bar chart, as shown in Figure 2.

Our method, CLG, compares 10 methods, including zero-shot, which is without any training data and just evaluates the model, and fine-tuning models, which use training data to provide the models with more information about the task and domain to help the model improve its ability. In addition, the bigger the base model, the more data are used, and the better the performance of the model. CLG reaches better accuracy than other methods. This shows that our method can improve the understanding and generation ability of the model by contrastive label generation with a knowledge graph for few-shot learning.

Table 9. The experimental result shows our method CLG achieves the best accuracy with other baselines. The bold accuracy represents the best accuracy in the experiment.

| No. | Methods | Acc. (%) |
|---|---|---|
| 1 | Zero-Shot RoBERTa [2] | 25.3 |
| 2 | Zero-Shot GPT [8] | 37.0 |
| 3 | Fine-Tuning RoBERTa [2] | 49.0 |
| 4 | Fine-Tuning ERIEN 1.0 [10] | 51.6 |
| 5 | EFL [57] | 52.1 |
| 6 | LM-BFF [37] | 53.0 |
| 7 | P-tuning RoBERTa [56] | 54.2 |
| 8 | PET [55] | 54.5 |
| 9 | P-Tuning ERIEN 1.0 [10] | 55.9 |
| 10 | EFL ERIEN 1.0 [10] | 56.3 |
| 11 | PET ERIEN 1.0 [10] | 56.4 |
| 12 | CLG (Ours) | **59.2** |

A heatmap is a visual tool to show the performance of the models. The diagonal line represents the ground truth, and the block color from white to red represents the accuracy from low to high.

The results of model classification are generally similar to the ground truth as shown in Figure 3, but some have high classification accuracies, and some have low classification accuracies. This may be due to the difference between the data of the different labels and the data of the other labels. The accuracy rate of label classification that is easy to distinguish is high, and the accuracy rate of label classification that is easy to confuse is low. To solve this problem, we can enhance the data of some labels with low accuracies, so that the model can better learn the features of such data.

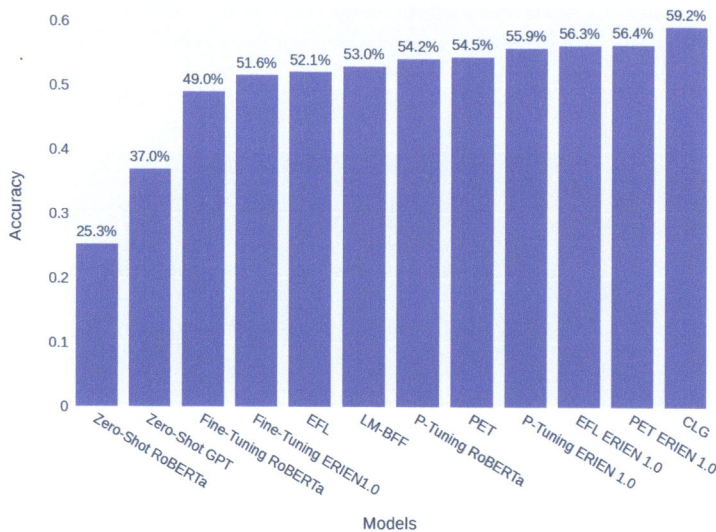

**Figure 2.** The accuracies of the models.

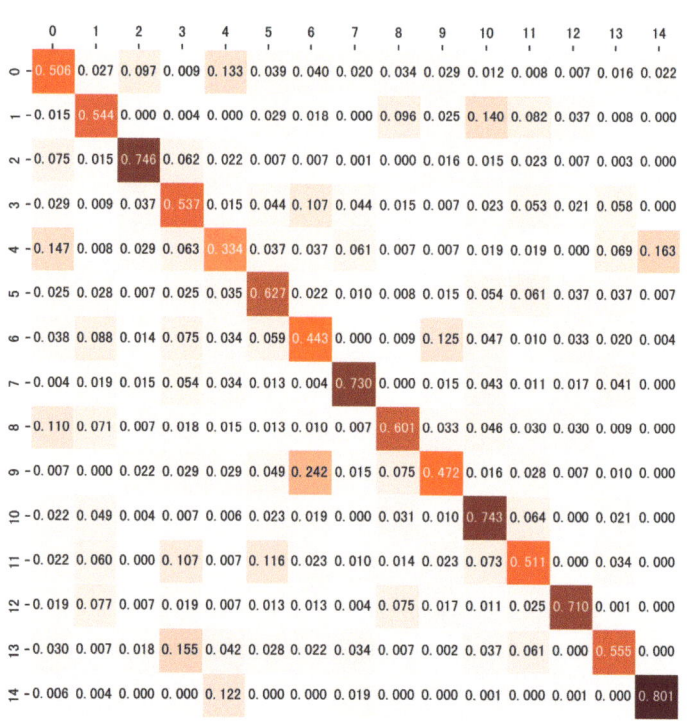

**Figure 3.** The heatmap shows the classification ability of each class.

*4.8. Ablation Study*

As the CLG consists of several key techniques, we probe and compare their effectiveness in this section. We use the control parameters method to remove each key part of the experiment, as shown in Table 10.

**Table 10.** The ablation experiment shows the contributions of each module in CLG. The bold accuracy represents the best accuracy in the experiment.

| No. | Function | Acc. (%) |
| --- | --- | --- |
| 1 | Prompts and Symbols | 52.344 |
| 2 | Block List | 58.513 |
| 3 | Text KG | 58.029 |
| 4 | Label KG | 58.638 |
| 5 | Logits and Labels Mask | 58.663 |
| 6 | Warmup | 55.978 |
| 7 | Learning Rate Scheduler | 58.967 |
| 8 | HCL SA | 58.219 |
| 9 | SIM SA | 58.847 |
| 10 | Early Stop | 58.992 |
| 11 | Dropout | 59.032 |
| 12 | Loss Weight | 57.610 |
| 13 | CLG | **59.237** |

For the ablation experiment, if the accuracy of a removed function is lower than the CLG accuracy, then it means that the removed relative function is useful to yield better results in CLG. In contrast, if the accuracy of a removed function is higher than the CLG accuracy that means the removed relative function is negative for the performance of the model. Thus, we should remove it. As shown in Table 10, we can see each function has a positive effect on the result and they are needed. The prompts and symbols convert the input task form, which improves the transfer learning effect. The block list avoids the unrelated triplet, which can prevent the noise. The label KG makes the label sentences align with the text sentences form, which reduces the difference between the text and label and improves the contrast learning effect. The logits and labels mask strategy avoids unimportant tokens, which narrows the search scope. The warmup trains the model with a small learning rate at the initial stage of training and then gradually restores the predetermined value so that the model can be fully explored in the early stage of training to find the appropriate gradient descent direction. The learning rate scheduler reduces the learning rate when the training slows down so that the model can approach the optimal point. The HCL SA and SIM SA are simulated annealing algorithms that help the model obtain a better update direction at the initial training stage. The early stop ends the training in advance under certain conditions, which avoids overfitting. Dropout inputs the same sentences twice to obtain additional different training features. The loss weight is the weight of the three losses, which makes the effective loss obtain more weight and improves the model's effect.

## 5. Conclusions

In this work, we propose CLG, a simple and efficient method that uses contrastive label generation with knowledge for few-shot learning.

CLG adds the prompt and injects knowledge into text and labels. Then, it tokenizes them to input token IDs. After that, it inputs the text and label to the model, including the embedding layers and encoder layer. In this phase, the text and label become feature vectors from token IDs. Then, it calculates the similarity between text features and label features in contrastive learning and predicts the masked word to obtain the logits and loss. Finally, it calculates the evaluation metric by logits and updates the model weights by loss.

CLG can obtain better feature vectors and not only augment data but also simplify the task. It can improve explainability and avoid knowledge noise. It can align the label with the text and shrink the search space. Apart from that, it can learn from the different perspectives of the training data. The experimental results demonstrate that the CLG is effective and can help to resolve the few-shot problem.

Although it is effective in resolving the few-shot problem, some situations need to be considered. Contrastive learning calculates the similarity scores between the feature vectors. It is worth finding a reasonable similarity function to achieve better features. Constructing the prompt manually is an easy and explicit method for creating the prompt and symbol. It is easy and effective to achieve, but the search area is small and limited, which may make it difficult to obtain the optimal solution. Matching the phrase in sentences with the head of triplets is an effective method for injecting the KG into sentences. However, there are some unrelated triplets that sentences should not inject into sentences. Although we set a block list to avoid matching the unrelated triplets, the performance also depends on the quality of the KG. The more homologous sources of the data and KG are, the better the models are.

In the future, we can explore further in these directions. Although our method performed well in many models at the time, the accuracy is still below 60%. We analyze that this is because the knowledge learned by the model from small samples is very limited, and the diversity of the samples in the test set is due to the training set. Therefore, we can consider exploring in further research how large the data volume needs to be, based on the model, to achieve good indicator values. In addition, we are also considering further improving the algorithm to enhance the efficiency of the model in learning samples.

**Author Contributions:** Conceptualization, H.M.; methodology, H.M.; software, H.M.; validation, H.M. and B.F.; formal analysis, H.M.; investigation, H.M. and B.F.; resources, B.K.N.; data curation, H.M. and B.F.; writing—original draft preparation, H.M.; writing—review and editing, H.M., B.F., B.K.N. and C.-T.L.; visualization, H.M. and B.F.; supervision, B.K.N. and C.-T.L.; project administration, B.K.N.; funding acquisition, B.K.N. All authors have read and agreed to the published version of the manuscript.

**Funding:** This research was funded by Macao Polytechnic University via grant number RP/ESCA-02/2021.

**Data Availability Statement:** Publicly available data sets were analyzed in this study. These data can be found here: https://github.com/CLUEbenchmark/FewCLUE/tree/main/datasets/tnews, accessed on 30 April 2021.

**Conflicts of Interest:** The authors declare no conflict of interest.

# References

1. Devlin, J.; Chang, M.W.; Lee, K.; Toutanova, K. BERT: Pre-training of Deep Bidirectional Transformers for Language Understanding. *arXiv* **2018**, arXiv:1810.04805.
2. Liu, Y.; Ott, M.; Goyal, N.; Du, J.; Joshi, M.; Chen, D.; Levy, O.; Lewis, M.; Zettlemoyer, L.; Stoyanov, V. Roberta: A robustly optimized bert pretraining approach. *arXiv* **2019**, arXiv:1907.11692.
3. Lan, Z.; Chen, M.; Goodman, S.; Gimpel, K.; Sharma, P.; Soricut, R. Albert: A lite bert for self-supervised learning of language representations. *arXiv* **2019**, arXiv:1909.11942.
4. Yang, Z.; Dai, Z.; Yang, Y.; Carbonell, J.; Salakhutdinov, R.R.; Le, Q.V. Xlnet: Generalized autoregressive pretraining for language understanding. *Adv. Neural Inf. Process. Syst.* **2019**, *32*, 670–681.
5. Lewis, M.; Liu, Y.; Goyal, N.; Ghazvininejad, M.; Mohamed, A.; Levy, O.; Stoyanov, V.; Zettlemoyer, L. Bart: Denoising sequence-to-sequence pre-training for natural language generation, translation, and comprehension. *arXiv* **2019**, arXiv:1910.13461.
6. Radford, A.; Narasimhan, K.; Salimans, T.; Sutskever, I. *Improving Language Understanding by Generative Pre-Training*; OpenAI: San Francisco, CA, USA, 2018.
7. Radford, A.; Wu, J.; Child, R.; Luan, D.; Amodei, D.; Sutskever, I. Language models are unsupervised multitask learners. *OpenAI Blog* **2019**, *1*, 9.
8. Brown, T.B.; Mann, B.; Ryder, N.; Subbiah, M.; Kaplan, J.; Dhariwal, P.; Neelakantan, A.; Shyam, P.; Sastry, G.; Askell, A.; et al. Language Models are Few-Shot Learners. *arXiv* **2020**, arXiv:2005.14165.
9. Raffel, C.; Shazeer, N.; Roberts, A.; Lee, K.; Narang, S.; Matena, M.; Zhou, Y.; Li, W.; Liu, P.J. Exploring the limits of transfer learning with a unified text-to-text transformer. *J. Mach. Learn. Res.* **2020**, *21*, 5485–5551.
10. Sun, Y.; Wang, S.; Li, Y.; Feng, S.; Chen, X.; Zhang, H.; Tian, X.; Zhu, D.; Tian, H.; Wu, H. Ernie: Enhanced representation through knowledge integration. *arXiv* **2019**, arXiv:1904.09223.

11. Sun, Y.; Wang, S.; Li, Y.; Feng, S.; Tian, H.; Wu, H.; Wang, H. Ernie 2.0: A continual pre-training framework for language understanding. In Proceedings of the AAAI Conference on Artificial Intelligence, New York, NY, USA, 7–12 February 2020; Volume 34, pp. 8968–8975.
12. Sun, Y.; Wang, S.; Feng, S.; Ding, S.; Pang, C.; Shang, J.; Liu, J.; Chen, X.; Zhao, Y.; Lu, Y.; et al. ERNIE 3.0: Large-scale Knowledge Enhanced Pre-training for Language Understanding and Generation. *arXiv* **2021**, arXiv:2107.02137.
13. Dosovitskiy, A.; Beyer, L.; Kolesnikov, A.; Weissenborn, D.; Zhai, X.; Unterthiner, T.; Dehghani, M.; Minderer, M.; Heigold, G.; Gelly, S.; et al. An image is worth 16x16 words: Transformers for image recognition at scale. *arXiv* **2020**, arXiv:2010.11929.
14. Ramesh, A.; Pavlov, M.; Goh, G.; Gray, S.; Voss, C.; Radford, A.; Chen, M.; Sutskever, I. Zero-shot text-to-image generation. In Proceedings of the International Conference on Machine Learning, Virtual, 18–24 July 2021; pp. 8821–8831.
15. Ramesh, A.; Dhariwal, P.; Nichol, A.; Chu, C.; Chen, M. Hierarchical text-conditional image generation with clip latents. *arXiv* **2022**, arXiv:2204.06125.
16. Alayrac, J.B.; Donahue, J.; Luc, P.; Miech, A.; Barr, I.; Hasson, Y.; Lenc, K.; Mensch, A.; Millican, K.; Reynolds, M.; et al. Flamingo: A visual language model for few-shot learning. *arXiv* **2022**, arXiv:2204.14198.
17. Wang, Y.; Yao, Q.; Kwok, J.T.; Ni, L.M. Generalizing from a few examples: A survey on few-shot learning. *ACM Comput. Surv.* **2020**, *53*, 1–34. [CrossRef]
18. Benaim, S.; Wolf, L. One-Shot Unsupervised Cross Domain Translation. *Adv. Neural Inf. Process. Syst.* **2018**, *31*, 2104–2114.
19. Lake, B.M.; Salakhutdinov, R.; Tenenbaum, J.B. Human-level concept learning through probabilistic program induction. *Science* **2015**, *350*, 1332–1338. [CrossRef] [PubMed]
20. Shyam, P.; Gupta, S.; Dukkipati, A. Attentive Recurrent Comparators. In Proceedings of the International Conference on Machine Learning, Sydney, Australia, 6–11 August 2017.
21. Qi, H.; Brown, M.; Lowe, D.G. Learning with Imprinted Weights. *arXiv* **2017**, arXiv:1712.07136.
22. Zhang, Y.; Tang, H.; Jia, K. Fine-Grained Visual Categorization using Meta-Learning Optimization with Sample Selection of Auxiliary Data. In Proceedings of the European Conference on Computer Vision (ECCV), Munich, Germany, 8–14 September 2018.
23. Edwards, H.; Storkey, A. Towards a Neural Statistician. *arXiv* **2016**, arXiv:1606.02185.
24. Kozerawski, J.; Turk, M. CLEAR: Cumulative LEARning for One-Shot One-Class Image Recognition. In Proceedings of the 2018 IEEE/CVF Conference on Computer Vision and Pattern Recognition (CVPR), Salt Lake City, UT, USA, 18–23 June 2018.
25. Qi, H.; Brown, M.; Lowe, D.G. Low-Shot Learning with Imprinted Weights. In Proceedings of the 2018 IEEE/CVF Conference on Computer Vision and Pattern Recognition, Salt Lake City, UT, USA, 18–23 June 2018.
26. Vinyals, O.; Blundell, C.; Lillicrap, T.; Kavukcuoglu, K.; Wierstra, D. Matching Networks for One Shot Learning. *Adv. Neural Inf. Process. Syst.* **2016**, *29*, 3637–3645.
27. Xie, Q.; Luong, M.T.; Hovy, E.; Le, Q.V. Self-Training With Noisy Student Improves ImageNet Classification. In Proceedings of the 2020 IEEE/CVF Conference on Computer Vision and Pattern Recognition (CVPR), Seattle, WA, USA, 13–19 June 2020; pp. 10684–10695. [CrossRef]
28. Sun, Z.; Fan, C.; Sun, X.; Meng, Y.; Wu, F.; Li, J. Neural semi-supervised learning for text classification under large-scale pretraining. *arXiv* **2020**, arXiv:2011.08626.
29. Kahn, J.; Lee, A.; Hannun, A. Self-training for end-to-end speech recognition. In Proceedings of the ICASSP 2020—2020 IEEE International Conference on Acoustics, Speech and Signal Processing (ICASSP), Barcelona, Spain, 4–8 May 2020; pp. 7084–7088.
30. Fan, B.; Liu, Y.; Cuthbert, L. Improvement of DGA Long Tail Problem Based on Transfer Learning. In *Computer and Information Science*; Lee, R., Ed.; Springer International Publishing: Cham, Switzerland, 2023; pp. 139–152. [CrossRef]
31. Liu, P.; Yuan, W.; Fu, J.; Jiang, Z.; Hayashi, H.; Neubig, G. Pre-train, prompt, and predict: A systematic survey of prompting methods in natural language processing. *arXiv* **2021**, arXiv:2107.13586.
32. Li, X.L.; Liang, P. Prefix-Tuning: Optimizing Continuous Prompts for Generation. *arXiv* **2021**, arXiv:2101.00190.
33. Hambardzumyan, K.; Khachatrian, H.; May, J. WARP: Word-level Adversarial ReProgramming. *arXiv* **2021**, arXiv:2101.00121.
34. Shin, T.; Razeghi, Y.; Logan IV, R.L.; Wallace, E.; Singh, S. Autoprompt: Eliciting knowledge from language models with automatically generated prompts. *arXiv* **2020**, arXiv:2010.15980.
35. Schick, T.; Schütze, H. Exploiting Cloze-Questions for Few-Shot Text Classification and Natural Language Inference. In Proceedings of the 16th Conference of the European Chapter of the Association for Computational Linguistics: Main Volume, online, 19–23 April 2021; pp. 255–269. [CrossRef]
36. Schick, T.; Schütze, H. Few-Shot Text Generation with Pattern-Exploiting Training. *arXiv* **2020**, arXiv:2012.11926.
37. Gao, T.; Fisch, A.; Chen, D. Making Pre-trained Language Models Better Few-shot Learners. *arXiv* **2020**, arXiv:2012.15723.
38. Cui, Y.; Liu, T.; Che, W.; Chen, Z.; Wang, S. Teaching machines to read, answer and explain. *IEEE/ACM Trans. Audio Speech Lang. Process.* **2022**, *30*, 1483–1492. [CrossRef]
39. Qin, L.; Xu, X.; Wang, L.; Zhang, Y.; Che, W. Modularized Pre-training for End-to-end Task-oriented Dialogue. *IEEE/ACM Trans. Audio Speech Lang. Process.* **2023**, *31*, 1601–1610. [CrossRef]
40. Peters, M.E.; Neumann, M.; Logan, R.L.; Schwartz, R.; Joshi, V.; Singh, S.; Smith, N.A. Knowledge Enhanced Contextual Word Representations. In Proceedings of the EMNLP, Hong Kong, China, 3–7 November 2019.
41. Ke, P.; Ji, H.; Liu, S.; Zhu, X.; Huang, M. SentiLR: Linguistic Knowledge Enhanced Language Representation for Sentiment Analysis. *arXiv* **2019**, arXiv:1911.02493.

42. Wang, X.; Gao, T.; Zhu, Z.; Liu, Z.; Li, J.; Tang, J. KEPLER: A Unified Model for Knowledge Embedding and Pre-trained Language Representation. *arXiv* **2019**, arXiv:1911.06136.
43. Sun, T.; Shao, Y.; Qiu, X.; Guo, Q.; Hu, Y.; Huang, X.; Zhang, Z. CoLAKE: Contextualized Language and Knowledge Embedding. *arXiv* **2020**, arXiv:2010.00309.
44. Liu, W.; Zhou, P.; Zhao, Z.; Wang, Z.; Ju, Q.; Deng, H.; Wang, P. K-BERT: Enabling Language Representation with Knowledge Graph. *arXiv* **2019**, arXiv1909.07606.
45. Ma, H.; Ng, B.K.; Lam, C.T. PK-BERT: Knowledge Enhanced Pre-trained Models with Prompt for Few-Shot Learning. In *Computer and Information Science*; Lee, R., Ed.; Springer International Publishing: Cham, Switzerland, 2023; pp. 31–44. [CrossRef]
46. Zhang, Z.; Han, X.; Liu, Z.; Jiang, X.; Sun, M.; Liu, Q. ERNIE: Enhanced language representation with informative entities. *arXiv* **2019**, arXiv:1905.07129.
47. Bai, J.; Yang, Z.; Yang, J.; Guo, H.; Li, Z. KIN ET: Incorporating Relevant Facts into Knowledge-Grounded Dialog Generation. *IEEE/ACM Trans. Audio Speech Lang. Process.* **2023**, *31*, 1213–1222. [CrossRef]
48. Liu, J.; Qin, X.; Ma, X.; Ran, W. FREDA: Few-Shot Relation Extraction Based on Data Augmentation. *Appl. Sci.* **2023**, *13*, 8312. [CrossRef]
49. Yang, L.; Huang, B.; Guo, S.; Lin, Y.; Zhao, T. A Small-Sample Text Classification Model Based on Pseudo-Label Fusion Clustering Algorithm. *Appl. Sci.* **2023**, *13*, 4716. [CrossRef]
50. Ma, J.; Cheng, J.; Chen, Y.; Li, K.; Zhang, F.; Shang, Z. Multi-Head Self-Attention-Enhanced Prototype Network with Contrastive–Center Loss for Few-Shot Relation Extraction. *Appl. Sci.* **2024**, *14*, 103. [CrossRef]
51. Radford, A.; Kim, J.W.; Hallacy, C.; Ramesh, A.; Goh, G.; Agarwal, S.; Sastry, G.; Askell, A.; Mishkin, P.; Clark, J.; et al. Learning transferable visual models from natural language supervision. In Proceedings of the International Conference on Machine Learning, Virtual, 18–24 July 2021; pp. 8748–8763.
52. Robinson, J.; Chuang, C.Y.; Sra, S.; Jegelka, S. Contrastive Learning with Hard Negative Samples. In Proceedings of the International Conference on Learning Representations, Virtual, 3–7 May 2021.
53. Xu, L.; Lu, X.; Yuan, C.; Zhang, X.; Xu, H.; Yuan, H.; Wei, G.; Pan, X.; Tian, X.; Qin, L.; et al. Fewclue: A chinese few-shot learning evaluation benchmark. *arXiv* **2021**, arXiv:2107.07498.
54. Xu, B.; Xu, Y.; Liang, J.; Xie, C.; Liang, B.; Cui, W.; Xiao, Y. CN-DBpedia: A Never-Ending Chinese Knowledge Extraction System. In Proceedings of the International Conference on Industrial, Engineering and Other Applications of Applied Intelligent Systems, Arras, France, 27–30 June 2017.
55. Schick, T.; Schütze, H. Exploiting Cloze Questions for Few-Shot Text Classification and Natural Language Inference. *arXiv* **2020**, arXiv:2001.07676.
56. Liu, X.; Zheng, Y.; Du, Z.; Ding, M.; Qian, Y.; Yang, Z.; Tang, J. GPT Understands, Too. *arXiv* **2021**, arXiv:2103.10385.
57. Wang, S.; Fang, H.; Khabsa, M.; Mao, H.; Ma, H. Entailment as few-shot learner. *arXiv* **2021**, arXiv:2104.14690.

**Disclaimer/Publisher's Note:** The statements, opinions and data contained in all publications are solely those of the individual author(s) and contributor(s) and not of MDPI and/or the editor(s). MDPI and/or the editor(s) disclaim responsibility for any injury to people or property resulting from any ideas, methods, instructions or products referred to in the content.

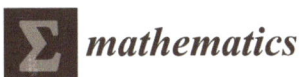

Article

# GA-CatBoost-Weight Algorithm for Predicting Casualties in Terrorist Attacks: Addressing Data Imbalance and Enhancing Performance

Yuxiang He, Baisong Yang and Chiawei Chu *

Faculty of Data Science, City University of Macau, Macau 999078, China; d21092100165@cityu.edu.mo (Y.H.); d22092100266@cityu.edu.mo (B.Y.)
* Correspondence: cwchu@cityu.edu.mo

**Abstract:** Terrorism poses a significant threat to international peace and stability. The ability to predict potential casualties resulting from terrorist attacks, based on specific attack characteristics, is vital for protecting the safety of innocent civilians. However, conventional data sampling methods struggle to effectively address the challenge of data imbalance in textual features. To tackle this issue, we introduce a novel algorithm, GA-CatBoost-Weight, designed for predicting whether terrorist attacks will lead to casualties among innocent civilians. Our approach begins with feature selection using the RF-RFE method, followed by leveraging the CatBoost algorithm to handle diverse modal features comprehensively and to mitigate data imbalance. Additionally, we employ Genetic Algorithm (GA) to finetune hyperparameters. Experimental validation has demonstrated the superior performance of our method, achieving a sensitivity of 92.68% and an F1 score of 90.99% with fewer iterations. To the best of our knowledge, our study is the pioneering research that applies CatBoost to address the prediction of terrorist attack outcomes.

**Keywords:** terrorist attack prediction; feature selection; CatBoost; sample imbalance

**MSC:** 68T09

**Citation:** He, Y.; Yang, B.; Chu, C. GA-CatBoost-Weight Algorithm for Predicting Casualties in Terrorist Attacks: Addressing Data Imbalance and Enhancing Performance. *Mathematics* **2024**, *12*, 818. https:// doi.org/10.3390/math12060818

Academic Editor: Florin Leon

Received: 25 February 2024
Revised: 4 March 2024
Accepted: 7 March 2024
Published: 11 March 2024

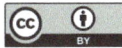

**Copyright:** © 2024 by the authors. Licensee MDPI, Basel, Switzerland. This article is an open access article distributed under the terms and conditions of the Creative Commons Attribution (CC BY) license (https:// creativecommons.org/licenses/by/ 4.0/).

## 1. Introduction

Terrorism, driven by motives such as political, economic, religious, or social aims, utilizes violence and illicit methods to intimidate, coerce, and instill fear [1] and remains a grave menace to international peace and security. Since the "9/11" attacks, efforts in counter-terrorism have been significantly intensified in the European and American regions to combat the development of terrorist forces. According to data from the Global Terrorism Database, there have been over 200,000 recorded terrorist attacks between 2010 and 2020, resulting in numerous casualties and property damage. Despite a decreasing trend in terrorist attacks since 2015, the future outlook on the risk of terrorist attacks remains concerning. The outbreak of COVID-19 at the end of 2019 not only severely disrupted people's lives, health, and travel routines but also dealt a heavy blow to market economies, nurturing negative emotions among the general populace and further fueling the unfavorable trends of terrorism [2]. In early 2022, the outbreak of the Russo–Ukrainian War significantly affected the development and security of neighboring countries and regions. Under the conflicts between nations and ethnicities, ordinary people are bound to harbor feelings of hatred, exacerbating the spread and escalation of terrorism [3]. With the ongoing escalation of the Israeli–Palestinian conflict, many countries are facing internal divisions, intensified opposition sentiments, posing threats to social stability and facing significant risks of terrorist attacks [4]. While many studies indicate that the purpose of terrorism is to advance specific political objectives, the act of terrorism itself not only spreads social panic but also results in infrastructure damage and the loss of innocent lives.

Due to the complexity of counter-terrorism measures and emergency controls, it is crucial to develop effective methods to predict the consequences of terrorist attacks.

Machine learning, as a robust computational tool, plays a pivotal role in decision-making processes for analyzing casualties in terrorist attacks. Research indicates that the incorporation of textual feature information derived from terrorism datasets can significantly improve the performance of models [5]. In previous studies, textual features in terrorism datasets were typically handled separately using text vectorization techniques and then combined with other types of features for analysis of terrorist attacks through machine learning algorithms. Hence, conventional data sampling techniques face challenges in addressing data imbalance within the aforementioned methods. However, no research has proposed a method that considers data imbalance while handling textual features of terrorist attacks. To fill this gap, we present a CatBoost-based model for predicting casualties in terrorist attacks, which can forecast whether terrorist attacks pose a threat to the safety of innocent civilians. The results of this study not only assist decision-makers in adjusting and deploying appropriate emergency measures but also provide valuable information support.

In the proposed algorithm, to eliminate feature redundancy and reduce computational complexity, we conducted feature selection by combining Random Forest (RF) and Recursive Feature Elimination (RFE) methods. Leveraging the advantages of CatBoost in handling numerical, categorical, and textual features simultaneously, we trained the model using CatBoost algorithm by combining textual features with the selected features obtained through screening to improve data imbalance issues. Additionally, hyperparameter tuning was performed using a genetic algorithm. Building on the GTD dataset, we compared the performance of our method with several state-of-the-art methods such as LR, DT, RF, Adaboost, XGBoost, and LightGBM. Experimental results demonstrate the superiority of our method over the aforementioned methods. Therefore, one can conclude that our approach is an efficient and effective algorithm for analyzing the risk of casualties in terrorist attacks.

The organization of the remaining sections of this paper is as follows: Section 2, we briefly review relevant literature. Section 3, we introduce the entire experimental process based on the CatBoost method proposed by us. Section 4, we conduct extensive numerical experiments to evaluate the performance of the proposed method. Finally, Section 5, we summarize the entire paper and analyze the advantages of our method.

## 2. Literature Review

Early statistical methods have been an efficient approach for analyzing terrorist attacks, with many studies conducting assessments of the consequences of terrorist attacks in real scenarios. Guo et al. constructed a risk assessment method for terrorist attacks on civil aviation airports using event trees and probabilistic risk assessment models, which evaluate the risk of various types of terrorist attacks on civil aviation airports [6]. Yang et al. utilized the FAHP-SWOT method to design a risk assessment model, analyzing various risk factors for terrorist attacks on religious sites [7]. The evaluation-based methods mentioned above allow for quantifiable analyses of specific scenarios but still suffer from high subjectivity.

With the increase in data volume and diversity of feature types, machine learning has provided algorithmic support for the analysis of consequences of terrorist attacks. Lanjun et al. aimed to select the most crucial indicators affecting the risk of terrorist attacks from various perspectives. They selected 28 indicators from several data sources and used the Random Forest algorithm to compute feature importance rankings, followed by a recursive process to obtain the most impactful set of features influencing the risk of terrorist attacks [8]. Zhang et al. considered 17 influencing factors in terrorist attack data and assessed the risk level of geographical regions in Southeast Asia using an improved location recommendation algorithm [9]. Feng et al. proposed a novel RP-GA-XGBoost algorithm to predict whether terrorist attacks would result in casualties [10].

While the aforementioned methods are single-model approaches, the complexity and quantity of data have led to the increasing advantages of hybrid models in analyzing terrorist attack issues. Shafiq et al. introduced a hybrid classifier to predict the type of attack in terrorist events, incorporating K-nearest neighbors, Naive Bayes, and decision trees [11]. Meng et al. proposed a hybrid classifier framework for terrorist attack prediction, comprising SVM, K-nearest neighbors (KNN), Bagging, and C4.5, and optimized the weights of individual classifiers using a genetic algorithm to enhance prediction accuracy [12].

Most current research on terrorist attacks focuses primarily on numerical and categorical features, with relatively limited studies exploring the inclusion of textual features to enhance model performance. Mohammed Abdalsalamde et al.'s study demonstrated that by using text representation techniques to process textual features and combining them with other types of features, the performance of predictive models for terrorist attack types can be improved [5]. However, they did not perform data cleaning on the text to remove redundant information and utilizing text representation techniques added processing steps and extra computational overhead to the model. Therefore, in future research, it may be beneficial to further investigate how to effectively handle textual features, optimize model performance, and reduce unnecessary computational costs.

If different terrorist attacks with varying levels of risk are treated equally in the context of terrorist attacks, it may lead decision-makers to make misjudgments and result in the waste of resources. Therefore, the issue of data imbalance is a crucial factor influencing terrorist attack models. Varun Teja Gundabathula et al. proposed using machine learning models to predict terrorist groups based on historical data and employing data sampling techniques to improve the accuracy of classification models [13]. Fahad Ali Khan and colleagues utilized the Particle Swarm Optimization (PSO) algorithm to determine the optimal weight distribution for Random Forest and Extreme Gradient Boosting Machine in accurately predicting whether terrorist activities would result in casualties. To address the issue of class imbalance, they applied the Synthetic Minority Oversampling Technique (SMOTE) to handle imbalanced data [14]. The aforementioned studies alleviate data imbalance issues through data sampling techniques. However, due to the structural nature of text data, these data sampling techniques are not suitable for directly processing textual information. Although text data can be first vectorized before data sampling, the conversion may result in the loss of some semantic information. Additionally, data sampling techniques are difficult to generate text information based on context. Currently, there is no research considering data sampling for terrorist attack texts, and text vectorization techniques independent of predictive models do not enhance model performance as effectively as end-to-end models.

Comparing with the above-mentioned studies, the main contributions of this article are as follows:

1. First, we propose an innocent civilian casualties prediction model named GA-CatBoost-Weight for terrorist attacks based on CatBoost. CatBoost is capable of directly handling numerical, categorical, and textual features, and its powerful computational capability has been widely applied in various fields. However, to our knowledge, there has been no research applying CatBoost to the issue of terrorist attacks. Therefore, we use the CatBoost algorithm combined with some strategies to enhance algorithm performance to predict whether terrorist attacks will result in casualties;

2. Secondly, we employ RF-RFE for feature selection. High-dimensional features not only increase the computational cost of models but also affect model performance. In this paper, we combine RF and RFE to reduce feature redundancy and effectively decrease computational costs. This method obtains importance scores for each feature using RF, reduces feature numbers based on feature importance ranking to generate a model performance curve, and obtains the optimal feature subset based on the trend of the curve;

3. Thirdly, we conduct hyperparameter tuning for CatBoost. In the case of data imbalance where traditional data sampling techniques struggle to handle textual information, we propose using CatBoost's built-in parameters to improve the data imbalance issue in terrorist attack scenarios. Instead of additional processing at the data level,

we address the data imbalance issue from the model perspective in an end-to-end manner to prevent the loss of excessive semantic information in textual features. GA is an excellent hyperparameter optimization algorithm that is not commonly combined with CatBoost for tuning. Hence, in this study, we choose genetic algorithm to effectively enhance the performance of our innocent civilian casualties prediction model for terrorist attacks.

## 3. Materials and Methods

In this paper, we have developed a casualty prediction algorithm for terrorist attacks based on CatBoost to predict whether terrorist attacks will result in casualties. The overall framework of the proposed method consists of four stages, as shown in Figure 1. Firstly, we preprocess the missing values, features, and labels in the dataset. Secondly, we conduct feature selection using the RF-RFE method. Subsequently, we employ GA to optimize the hyperparameters of CatBoost. Finally, we evaluate the trained model on the test set using evaluation metrics. The following sections provide detailed information on the primary steps.

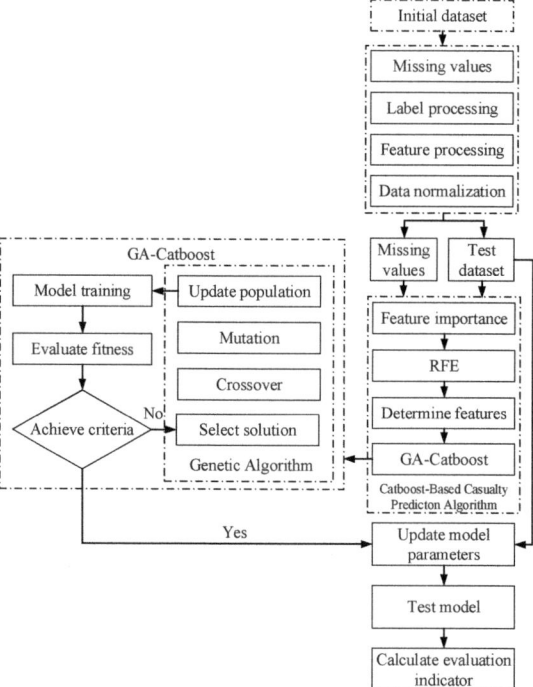

**Figure 1.** A flowchart of the proposed method.

### 3.1. Data Preprocessing

The data used in this study are from the Global Terrorism Database (GTD) maintained by the National Consortium for the Study of Terrorism and Responses to Terrorism (START) (https://www.start.umd.edu/gtd) (accessed on 28 August 2022). The database collects information on global terrorist events from 1970 to 2020, including data from sources such as news, books, and legal documents. It consists of 135 features and over 200,000 samples.

To ensure the quality and reliability of the data, we first removed features with missing values exceeding 70%. We then further eliminated irrelevant features for predictions such as event number, event summary, event source, and similar. We also directly eliminated event records with outliers. The data was then normalized using the Min-Max scaling method to scale the data to the [0, 1] interval [15]. The transformation formula is defined as follows:

$$x'(k) = \frac{x(k) - \min x(k)}{\max x(k) - \min x(k)} \quad (1)$$

After preprocessing, we have obtained 98,508 samples and 24 features. For the selected event records, we use "nkill" to represent the number of fatalities in the event and "nwound" to represent the number of wounded individuals in the event. An attack event is considered to have resulted in casualties only when the sum of fatalities and injuries is greater than 0. Since the focus is on civilian casualties in each attack event, casualties caused by terrorists themselves, such as in suicide attacks or due to being killed, are excluded from the event. We define "risk" as a binary label related to the casualty situation. Among the 98,508 samples, there are 33,499 samples where no casualties occurred and 65,009 samples where casualties occurred.

*3.2. Feature Processing*

The Global Terrorism Database (GTD) contains numerical, categorical, and text features. In order to fully leverage the performance of the model, feature preprocessing is necessary.

While some studies on terrorist attacks have shown that time variable features have less importance in the analysis of terrorist attacks, it is important to consider that the consequences of terrorist attacks may not solely depend on a single time variable but may be related to specific dates within a week. Therefore, for the specific time variable features "iyear", "imonth", and "iday" that represent the occurrence of events, these three individual time variable features are transformed into a new time variable feature "date" representing the day of the week, defined within the interval [1,7]. This can provide additional context related to the day of the week.

The text feature "summary" provides a brief description of terrorist events, including specific details such as the time, location, individuals involved, and the method of the attack. Current studies on terrorist attacks that consider text features typically extract information from text through text vectorization techniques. With the advantage of CatBoost's text processing technology, it can directly compute text features without the need for additional natural language processing (NLP) steps. However, in this experiment, the "summary" feature contains information about the date of the attack and the consequences of the attack, which conflicts with the prediction target of this study. Therefore, it needs to be removed.

To avoid introducing high subjectivity during feature selection, common feature selection methods include filter, embedded, and wrapper methods [16]. However, many studies on terrorist attacks often subjectively determine the number of features [12,17]. In order to effectively eliminate redundant features, reduce computational costs, and manage feature dimensions, this study utilizes a method combining RF with RFE to determine a subset of features.

Random Forest can be considered as an ensemble learning model consisting of multiple decision trees, widely used for classification and regression analysis. Due to its inherent randomness, Random Forest retains some sample data through random sampling with replacement during training, known as Out of Bag (OOB) data. These OOB samples are often used to measure the importance of features [18]. In essence, Random Forest calculates the corresponding Out of Bag score (OOB score) through the OOB data. If adding noise to a particular feature significantly decreases the OOB score, it indicates that this feature is important for influencing the outcome.

In this experiment, the importance of features is evaluated based on the OOB score of Random Forest, which helps in ranking the features based on their importance. The OOB scores are used to assess the importance of features, as shown in Figure 2, where the horizontal axis represents the score of each feature and the vertical axis represents the feature names.

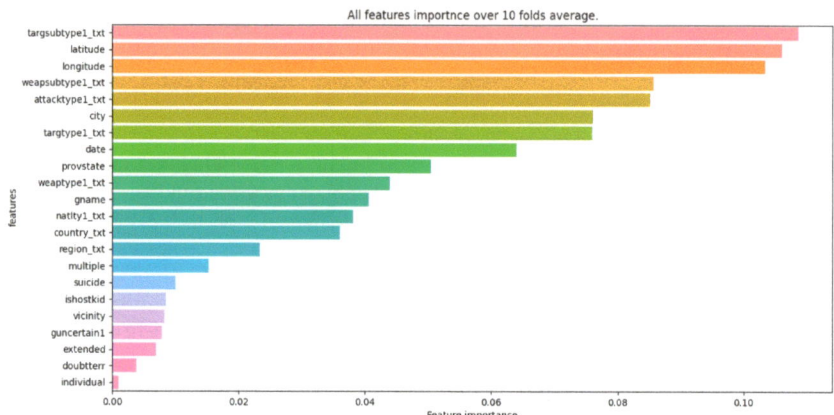

**Figure 2.** Feature importance ranking.

After obtaining the importance ranking of the original features, in order to objectively determine the number of features, we utilize RFE to analyze the performance of RF with different subsets of features. RFE works by iteratively constructing different subsets of features based on their importance, starting with the most important features determined earlier. This process involves incrementally adding individual features in order of importance to form various feature subsets. Using RF, the performance of the model is validated with different feature subsets, and the optimal feature subset is identified based on the trend of performance changes.

Figure 3 illustrates the model performance curve based on RF, where the horizontal axis represents the number of features, and the vertical axis represents the model evaluation metric. By analyzing this curve, we can determine the optimal number of features that maximize the model's performance. Based on Figure 3, we observe that by continuously adding features based on their importance ranking, the ROC, accuracy, F1, and sensitivity model evaluation curves continue to increase until reaching a peak when the feature subset contains eight features. After that, the model performance starts to decline and reaches a balance. While there is some incremental improvement afterwards, it is not significant. The precision model evaluation curve reaches its peak when the number of features reaches seven.

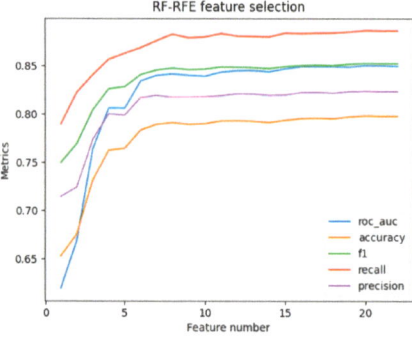

**Figure 3.** RF performance curve.

Therefore, we have selected the top 8 features according to their importance ranking as the feature subset for our method: 'city', 'latitude', 'longitude', 'attacktype1_txt', 'targtype1_txt', 'targsubtype1_txt', 'weapsubtype1_txt', 'date'. At this point, the model not only exhibits high reliability but also significantly reduces computational cost. It is worth noting that our custom time variable feature "date" is also included in the selected feature subset, validating the rationality of the features we constructed.

### 3.3. Hyperparameter Tuning Method Based on CatBoost

The CatBoost algorithm is a new gradient boosting algorithm that improves model performance by having each decision tree learn from the previous tree and influence the next tree. In traditional Gradient Boosting Decision Tree (GBDT) algorithms, the ensemble of weak classifiers for each round is used as the final result. Representing a decision tree as $T(\cdot)$, the model can be expressed as follows:

$$f_D(x) = \sum_{d=1}^{D} T(x; \Theta_d) \tag{2}$$

Here, $D$ represents the number of decision trees, and $\Theta_d$ denotes the parameters of each decision tree. Each decision tree continuously minimizes the empirical risk of the parameters $\Theta_d$ by training on the residuals from the previous round's decision tree to obtain:

$$\Theta_d = \underset{\Theta_d}{\text{argmin}} \sum_{s=1}^{S} L(y_i, f_{d-1}(x_i) + T(x; \Theta_d)) \tag{3}$$

Here, s represents the number of parameters $x_i$, and $y_i$ represents the target value that needs to be fitted. During the process of estimating residuals, GBDT mainly uses the negative gradient of the loss function to iteratively fit each decision tree in every round. The overall basic workflow of the algorithm is as follows:

1. Initialize the first decision tree:

$$f_0(x) = \text{argmin} \sum_{s=1}^{S} L(y_i, c) \tag{4}$$

where $L(y_i, c)$ is the loss function, and c is the initialized constant value.

2. For each iteration $d = 1, 2, \ldots, D$:

   (a) Compute the negative gradient of the loss function to fit the residual values in the current iteration of the model:

$$r_{di} = \left[\frac{\partial L(y_i, f(x_i))}{\partial f(x_i)}\right]_{f(x)=f_{d-1}(x)} \tag{5}$$

   (b) In the leaf node region of the current iteration $R_{mj}, j = 1, 2, \ldots, J$ of the model, fit a decision tree for $r_{di}$ (using CART regression tree as an example) using $(x_i, y_{it})$. Here, t represents the index of $y_i$. Calculate the optimal value within the leaf node region:

$$C_{dj} = \underset{x_i \in R_{mj}}{\text{argmin}} \sum L(y_i, f_{m-1}(x_i) + c) \tag{6}$$

   (c) Update the model:

$$f_m(x_i) = f_{m-1}(x_i) + \sum_{j=1}^{j} c_{dj} I(x_i \in R_{mj}) \tag{7}$$

3. Output the final strong learner $f_M(x)$.

CatBoost has made several improvements over traditional GBDT, with key characteristics in the following areas:

1.  Feature handling: CatBoost introduces the Ordered Target Statistic method to handle categorical features. This method sorts each category feature value based on its relationship with the target variable and performs corresponding statistical calculations. This technique can be used to encode category features, helping the model better understand the meaning of category features. The formula is as follows:

$$x_{\sigma_p,z} = \frac{\sum_{n=1}^{p-1} \left[ x_{\sigma_n,z} = x_{\sigma_p,z} \right] Y_{\sigma_r} + ap}{\sum_{n=1}^{p-1} \left[ x_{\sigma_n,z} = x_{p,z} \right] + a} \tag{8}$$

Here, $\left( x_{\sigma_p,z}, Y_{\sigma_p} \right)$ represents the sample representation of example $\sigma_p$ in the sample sequence $\sigma$. $p$ is the prior; $a$ is the weight; $z$ is the category to which the sample belongs.

For text features, CatBoost first maps text features to a fixed-length feature vector through feature hashing, compressing different text features into vectors of the same length. Subsequently, CatBoost processes the feature vectors obtained from feature hashing by combining them. This combination enables the model to capture relationships and interactions between features more effectively. This processing method can effectively process text features, making CatBoost more convenient and efficient in handling text data. In addition, CatBoost provides various additional methods to handle text features, including converting text features to numerical features using category encoding, representing text features as bag-of-words models such as word frequency or TF-IDF, transforming text features into vector representations of fixed length as text embeddings, and extracting n-gram features based on text features for feature derivation. Depending on the specific problem and characteristics of the data, appropriate methods can be chosen for feature processing and model training. In this study, we use the default handling method.

During the second split of trees, CatBoost combines features within the tree to enrich the feature dimensions of the model, thereby further learning the nonlinear relationships between features.

2.  Addressing Gradient Bias: Traditional GBDT methods estimate gradients using the same dataset for model training, which can lead to cumulative bias and overfitting due to incomplete consistency in data distribution. To address this issue, CatBoost introduces the Ordered Boosting method. The approach involves first shuffling the sample data. For each sequence $\sigma$, $t$ models $M_1, \ldots, M_t$ are trained, where $t$ represents the number of samples. Each model $M_q (q = 1, 2, \ldots, t)$ is trained using data preceding the current sample sequence.

3.  Symmetric Trees. Compared to conventional decision trees, CatBoost uses a lower-degree symmetric tree structure, which has the following characteristics:

    (a) Symmetric Splitting: In contrast to traditional decision tree algorithms that split nodes based on a single optimal feature dimension, the symmetric tree in CatBoost splits nodes based on two feature dimensions simultaneously. This symmetric splitting allows for more effective utilization of relationships and interactions between features, enhancing the model's training efficiency and generalization capability;

    (b) Feature Interaction: In a symmetric tree, decision tree nodes at the same level consider the mutual influence of multiple features simultaneously. This feature interaction helps the model capture feature interactions better, enhancing accuracy and robustness.

These features of the symmetric tree enhance CatBoost's understanding of feature interactions, thereby improving the model's generalization capability and reducing overfitting to noise and irrelevant features in training data. Additionally, the classification method of the symmetric tree during predictions eliminates the need for traversal from the root node; instead, it can be implemented simply through array indexing, reducing computation during prediction and improving prediction speed.

CatBoost is composed of multiple hyperparameters, each controlling different functions, which makes hyperparameter optimization extremely complex. Firstly, there are interactions and influences between hyperparameters; changing one hyperparameter may affect the optimal values of other hyperparameters, making the optimization process complex and challenging. Secondly, a larger hyperparameter search space requires trying more different combinations of hyperparameter values, leading to high computational costs. Additionally, the large number and wide range of hyperparameters create a high-dimensional search space that demands significant time and computational resources. Lastly, excessive or frequent searching may result in overfitting on the training set, compromising the model's generalization ability. Therefore, hyperparameter optimization is seen as a complex and challenging task.

Genetic algorithms simulate the theory of survival of the fittest, allowing the initial population to evolve towards better solutions and eventually converge to the most suitable individual for the environment [19]. In genetic algorithms, chromosomes are typically represented as binary strings in the solution space, with a fitness function indicating the quality of individuals or solutions. Genetic operators typically include selection, mutation, and crossover. The selection operator involves selecting good individuals from the old population with a certain probability to form a new population. The mutation operator helps prevent the algorithm from getting stuck in local optimal solutions during optimization. The crossover operator randomly selects two individuals' chromosomes for exchange and recombination to create new individuals. Genetic algorithms have good robustness and simplicity, which can make CatBoost more stable and efficient. In this study, the Uniform Crossover genetic operator is used to enhance the algorithm's search capability, while model performance evaluation metrics are used as the fitness function.

The pseudo of GA-CatBoost is shown in Algorithm 1.

---

**Algorithm 1.** GA-CatBoost hyperparameters tuning mechanism.

Input: cross-validation fold K, mutation type MT, fitness function Func, crossover type CT, total iterations I, Dataset D, crossover probability C, mutation probability M
Output: The optimal hyperparameter values for CatBoost
1. Initialize i to 0
2. Initialize population randomly
3. Execute the following loop until i < I:
4.     For each solution in the population do
5.     Extract hyperparameters for CatBoost from solution
6.     Split D into K parts, one part as testing set and the rest as training set
7.         For each fold from 1 to K do
8.         Training CatBoost on the training set
9.         Predict values using CatBoost on the testing set
10.        Calculate fitness value based on Func
11.        End for
12.     Compare and select the optimal model performance parameters
13.     End for
14. Select solutions using roulette wheel selection
15. Apply crossover on the selected solutions with CT and C
16. Mutate of the new solutions with MT and M
17. Generate the new population
18. End loop
19. Return the optimal hyperparameter values of CatBoost

---

Due to the imbalance in the number of samples between the category of personnel deaths and other categories in the dataset, there is a problem of data imbalance. This imbalance may lead to classification models that overly rely on limited data samples, resulting in overfitting and reduced accuracy and robustness of the model. In the classification of casualties in terrorist attacks, misclassification of major casualty events can lead to unreasonable resource allocation and decision-making errors, resulting in significant costs. Since the dataset involves textual features, traditional sampling methods at the data level may not be suitable for sampling textual information.

Therefore, our method addresses the issue of data imbalance by leveraging the built-in parameter of CatBoost. We need to optimize key hyperparameters in CatBoost, including learning rate, depth, l2_leaf_reg, min_data_in_leaf, and max_ctr_complexity. These hyperparameters affect the performance and generalization ability of the CatBoost model during training. Additionally, by setting the "auto_class_weights" parameter to "Balanced", we enable CatBoost to automatically handle the issue of data imbalance. In other words, by ensuring that the "auto_class_weights" parameter is set to "Balanced", CatBoost optimizes the aforementioned five parameters. Specifically, CatBoost achieves data balancing by comprehensively adjusting the frequency of each class in the training data, the gradient of the loss function on samples in each iteration, and the splitting of tree nodes. Our method utilizes the parameter tuning functionality of genetic algorithms, setting the crossover probability of the genetic algorithm to 0.6, and the mutation probability to 0.01. The tuning range for each hyperparameter of CatBoost is as shown in Table 1.

**Table 1.** Experimental hyperparameters tuning range.

| Hyperparameter Name | Interval | Explain |
| --- | --- | --- |
| learning_rate | [0.01, 1] | Weight of each step |
| depth | [1, 16] | Limiting the maximum depth of the tree model |
| l2_leaf_reg | [0, 10] | Penalizing the model complexity. |
| min_data_in_leaf | [1, 1000] | Making the model more robust. |
| max_ctr_complexity | [1, 10] | Controlling the complexity of feature combinations. |
| auto_class_weights | Balanced | Automatically adapt to the data imbalance issue. |

## 4. Results

*4.1. Model Training*

After data preprocessing, we compared our method with traditional machine learning methods in terms of model performance. In this experiment, the feature selection part using RF-RFE with three-fold cross-validation to obtain intermediate results, while the main machine learning algorithms employed ten-fold cross-validation to prevent overfitting and better evaluate the model's generalization ability. The iteration number for CatBoost was set at 150 for the main experiment, with some comparative experiments using 50 iterations. The final results were evaluated using metrics such as accuracy, sensitivity, precision, F1 score, and AUC. The experimental setup included an Intel Core i7 processor @2.80 GHz, 16 GB of memory, and Windows 10 operating system. Python environment was constructed using Anaconda, and coding was performed using Python third-party libraries such as numpy and pandas.

*4.2. Comparison among CatBoost and Other Classifcation Methods*

We analyzed the proposed method and compared its model performance with other commonly used machine learning methods. When data preprocessing and feature selection were the same, we comprehensively analyzed the performance of the models from different categorical feature processing and different machine learning methods. Table 2 summarizes the experimental results of LR, Adaboost, DT, RF, XGBoost, LightGBM, and CatBoost. Since only LightGBM and CatBoost have the ability to handle categorical features, the input features for these two algorithms do not require further processing, while the input features for the remaining algorithms are processed using LabelEncoder. We can see that CatBoost without text features performs similarly to LightGBM, but after adding text features, all evaluation metrics show significant improvement. After further tuning with GA, the performance of the GA-CatBoost model further improved. Building upon the GA-CatBoost model, we addressed the data imbalance issue by setting data balance parameters, and our proposed model outperformed other algorithms in terms of accuracy (87.87), sensitivity (92.68), precision (89.35), F1 score (90.99), and AUC (85.59). Additionally, we found that the performance of Adaboost and RF surpassed that of LR and DT. Adaboost and RF belong to ensemble learning algorithms, indicating that ensemble learning methods outperform single learning classifiers.

**Table 2.** Performance comparison of different classification methods.

| Feature Processing | Training Models | AUC | Accuracy | F1 | Sensitivity | Precision |
|---|---|---|---|---|---|---|
| LabelEncoder | Logistics regression | 61.54 | 70.93 | 80.48 | 90.74 | 72.31 |
| | Adaboost | 72.62 | 78.55 | 84.87 | 91.07 | 79.46 |
| | Decision tree | 74.98 | 77.25 | 82.65 | 82.04 | 83.27 |
| | Random forest | 79.22 | 82.65 | 87.26 | 89.90 | 84.76 |
| | XGBoost | 78.56 | 82.52 | 87.29 | 90.87 | 83.98 |
| Built-in category processing | LightGBM | 78.87 | 82.60 | 87.29 | 90.48 | 84.32 |
| | CatBoost | 78.24 | 82.24 | 87.09 | 90.69 | 87.37 |
| | CatBoost(text) | 84.06 | 86.79 | 90.25 | 92.56 | 88.06 |
| | GA-CatBoost | 85.50 | 87.77 | 90.91 | 92.59 | 89.29 |
| | GA-CatBoost-weight | 85.59 | 87.87 | 90.99 | 92.68 | 89.35 |

*4.3. Comparison between Training Models with Different Fitness Evaluations*

After obtaining the optimal feature subset through RFE feature selection, we evaluated the impact of different fitness functions on the model results, as GA requires specifying a specific fitness function. We introduced the optimal fitness function into CatBoost. Table 3 displays the model performance with different fitness functions.

**Table 3.** Experimental results of GA-CatBoost with different fitness functions.

| Training Model | AUC | Accuracy | F1 | Sensitivity | Precision |
|---|---|---|---|---|---|
| GA-CatBoost-Accuracy | 84.92 | 87.39 | 90.65 | 92.59 | 88.80 |
| GA-CatBoost-Sensitivity | 84.92 | 87.39 | 90.65 | 92.59 | 88.80 |
| GA-CatBoost-Precision | 84.91 | 87.38 | 90.65 | 92.59 | 88.78 |
| GA-CatBoost-F1 | 84.92 | 87.39 | 90.65 | 92.59 | 88.80 |
| GA-CatBoost-AUC | 84.91 | 87.38 | 90.65 | 92.59 | 88.78 |

We can observe that the model performance is very similar under different fitness functions, with GA-CatBoost showing the best performance in accuracy, sensitivity, and F1 score functions. However, we are more focused on the performance of sensitivity, as from the definition of sensitivity, we understand that sensitivity refers to the proportion of correctly predicting positive samples among all actual positive samples, indicating the model's ability to identify all terrorist attacks with casualties. In the context of terrorist attacks, the model may accidentally predict events with no casualties as events with casualties, as decision-makers may prepare for the worst-case scenario by allocating sufficient resources. However, even if a terrorist attack with casualties is not accurately predicted, it could lead to severe consequences due to insufficient preparedness for terrorist attacks. Therefore, in this study, we selected sensitivity as the fitness function for GA.

*4.4. Comparison between Different Hyperparameter Tuning Methods*

In this section, we analyzed the model performance comparison of our hyperparameter optimization method with other commonly used hyperparameter optimization methods. Table 4 lists the comparison of the results of CatBoost after parameter tuning using manual hyperparameter adjustment, grid search algorithm, random search algorithm, Bayesian hyperparameter optimization algorithm, and genetic hyperparameter optimization algorithm.

Table 4. Results of different hyperparameter tuning methods.

| Training Model | AUC | Accuracy | F1 | Sensitivity | Precision |
|---|---|---|---|---|---|
| Manual | 78.52 | 82.22 | 87.00 | 90.04 | 84.16 |
| Grid search | 84.64 | 87.13 | 90.46 | 92.38 | 88.62 |
| Random search | 81.82 | 84.93 | 88.91 | 91.49 | 86.48 |
| Bayesian | 83.81 | 86.51 | 90.03 | 92.19 | 87.96 |
| Genetic algorithm | 84.92 | 87.39 | 90.65 | 92.59 | 88.80 |

Through comparison, we can draw the following conclusions. Firstly, manual hyperparameter optimization methods not only incur significant human costs but also make it difficult to manually grasp the regularities of hyperparameters, hence resulting in the poorest model performance. Secondly, the grid search algorithm outperforms the random search algorithm and the Bayesian hyperparameter optimization algorithm. This is because the grid search algorithm traverses candidate hyperparameter combinations in a polling manner, which allows for testing the performance of more hyperparameter combinations. However, the computation cost increases with the number of hyperparameters. Therefore, the efficiency of the grid search algorithm is lower compared to the random search algorithm and the Bayesian hyperparameter optimization algorithm. Additionally, when the search iterations of the random search algorithm and Bayesian hyperparameter optimization algorithm are sufficiently large, the performance results of these two optimization algorithms tend to approach the results of the grid search algorithm. Lastly, the results of genetic hyperparameter optimization algorithm are superior to other hyperparameter optimization algorithms, indicating that the genetic algorithm is a more effective hyperparameter optimization algorithm, particularly for CatBoost.

## 5. Conclusions

Rapid and effective assessment of the potential severe consequences of terrorist attacks can provide valuable information support for decision-makers to formulate emergency measures and counter-terrorism plans. This paper proposes a terrorist attack casualty prediction algorithm named GA-CatBoost-Weight based on CatBoost, aiming to predict whether a terrorist attack will cause harm to innocent civilians.

In the proposed algorithm, to address the data imbalance issue of traditional data sampling methods in handling textual information, the performance of the model is further improved on balanced data basis through the inherent functions and superior feature analysis capabilities of CatBoost. Additionally, genetic algorithm is utilized to optimize various parameters of CatBoost. The algorithm is evaluated on a terrorist attack dataset, demonstrating superior performance compared to several commonly used machine learning methods.

Using machine learning methods to predict the consequences of terrorist attacks can effectively reduce the harm caused by attacks. This study is the first to use the CatBoost algorithm for predicting terrorist attacks, which holds multiple significances. Firstly, CatBoost can directly handle textual information without the need for intermediate steps such as text vectorization, preserving semantic information of the text and reducing time complexity. Secondly, traditional data sampling struggles to handle data imbalance issues with textual features directly, while CatBoost can address sample balance for various modal data through its inherent hyperparameters. Lastly, CatBoost can achieve superior model performance with a small number of iterations, paving the way for new research avenues.

**Author Contributions:** Conceptualization, Y.H.; methodology, Y.H. and B.Y.; software, Y.H. and B.Y.; validation, Y.H. and B.Y.; formal analysis, Y.H.; investigation, Y.H.; resources, Y.H.; data curation, Y.H.; writing—original draft preparation, Y.H.; writing—review and editing, C.C.; supervision, C.C. All authors have read and agreed to the published version of the manuscript.

**Funding:** This research received no external funding.

**Data Availability Statement:** The open-source data used in this study comes from the Global Terrorism Database, which can be obtained from https://www.start.umd.edu/gtd (accessed on 28 August 2022).

**Acknowledgments:** The authors declare any support not covered by the author's contribution or funding section.

**Conflicts of Interest:** The authors declare no conflicts of interest.

## References

1. LaFree, G.; Dugan, L. Introducing the Global Terrorism Database. *Terror. Political Violence* **2007**, *19*, 181–204. [CrossRef]
2. Li, W.; Guo, L. The Impact of COVID-19 on International Terrorism and Its Counter-measures. *Glob. Gov.* **2021**, *3*, 65–77+157.
3. Han, X. Kremlin Drone Attack Raises Concerns of Escalating Russia-Ukraine Conflict. *Guangming Dly.* **2023**, *008*. [CrossRef]
4. Lu, Y. Intensification of Israel-Palestine Conflict Exacerbates Social Division, Europe Faces High Risk of Major Terrorist Attacks. *Lib. Dly.* **2023**, *007*.
5. Abdalsalam, M.; Li, C.; Dahou, A.; Noor, S. A Study of the Effects of Textual Features on Prediction of Terrorism Attacks in GTD Dataset. *Eng. Lett.* **2021**, *29*, 416–443.
6. Guo, X.; Wu, W.; Xiao, Z. Civil aviation airport terrorism risk assessment model based on event tree and PRA. *Appl. Res. Comput.* **2017**, *34*, 1809–1811.
7. Yang, Y. Research on the Risk Assessment and Prevention of Terrorist Attacks in Religious Site Based on FAHP-SWOT. *J. Hunan Police Acad.* **2019**, *31*, 99–106.
8. Luo, L.; Qi, C. An analysis of the crucial indicators impacting the risk of terrorist attacks: A predictive perspective. *Saf. Sci.* **2021**, *144*, 105442. [CrossRef]
9. Zhang, D.; Qian, L.; Mao, B.; Huang, C.; Huang, B.; Si, Y. A Data-Driven Design for Fault Detection of Wind Turbines Using Random Forests and XGboost. *IEEE Access* **2018**, *6*, 21020–21031. [CrossRef]
10. Feng, Y.; Wang, D.; Yin, Y.; Li, Z.; Hu, Z. An XGBoost-based casualty prediction method for terrorist attacks. *Complex Intell. Syst.* **2020**, *6*, 721–740. [CrossRef]
11. Shafiq, S.; Haider Butt, W.; Qamar, U. Attack type prediction using hybrid classifier. In *Advanced Data Mining and Applications, Proceedings of the 10th International Conference, ADMA 2014, Guilin, China, 19–21 December 2014*; Springer International Publishing: Berlin/Heidelberg, Germany,, 2014; pp. 488–498.
12. Meng, X.; Nie, L.; Song, J. Big data-based prediction of terrorist attacks. *Comput. Electr. Eng.* **2019**, *77*, 120–127. [CrossRef]
13. Gundabathula, V.T.; Vaidhehi, V. An Efficient Modelling of Terrorist Groups in India Using Machine Learning Algorithms. *Indian J. Sci. Technol.* **2018**, *11*, 1–10. [CrossRef]
14. Khan, F.A.; Li, G.; Khan, A.N.; Khan, Q.W.; Hadjouni, M.; Elmannai, H. AI-Driven Counter-Terrorism: Enhancing Global Security Through Advanced Predictive Analytics. *IEEE Access* **2023**, *11*, 135864–135879. [CrossRef]
15. Zhang, L.; Qiao, F.; Wang, J.; Zhai, X. Equipment Health Assessment Based on Improved Incremental Support Vector Data Description. *IEEE Trans. Syst. Man Cybern. Syst.* **2021**, *51*, 3205–3216. [CrossRef]
16. Rodriguez-Galiano, V.F.; Luque-Espinar, J.A.; Chica-Olmo, M.; Mendes, M.P. Feature selection approaches for predictive modelling of groundwater nitrate pollution: An evaluation of filters, embedded and wrapper methods. *Sci. Total Environ.* **2018**, *624*, 661–672. [CrossRef] [PubMed]
17. Zhang, X.; Jin, M.; Fu, J.; Hao, M.; Yu, C.; Xie, X. On the Risk Assessment of Terrorist Attacks Coupled with Multi-Source Factors. *ISPRS Int. J. Geo-Inf.* **2018**, *7*, 9. [CrossRef]
18. Jiang, L.; Kong, G.; Li, C. Wrapper Framework for Test-Cost-Sensitive Feature Selection. *IEEE Trans. Syst. Man Cybern. Syst.* **2021**, *51*, 1747–1756. [CrossRef]
19. Michalewicz, Z.; Schoenauer, M. Evolutionary Algorithms for Constrained Parameter Optimization Problems. *Evol. Comput.* **1996**, *4*, 1–32. [CrossRef]

**Disclaimer/Publisher's Note:** The statements, opinions and data contained in all publications are solely those of the individual author(s) and contributor(s) and not of MDPI and/or the editor(s). MDPI and/or the editor(s) disclaim responsibility for any injury to people or property resulting from any ideas, methods, instructions or products referred to in the content.

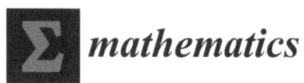 

Article

# SSGCL: Simple Social Recommendation with Graph Contrastive Learning

Zhihua Duan [1], Chun Wang [1,*] and Wending Zhong [2]

[1] Faculty of Data Science, City University of Macau, Macau 999078, China; d22091101472@cityu.edu.mo
[2] Faculty of Applied Sciences, Macao Polytechnic University, Macau 999078, China; p2209473@mpu.edu.mo
* Correspondence: chunwang@cityu.edu.mo

**Abstract:** As user–item interaction information is typically limited, collaborative filtering (CF)-based recommender systems often suffer from the data sparsity issue. To address this issue, recent recommender systems have turned to graph neural networks (GNNs) due to their superior performance in capturing high-order relationships. Furthermore, some of these GNN-based recommendation models also attempt to incorporate other information. They either extract self-supervised signals to mitigate the data sparsity problem or employ social information to assist with learning better representations under a social recommendation setting. However, only a few methods can take full advantage of these different aspects of information. Based on some testing, we believe most of these methods are complex and redundantly designed, which may lead to sub-optimal results. In this paper, we propose SSGCL, which is a recommendation system model that utilizes both social information and self-supervised information. We design a GNN-based propagation strategy that integrates social information with interest information in a simple yet effective way to learn user–item representations for recommendations. In addition, a specially designed contrastive learning module is employed to take advantage of the self-supervised signals for a better user–item representation distribution. The contrastive learning module is jointly optimized with the recommendation module to benefit the final recommendation result. Experiments on several benchmark data sets demonstrate the significant improvement in performance achieved by our model when compared with baseline models.

**Keywords:** recommendation system; collaborative filtering; social recommendation; contrastive learning; graph neural networks

**MSC:** 68T07

## 1. Introduction

With the rapid evolution of internet technology, users are inundated with exponential amounts of information every day. This leads to a situation where, although users seem to receive a greater volume of it, it becomes challenging to extract useful information from the large volume of redundant data. Recommendation systems play a crucial role in addressing this issue. At present, recommendation systems have already become a common solution to provide information filtering and prediction in various domains, such as social networks and short videos [1–3]. The critical function of recommendation systems is to provide users with items they may find interesting while avoiding recommending items that they do not, thereby saving them time and effort while boosting the revenue of various companies.

Collaborative filtering (CF) is one of the most popular technologies for recommendation which predicts users' interest in items by analyzing collaborative behaviors between users [4]. Many of the early CF models are based on matrix factorization (MF) [5–11]. These methods decompose the user–item matrix into two lower-dimensional latent representation matrices to capture the features of users and items. However, due to the inherent sparsity of data (a user is usually associated with only a few items, resulting in very few non-zero

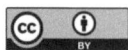

Citation: Duan, Z.; Wang, C.; Zhong, W. SSGCL: Simple Social Recommendation with Graph Contrastive Learning. *Mathematics* **2024**, *12*, 1107. https://doi.org/10.3390/math12071107

Academic Editor: Andrea Scozzari

Received: 7 March 2024
Revised: 3 April 2024
Accepted: 5 April 2024
Published: 7 April 2024

**Copyright:** © 2024 by the authors. Licensee MDPI, Basel, Switzerland. This article is an open access article distributed under the terms and conditions of the Creative Commons Attribution (CC BY) license (https://creativecommons.org/licenses/by/4.0/).

entries in the matrix), models based on MF often struggle to effectively capture feature embeddings for users and items.

To address this issue, some studies have aimed to involve social information and perform social recommendations. These methods are based on the idea that users in a social network may influence each other and share their preferences toward items. Therefore, the user–user interactions in the social network are worth exploring and are usually jointly learned with the user–item interactions in the network of interest. Through introducing social information, the sparsity issue is mitigated, and the efficiency and effectiveness of recommendations are enhanced.

In recent years, graph neural networks (GNNs) have emerged as effective methods for handling networked data. To learn better feature embedding, GNNs have also been successfully introduced into the recommendation task [12,13]. One of the reasons for the popularity of GNNs is their ability to capture high-order connectivity [14]. In GNN-based social recommendation systems, the user–item interactions form a bipartite graph, allowing for users to have two types of neighbors: directly associated items and two-step neighbor users sharing the same preferences. The user–user social interactions can also be easily turned into a graph. This property enables GNN-based recommendation system models [15–17] to extract collaboration signals from numerous interactions and obtain powerful node representations from high-order neighbor information.

Furthermore, some GNN-based recommendation systems have also aimed to employ self-supervision signals from autoencoders [18–20] or contrastive learning-based approaches [21,22]. Contrastive learning typically constructs pairs of positive and negative samples through data augmentation methods and then forces positive samples closer to and negative samples further from each other, thereby maximizing the discrimination between positive and negative pairs for representation learning. The contrastive loss is usually jointly optimized with the GNN loss to manipulate the embedding learning.

Although existing GNN-based social recommendation systems have combined social, interest, and even self-supervised information, achieving satisfactory results, some problems still limit the performance of these algorithms.

**Sparse and unbalanced data sets:** In practical applications, there is often a disparity in the number of users and items in the graph or the sparsity of the data set. Taking the Yelp data set as an example, the number of items is more than twice the number of users. This means that information related to a single item is sparser than that related to a user. Therefore, achieving the same high quality in learning item representations as in user representations is challenging. The inclusion of social information has made this inclination even worse. Unbalanced user and item representation learning will, without doubt, degrade the recommendation performance.

**Complex and inefficient augmentation:** Many social recommendation systems that incorporate graph neural networks (GNNs) tend to employ overly complex graph augmentation methods for contrastive learning, such as randomly dropping nodes or edges in the graph [23]. Research has shown that this type of operation can alter the original structure of the graph, leading to changes in the semantics of the user–item interactions [24]. Existing social recommendation models lack direct and simple ways of extracting information from the interactions. This dramatically affects the effectiveness and efficiency of the social recommendation.

Motivated by these observations, we address the following challenges in performing satisfactory social recommendations:

- In social recommendation, we have both social and interest information, which is sparse and unbalanced. How can we effectively learn useful user and item embedding from such complex information?
- Contrastive learning is a promising path toward better recommendation performance. How can we design a practical graph augmentation approach for contrastive learning?

To deal with the first challenge, we propose a diffusion module to effectively learn user and item embedding. Instead of the traditional GCN [25], a more straightforward

GNN-based strategy is designed to perform influence diffusion and learn informative user and item representation separately from the social and interest graph. Instead of aggregating and updating the user embedding learned from the interest and social graph at each GNN layer, we choose to update the user embedding from the two graphs separately by themselves and simply sum up the final embedding from the two networks. We argue that this method sufficiently extracts information related to both users and items without disturbing each other and obtains better embedding.

For the second challenge, we abandon complex graph enhancement methods and simply generate positive and negative samples for self-supervision by adding noise to the embedding. The experimental results suggest that such graph augmentation improves the model performance without compromising the original semantics of the graph. In such a simple way, our contrastive learning component can manipulate the embedding learning toward a smoother distribution, thereby improving the recommendation performance.

To summarize, in this paper, we propose a model called SSCGL specifically designed for social recommendation. SSCGL consists of three main modules: a diffusion module, a contrastive learning module, and a prediction module. The diffusion module learns informative user and item embedding separately from the social and interest information with a specially designed GNN-based architecture. Then, a contrastive learning module that generates contrastive views by adding noise to the graph is incorporated to further manipulate the embedding learning. Finally, the contrastive learning and the recommendation are jointly optimized to predict the final recommendation results. Experimental results on real-world social recommendation data sets validate the effectiveness of our designs.

Our work significantly contributes in the following aspects:

- We successfully integrate social information and self-supervised signals into the recommendation system, significantly improving the performance.
- While existing social recommendation works tend to design complex attention mechanisms to fuse the social and interest information during the GNN propagation, we abandon traditional GCN encoding and opt for a more straightforward encoder for layer-wise embedding updating. The representations from the interest and social networks are separately updated and, at last, combined with a simple sum. Our design demonstrates simple and powerful acquisition of better item and user representations.
- We abandon complex graph enhancement methods commonly used in traditional contrastive learning approaches and employ a simpler and more effective approach by adding noise to embeddings, further improving the model's performance.
- We evaluate our model on three real-world publicly available data sets. Our SSGCL demonstrates superior performance, compared with eight state-of-the-art baselines, in terms of social recommendations.

## 2. Related Work

In this section, we provide a brief overview of recommendation systems based on different kinds of approaches.

### 2.1. Matrix Factorization (MF)-Based Recommendation Systems

In the current field of recommendation systems, many classic collaborative filtering algorithms adopt the matrix factorization (MF) approach [26–28]. Models based on MF map users and items to a lower-dimensional space using vector representations [29]. Satisfaction is then evaluated by computing the inner product of the vectors representing users and items. However, MF-based models struggle to effectively encode features of the user–item matrix, meaning that MF cannot capture more implicit factors. Moreover, traditional matrix factorization methods based on MF typically only leverage relationships between users and items for recommendations, neglecting user–user relationships. This implies that the model cannot capture information about higher-order neighbors, as simple matrix factorization essentially considers only first-order neighbor information and ignores potential relationships between users. These limitations result in sub-optimal recommendation performance for traditional MF models.

Early social recommendation models based on MF include SocialMF [26], TrustMF [27], and BPR-MF [28]. SocialMF is a recommendation approach based on social networks that assumes the existence of social networks between users and making recommendations based on direct or indirect social relationships between users. TrustMF moves a step further by considering the impact of social trust propagation. In TrustMF, the configuration of trust networks and trust matrices allows for a thorough analysis of the mutual influence between trustors and trustees. In contrast to the previous two models, BPR-MF introduces a pairwise BPR loss, leading to improved optimization of the model.

However, most of the aforementioned MF-based models are no longer effective in handling large-scale data sets and sparsely rated data sets compared with GNN-based methods.

### 2.2. Recommendation Systems Based on Graph Neural Networks

Methods based on graph neural networks (GNNs) have gradually become mainstream in the field of recommendation systems. The inherent structure of GNNs can effectively represent the graph between users and users, as well as between users and items, which aligns well with the high connectivity observed in social networks. The core objective of GNN-based recommendation systems is to learn representations for each node.

NGCF [30], for instance, aims to further learn embeddings for users and items in the latent space by exploring high-order connectivity relationships to refine the embedding representations. The refined user and item representations are then used for predictions. Diffnet++ [31] constructs a powerful and efficient diffusion network that combines the user–user graph and user–item graph to address the shortcomings of traditional MF-based methods in capturing high-order neighbor information. It incorporates carefully designed attention mechanisms in the model to resolve the inconsistency between the user–user graph and user–item graph relationships.

Approaching the issue of social inconsistency from a different angle, the authors of ref. [32] introduce the concept that social relationships may not necessarily align with rating predictions to create ConsisReg. Based on this insight, they propose a new framework to address this problem.

In many GNN-based models [31,32], graph convolutional networks (GCNs) are commonly used for embedding. However, the GCN was initially designed for homogeneous graphs and may not be suitable for GNN-based social models. LightGCN [33] improved upon the GCN by removing unnecessary non-linear activation functions and feature transformation matrices, making it more suitable for recommendation systems and achieving more advanced recommendation performance.

To further enhance the performance and robustness of recommendation systems, these GNN-based models strive to innovate and address specific challenges, showcasing the ongoing evolution in this area.

### 2.3. Recommendation System with Graph Contrastive Learning

A highly promising approach recently used in research involves integrating contrastive learning methods into graph-based recommendation systems to address challenges such as insufficient collaboration signals and data sparsity. In particular, SGL [23] combines contrastive learning with recommendation systems, employing three strategies—node dropping, edge dropping, and random walks—to enhance the graph. Contrastive learning is then utilized to obtain diverse self-supervised signals. The model is subsequently jointly trained with these signals as auxiliary modules, leading to improved performance.

SimGRACE [34] introduces perturbations to GCN encoders to generate new views for contrastive learning, while LightGCL [35] employs singular value decomposition to reconstruct different views for contrastive learning. These new views are then jointly optimized with the main model. SimGCL [36], on the other hand, recognizes that complex graph augmentation strategies may adversely affect the model. SimGCL opts for a simpler and more efficient approach by introducing noise into the embedding representations for contrastive learning.

Nevertheless, there is still a lack of a contrastive learning enhanced social recommendation method, where the self-supervision signal can effectively manipulate the learning toward better recommendation.

## 3. Methodology

This section presents our proposed recommendation model, SSGCL, which consists of four components. We first introduce some essential notation. In the second and third parts, the diffusion module and prediction layer employed in our model are introduced, respectively. The training approach of the model is presented in the last part. The framework of SSGCL is illustrated in Figure 1.

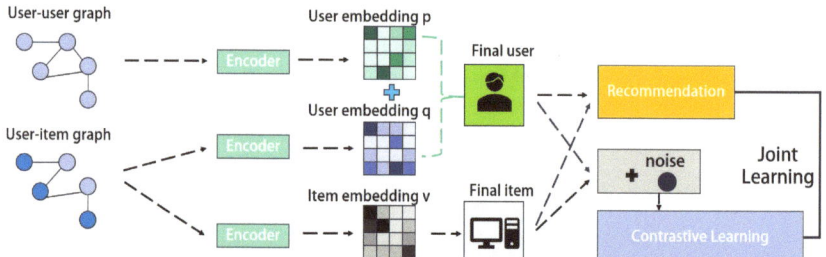

**Figure 1.** The conceptual framework of our proposed social recommendation system SSGCL. Through a GNN-based encoder, it learns a user embedding $p$ from the user–user graph representing social information, a user embedding $q$, and an item embedding $v$ from the user–item graph representing interest information. The two user embeddings $p$ and $q$ are summed to provide the final user embedding. Based on these, a contrastive learning module is jointly optimized with the recommendation task to learn the final embedding and recommendation result.

### 3.1. Notation

This study focuses on the social recommendation problem. Social recommendation systems generally have two sets of entities: a user set $U$ consisting of $m$ users and an item set $V$ consisting of $n$ items. Users may form two types of relationships: social connections between users and interest relationships toward items. These behaviors can be represented as a social graph and an interest graph: the social graph $G_s$ contains nodes denoting users and edges denoting social connections, while the interest graph $G_i$ contains nodes denoting both users and items, and edges denoting user preference toward the items.

These two graphs can be defined by two matrices: a user–user social relationship matrix $S \in \mathbb{R}^{M \times M}$ and a user–item interest relationship matrix $R \in \mathbb{R}^{M \times N}$.

In the user–user social relationship matrix $S$, if user $a$ trusts user $b$ or, in other words, user $a$'s decision may be influenced by user $b$, $s_{ab} = 1$; otherwise, $s_{ab} = 0$. We use $S_a$ to represent the set of all users that user $a$ follows or trusts, i.e., $S_a = [b|s_{ab} = 1]$.

Similarly, in the user–item interest matrix $R$, $r_{ac} = 1$ means user $a$ is interested in item $c$, and $r_{ac} = 0$ otherwise. $R_a$ represents the set of items that user $a$ is interested in, i.e., $R_a = [c|r_{ac} = 1]$, and $R_c$ represents the set of users that voted for item $c$, i.e., $R_c = [a|r_{ca} = 1]$.

Our goal is to find unknown preferences from users toward items; that is, a predicted new user–item matrix $\hat{R}$ from $R$, with new preferences added.

### 3.2. Diffusion Module

As mentioned before, we design a diffusion module to learn comprehensive representations of users and items based on social and interest information. It has two parts, which acquire the representations from $G_s$ and $G_i$.

First, representations are acquired from the user–item graph (interest graph $G_i$). While most GNN-based recommendation systems [12,31] commonly employ traditional GCN encoders to aggregate various information in the social and interest graphs, in this study, we follow [33] and employ a simple but efficient aggregation strategy.

Specifically, both user and item representations are acquired from the interest graph. The diffusion process of the interest graph $G_i$ can be defined as

$$q_i^{(L)} = AGG_{items}(v_j^{(L-1)}, \forall j \in R_i) = \sum_{j \in N_i} \frac{v_j^{(L-1)}}{\sqrt{|R_i||R_j|}}, \quad (1)$$

$$v_j^{(L)} = AGG_{users}(q_i^{(L-1)}, \forall i \in R_j) = \sum_{i \in N_j} \frac{q_i^{(L-1)}}{\sqrt{|R_j||R_i|}}. \quad (2)$$

Here, $L$ is the number of stacked diffusion layers. $q_i^{(L)}$ is the representation of user $i$ obtained from the interest graph. Similarly, $v_j^{(L)}$ is the representation of item $j$ from the interest graph. $R_i$ represents the set of items $j$ that user $i$ is interested in, and $R_j$ is the set of users $i$ that voted for item $j$. It is worth mentioning that the input of the first layer $q_i^{(0)}$ and $v_j^{(0)}$ are randomly initialized.

Such an encoder is better suited for GNN-based recommendation systems, as it abandons the redundant non-linear transformations of traditional GCN encoders.

The second part involves learning representations from the social graph $G_s$. Unlike the user–item graph $G_i$, the social graph only contains nodes representing users, and we can learn only user representations from it. The propagation of user $i$ based on the social graph $G_s$ at the Lth layer could be defined as

$$p_i^{(L)} = AGG_{users}(p_t^{(L-1)}, \forall t \in S_i) = \sum_{t \in S_i} \frac{p_t^{(L-1)}}{\sqrt{|S_i||S_t|}}, \quad (3)$$

where $p_i^{(L)}$ is the embedding for user $i$ at layer $L$ and $S_i$ is the set of socially connected neighbor users of user $i$.

Upon completion of the aggregation through Equations (1) and (2), representations $q_i^{(L)}$ are obtained for user $i$ after $L$ layers of iterations and $v_j^{(L)}$ for item $j$ after $L$ layers of iterations based on the user–item graph. Through Equation (3), the social-relation-based user representation denoted as $p_i^{(L)}$ is obtained. To aggregate user representation learned from the social graph and the interest graph, previous works [31] designed complex attention mechanisms and combined the two view information from every layer. However, we opt for a simple yet effective sum aggregation function to obtain the final user representation:

$$u_i^{(L)} = q_i^{(L)} + p_i^{(L)} \quad (4)$$

With our aggregation approach, both $q_i^{(L)}$ and $p_i^{(L)}$ effectively learn user representations from their respective views, making full use of the information in each graph without being subject to additional interference.

### 3.3. Prediction Layer

In the previous section, it is shown that the final user embedding $u_i^{(L)}$ and the final item embedding $v_j^{(L)}$ are obtained from Equations (2) and (4). Then, the prediction results of our model are calculated by taking the inner product of the final user embedding and item embedding:

$$\hat{y}_{ij} = <u_i^{(L)}, v_j^{(L)}>. \quad (5)$$

where $\hat{y}_{ij}$ is user $i$'s predicted preference score for item $j$, according to our model.

### 3.4. Model Training

In order to capture more collaborative signals, we employed two types of losses for joint learning to optimize the model: a supervised loss suitable for recommendation systems and a self-supervised loss to capture more collaborative signals.

#### 3.4.1. Supervised Loss

We opted not to use point-wise loss functions [37] which are widely used for recommendation, and instead chose the Bayesian personalized ranking (BPR) pairwise loss function instead. The BPR loss function is specialized for the ranking task. In Bayesian personalized ranking, instances with an interaction are considered positive samples, while those without interaction are considered negative samples. The objective is to maximize the margin between positive and negative samples, which is similar to contrastive learning in principle. This matches our need to determine which items are more worthy of recommendation to the users (potential positive samples with high ranking). Additionally, recommendation data are sparse, with positive samples (instances where users interact with items) being far fewer than negative samples. The sampling-based BPR loss can satisfactorily resolve this problem and lead to better performance. The BPR loss is defined as

$$L_{bpr} = \sum_{(i,j^+,j^-) \in O} -\log \sigma(\hat{y}_{ij^+} - \hat{y}_{ij^-}), \tag{6}$$

where $O = [(i, j^+, j^-) | (i, j^+) \in O^+, (i, j^-) \in O^-]$ is the training data, $O^+$ represents the observed interaction information, and $O^-$ denotes unobserved interactions. $\sigma$ is the sigmoid function. The BPR loss provides positive and negative signals to model the user–item interaction but still lacks the ability to enhance the embedding based on the nodes themselves. This could potentially result in sub-optimal representations. To address this issue, we employed a specially designed contrastive loss as assistance.

#### 3.4.2. Self-Supervised Loss

To create contrastive views, traditional GNN-based contrastive learning involves preprocessing steps, such as randomly dropping nodes or edges, performing random walks, or even constructing an entirely new graph [23]. Such strategies tend to be over-designed. According to the findings of previous work, steps such as randomly dropping nodes and edges are likely to result in the loss of important information [36]. Moreover, enhancing the graph in these ways can be very time-consuming.

Therefore, here, we adopt a simpler and more efficient contrastive learning approach. Inspired by [36], traditional graph enhancement methods are abandoned and instead positive and negative samples are constructed by adding noise to the learned embedding of users and items. In particular, for a user embedding $u_i$, samples $u_i'$ and $u_i''$ are generated as follows:

$$u_i' = u_i + \beta_i', \quad u_i'' = u_i + \beta_i''. \tag{7}$$

Here, for user $i$ with learned representation $u_i$, $\beta'$ and $\beta''$ represent the added vector noises. These noises are constrained by $||\beta||_2 = \varepsilon$ and $\beta = \bar{\beta} \odot sign(u_i)$, $\bar{\beta} \in \mathbb{R}^d \sim U(0,1)$. $\varepsilon$ is a hyperparameter and $\odot$ is the Hadamard product. These constraints control the magnitude and the orthant of the noise, which could otherwise lead to significant biases and disrupt the original semantics of the node. Figure 2 briefly illustrates our contrastive learning method described in Equation (7).

We consider samples generated from the same node as positive pairs and samples from different nodes as negative ones for contrastive learning. This simple strategy can smoothly manipulate the learned representation toward a better distribution. The InfoNCE contrastive loss [38] is employed to force positive pairs close to each other and negative pairs distant from each other,

$$L_{cl}^{user} = \sum_{i \in U} -\log \frac{\exp(cos < u_i', u_i'' > /\tau)}{\sum_{k \in U} \exp(cos < u_i', u_k > /\tau)}. \tag{8}$$

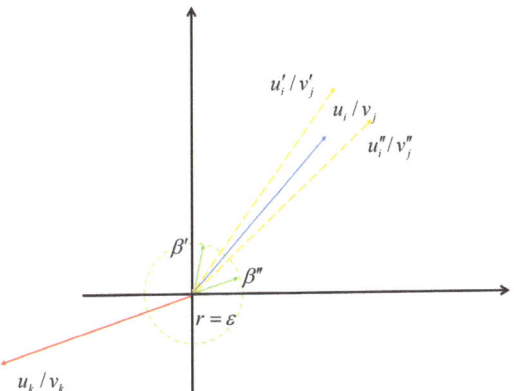

**Figure 2.** Illustration of data augmentation with added noise. $\beta'$ and $\beta''$ are the noises we add to the learned representations, constrained by hyperparameter $\varepsilon$. $u_i'/v_j'$ and $u_i''/v_j''$ are the samples generated from $u_i/v_j$ with the noises. They are close to the original representation and can be regarded as positive samples, compared with the representations of other nodes $u_k/v_k$.

Here, $cos <,>$ denotes the cosine similarity between two vectors. $\tau$ is a temperature hyperparameter. The denominator is summed over all possible users $k$ in the user set $U$. This contrastive loss can be regarded as a softmax classifier that classifies $u'$ to $u''$.

Similarly, for item embedding $v_j$, the following is the item-based noised samples and contrastive loss:

$$v_j' = v_j + \beta_j', v_j'' = v_j + \beta_j''. \tag{9}$$

$$L_{cl}^{item} = \sum_{j \in V} -\log \frac{\exp(cos < v_j', v_j'' > /\tau)}{\sum_{k \in V} \exp(cos < v_j', v_k > /\tau)}. \tag{10}$$

The final self-supervised loss is the sum of the user-based contrastive loss and the item-based contrastive loss:

$$L_{ssl} = L_{cl}^{item} + L_{cl}^{user} \tag{11}$$

3.4.3. Final Loss

We incorporated our supervised BPR loss (refer to Equation (6)) with our self-supervised contrastive loss (refer to Equation (11)) for joint learning and to optimize our model. The final loss function is defined as

$$L_{final} = L_{bpr} + \lambda_1 L_{ssl} + \lambda_2 ||\theta||_2, \tag{12}$$

where $||\theta||_2$ is the regularization term of $L_{final}$ introduced to prevent model overfitting. $\lambda_1$ and $\lambda_2$ are two hyperparameters used to control the balance. The learning process is conducted in a supervised manner. The BPR loss is the primary supervised component that optimizes the user and item embedding, while the self-supervised learning module merely serves as an auxiliary part that manipulates the learned embedding toward a better distribution.

## 4. Experiments

In this section, to demonstrate the effectiveness and superiority of our model, we conducted extensive experiments and addressed the following questions from various perspectives:

- **RQ1:** How does our model perform compared with various state-of-the-art (SOTA) models on different data sets?
- **RQ2:** How do the self-supervised learning module and diffusion modules' propagation mechanisms impact the model?
- **RQ3:** How do different parameter settings affect the model?

### 4.1. Benchmark Data Sets

We utilized three real-world publicly available data sets: Yelp [23], Last.fm [39], and Douban-book [36]. Below, detailed information about the data sets is provided.

- **Yelp**: Yelp is a geographically based online review platform that encourages users to share their perspectives and experiences by writing reviews and providing ratings. The data set encompasses interactions between users and various locations, including visits and comments. Additionally, by leveraging user friend lists, we can infer user relationships, enabling further analysis of influencing factors within the social network.
- **Douban-book**: Douban-book is a highly influential book-related online social platform in China that gathers extensive information on books and user reviews. This platform enables users to search for books, share their book reviews, rate works, and create personal booklists. Additionally, users can follow other readers, thereby establishing a social network to receive more book recommendations and enhance their interactive experiences.
- **Last.fm**: Last.fm is a music-related data set that includes user, artist, song, and social relationship data. It is widely used in research on music recommendation systems, social network analysis, and music data mining. The data set comprises information such as users' listening histories, social relationships, tags, and events, providing valuable resources for studying music consumption behavior and music social networks.

The three data sets are publicly available for download. All processed data sets were obtained from https://recbole.io/cn/dataset_list.html (accessed on 6 March 2024). A summary of the data set details is provided in Table 1. The data sets were all preprocessed [40] and have been widely used for the recommendation task. Our focus was solely on the social interest information within the data sets, while other user attributes and item details were not within the scope of our consideration.

**Table 1.** Benchmark graph data sets.

| Data Set | Users | Avg. Actions of Users | Items | Avg. Actions of Items | Interactions | Sparsity |
|---|---|---|---|---|---|---|
| Yelp | 17,236 | 12.065 | 37,379 | 5.563 | 207,945 | 99.968 |
| Douban-book | 13,025 | 60.812 | 22,348 | 35.443 | 792,062 | 99.728 |
| Last.fm | 1893 | 49.067 | 17,633 | 5.265 | 92,834 | 99.722 |

### 4.2. Baseline Methods

In the experiments, we compared a total of eight recommendation system models with our proposed SSGCL. The main differences between these baselines are summarized in Table 2.

- **MF-BPR** [28] is a recommendation system model. Built upon the idea of matrix factorization, it aims to learn latent representations of users and items for personalized item recommendations. The model is optimized using Bayesian personalized ranking (BPR) loss.

- **Social-MF** [26] is a model designed for recommendation systems. It is also based on the idea of matrix factorization, integrating social information with purchase data to provide personalized recommendations.
- **NGCF** [30] is a deep learning model for recommendation systems, combining traditional collaborative filtering methods with graph neural networks to enhance the effectiveness of personalized recommendations. The core idea involves representing users and items as nodes in a graph and using graph neural networks to learn their latent relationships. Through multiple layers of neural networks, NGCF can better capture the complex interactions between users and items, thereby improving the model performance.
- **Diffnet++** [31] is a graph diffusion model for social recommendations. It combines social and interest information in a recursive manner and employs an attention mechanism during the propagation and aggregation process to enhance the model's performance.
- **MHCN** [41] is a model based on hyper-graph convolutional networks for recommendation systems. The model utilizes social and other information to model edges in the hyper-graph, thereby enhancing the recommendation performance of the model.
- **LightGCN** [33] is a lightweight graph convolutional model. In comparison with traditional graph convolutional networks (GCNs), it simplifies the structure and parameters. By directly updating user and item embedding vectors, it enhances the learning efficiency and effectiveness in social networks and recommendation systems.
- **SGL** [23] is a graph convolutional model that incorporates self-supervised learning for recommendation systems. The algorithm enhances the graph to transform the original graph and create different views by using uniform node and edge dropout strategies. Subsequently, it employs contrastive learning methods to learn from these views. The losses are jointly optimized to obtain the final representations of nodes.
- **SEPT** [42] is a recommendation system model that incorporates self-supervised learning. By constructing complementary views of the graph, pseudo-labels are obtained, and triplet training is employed to assist the training process.

**Table 2.** Algorithm comparison.

|  | Interest Information | Social Information | GNN | Self-Supervised Learning | Diffusion Module | BPR |
|---|---|---|---|---|---|---|
| MF-BPR | ★ |  |  |  |  | ★ |
| Social-MF | ★ | ★ |  |  |  |  |
| NGCF | ★ |  | ★ |  |  | ★ |
| Diffnet++ | ★ | ★ | ★ |  | ★ | ★ |
| MHCN | ★ | ★ |  | ★ |  | ★ |
| LightGCN | ★ |  | ★ |  |  | ★ |
| SGL | ★ |  | ★ | ★ |  | ★ |
| SEPT | ★ | ★ | ★ | ★ |  | ★ |
| SSCGL | ★ | ★ | ★ | ★ | ★ | ★ |

*4.3. Experimental Setup*

For the effectiveness and fairness of the experiments, we adjusted the hyperparameters for all baselines following the strategies in the original papers. We ran all experiments with the Adam optimizer. The data sets were randomly divided into training, validation, and test sets in an 8:1:1 ratio. Meanwhile, we employed two advanced and effective evaluation metrics that are widely used in top conferences [31,33,36,43]—namely Recall@K and NDCG@K (normalized discounted cumulative gain)—to assess the model performance. In our SSGCL model, we stacked three GNN layers for the influence diffusion, and the embedding size for both users and items was set to 64. The L2 norm was employed for the regularization. The trade-off hyperparameters of the contrastive learning module $\lambda_1$ and the regularization term $\lambda_2$ were set to $1 \times 10^{-5}$ and $1 \times 10^{-2}$, respectively. The learning rate $\alpha$ was set to $1 \times 10^{-3}$. The temperature coefficient $\tau$ was 0.15. The noise radius $\varepsilon$ is 0.1. Additionally, all our experiments were conducted on an RTX 2070 (8 GB) GPU, and the results of the first 50 epochs are illustrated in Figure 3.

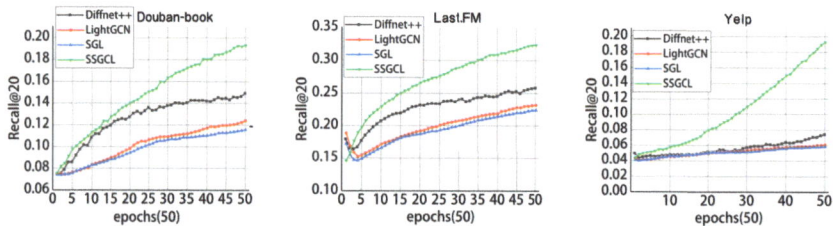

**Figure 3.** The performance curves in the first 50 epochs.

### 4.4. Performance Comparison (RQ1)

This study compared eight baseline models with two variants of SSGCL, namely SSGCL-M and SSGCL-L, across three public data sets and two evaluation metrics. SSGCL-M was the model that only aggregated the user representation of the two graphs in the last GNN layer, as described in our Methodology section. SSGCL-L was a variant of our model in which we followed previous works and aggregated the user representation at each layer of the GNN influence diffusion. The learned user representation that combined two sides of information was then updated into the two graphs for the influence diffusion of the next GNN layer.

We conducted the experiment by evaluating the rankings for the top 10, top 20, and top 30 recommendations. As shown in Tables 3–5, our SSGCL-M (final aggregation) consistently outperformed the optimal baseline in the top@k experiments, while SSGCL-L (intermediate aggregation) achieved a performance close to the baseline. We summarize our findings as follows:

1. **The exploration of social information could benefit the recommendation system.**

    The tables show that many recommendation systems that incorporate social information performed better than other methods proposed during the same time period, such as Diffnet++, SEPT, and our method. However, the advantages of social information were not apparent when compared with more up-to-date methods. This was probably because taking full advantage of social information is difficult. Early approaches lack effective ways to jointly learn social interactions with the interest information.

2. **The approaches based on GNNs exhibited excellent performance.**

    From the tables, it is evident that GNN-based models generally exhibited a significant improvement over traditional approaches, such as matrix factorization-based recommendation systems. For example, LightGCN and SGL performed quite well without social information, and mainly benefited from their well-designed GNN layers. MHCN involves both social information and self-supervised signals but has yet to achieve satisfactory results, which may be because it fails to model multifaceted information sufficiently without the assistance of GNNs. This demonstrates a GNN's effectiveness in handling such interest and social networks, as well as modeling the complex interactions in the recommendation task.

3. **Self-supervised learning shows great potential in recommendation system tasks.**

    It can be observed from the tables that recent recommendation system approaches, such as SGL and SEPT, tended to employ self-supervised learning and obtained satisfactory performance. This was because the self-supervised learning module could help to learn more informative representations and make the user and item representation uniform, thereby helping to achieve better recommendation results.

4. **The superiority of our SSGCL.**

Our SSGCL sufficiently explored the social and interest network with a GNN-based influence diffusion layer. The learned representation was further optimized with a contrastive learning module that extracts self-supervised signals. This should be the reason why our SSGCL performed well compared with the baseline methods.

**Table 3.** Experimental results for the Douban-book data set.

| Model | Recall@10 | Recall@20 | Recall@30 | NDCG@10 | NDCG@20 | NDCG@30 |
|---|---|---|---|---|---|---|
| MF-BPR | 0.0901 | 0.1362 | 0.1685 | 0.0706 | 0.0838 | 0.1059 |
| Social-MF | 0.0246 | 0.0399 | 0.0534 | 0.0122 | 0.0162 | 0.0192 |
| NGCF | 0.1061 | 0.1559 | 0.1905 | 0.0831 | 0.0968 | 0.1068 |
| Diffnet++ | 0.1285 | 0.1822 | 0.2181 | 0.0998 | 0.1151 | 0.1251 |
| MHCN [1] | - | - | - | - | - | - |
| LightGCN | 0.1962 | 0.2576 | 0.3306 | 0.1666 | 0.1828 | 0.1947 |
| SGL | 0.1941 | 0.2581 | 0.3025 | 0.1681 | 0.1828 | 0.1972 |
| SEPT | 0.2370 | 0.3046 | 0.3523 | 0.1957 | 0.2138 | 0.2271 |
| SSGCL-L | 0.2407 | 0.3042 | 0.3468 | 0.1961 | 0.2129 | 0.2248 |
| SSGCL-M [2] | **0.2765** | **0.3367** | **0.3757** | **0.2298** | **0.2460** | **0.2572** |

[1] The Douban-book data set was too large for the MHCN algorithm. [2] In the table, data in bold indicates optimal performance.

**Table 4.** Experimental results for the Last.fm data set.

| Model | Recall@10 | Recall@20 | Recall@30 | NDCG@10 | NDCG@20 | NDCG@30 |
|---|---|---|---|---|---|---|
| MF-BPR | 0.1786 | 0.2438 | 0.2958 | 0.1681 | 0.1958 | 0.2145 |
| Social-MF | 0.1510 | 0.2196 | 0.2676 | 0.1400 | 0.1690 | 0.1863 |
| NGCF | 0.1958 | 0.2738 | 0.3261 | 0.1854 | 0.2185 | 0.2372 |
| Diffnet++ | 0.2545 | 0.3521 | 0.4184 | 0.2512 | 0.2921 | 0.3159 |
| MHCN | 0.3357 | 0.4684 | 0.5499 | 0.2995 | 0.3557 | 0.3848 |
| LightGCN | 0.3929 | 0.5097 | 0.5823 | 0.3808 | 0.4308 | 0.4571 |
| SGL | 0.3831 | 0.4991 | 0.5741 | 0.3739 | 0.4231 | 0.4501 |
| SEPT | 0.3774 | 0.4818 | 0.5562 | 0.3753 | 0.4195 | 0.4463 |
| SSGCL-L | 0.4844 | 0.6092 | 0.6770 | 0.4669 | 0.5202 | 0.5448 |
| SSGCL-M | **0.5495** | **0.6650** | **0.7241** | **0.5510** | **0.6005** | **0.6219** |

**Table 5.** Experimental results for the Yelp data set.

| Model | Recall@10 | Recall@20 | Recall@30 | NDCG@10 | NDCG@20 | NDCG@30 |
|---|---|---|---|---|---|---|
| MF-BPR | 0.0222 | 0.0367 | 0.0512 | 0.0112 | 0.0151 | 0.0182 |
| Social-MF | 0.0240 | 0.0400 | 0.0543 | 0.0122 | 0.0163 | 0.0195 |
| NGCF | 0.0327 | 0.0571 | 0.0747 | 0.0164 | 0.0227 | 0.0265 |
| Diffnet++ | 0.2077 | 0.2678 | 0.3081 | 0.1456 | 0.1613 | 0.1702 |
| MHCN | 0.1368 | 0.1996 | 0.2470 | 0.0787 | 0.0951 | 0.1055 |
| LightGCN | 0.5721 | 0.6631 | 0.7136 | 0.4318 | 0.4561 | 0.4674 |
| SGL | 0.5832 | 0.6695 | 0.7194 | 0.4478 | 0.4708 | 0.4822 |
| SEPT | 0.4101 | 0.5065 | 0.5638 | 0.2816 | 0.3068 | 0.3195 |
| SSGCL-L | 0.6772 | 0.7690 | 0.8143 | 0.5050 | 0.5296 | 0.5505 |
| SSGCL-M | **0.7143** | **0.7910** | **0.8296** | **0.5546** | **0.5755** | **0.5846** |

*4.5. Ablation Study (RQ2)*

Ablation experiments helped us gain a deeper understanding of the contributions of different components of the model to the overall performance. Through gradually removing specific parts of the model or altering their configurations, we assessed the impacts of these parts on the model's performance, thus revealing key factors in the model design.

From the above experiments, we could observe that both SSGCL-L and SSGCL-M performed well. The variant SSGCL-L adopts a more complicated influence diffusion strategy that aggregates the user representation at each layer like in many other algorithms that take social information into account. However, it cannot beat SSGCL-M, which has a simple final aggregation strategy.

In this subsection, to further investigate the effectiveness of the model's simple influence diffusion strategy and the contrastive learning module, we conducted ablation experiments to address the question of whether simpler aggregation mechanisms and contrastive learning make sense. For this purpose, we compared four variants of the model, namely SSGCL-M utilizing final layer aggregation with contrastive learning, SSGCL-L employing intermediate layer aggregation with contrastive learning, SSGCL-N using final layer aggregation without contrastive learning, and SSGCL-O using intermediate layer aggregation without contrastive learning. To ensure the fairness of the ablation experiments, we used the same optimizer and other parameters as mentioned before.

From Tables 6–8, it is evident that SSGCL-M achieved the best performance on all three public data sets. This further shows the effectiveness of our simple final layer aggregation and the contrastive learning module. SSGCL-M performed better than SSGCL-L, and SSGCL-N performed better than SSGCL-O, both of which demonstrated that the precisely designed propagation of previous social recommendation systems did not have much of an effect on the final performance; furthermore, our final aggregation strategy was simple and effective, and it lead to better representations and recommendation results. SSGCL-M and SSGCL-L clearly outperformed the other two variants, which shows the superiority of our contrastive learning module.

**Table 6.** Ablation study of the Douban-book data set.

| Model | Recall@10 | Recall@20 | Recall@30 | NDCG@10 | NDCG@20 | NDCG@30 |
|---|---|---|---|---|---|---|
| SSGCL-M | **0.2765** | **0.3367** | **0.3757** | **0.2298** | **0.2460** | **0.2572** |
| SSGCL-L | 0.2407 | 0.3042 | 0.3468 | 0.1961 | 0.2129 | 0.2248 |
| SSGCL-N | 0.1947 | 0.2613 | 0.3053 | 0.1619 | 0.1792 | 0.1914 |
| SSGCL-O | 0.1717 | 0.2335 | 0.2796 | 0.1400 | 0.1560 | 0.1856 |

**Table 7.** Ablation study of the Last.fm data set.

| Model | Recall@10 | Recall@20 | Recall@30 | NDCG@10 | NDCG@20 | NDCG@30 |
|---|---|---|---|---|---|---|
| SSGCL-M | **0.5495** | **0.6650** | **0.7241** | **0.5510** | **0.6005** | **0.6219** |
| SSGCL-L | 0.4844 | 0.6092 | 0.6770 | 0.4669 | 0.5202 | 0.5448 |
| SSGCL-N | 0.3162 | 0.4321 | 0.5100 | 0.3049 | 0.3541 | 0.3821 |
| SSGCL-O | 0.2997 | 0.4115 | 0.4897 | 0.2893 | 0.3370 | 0.3648 |

**Table 8.** Ablation study of the Yelp data set.

| Model | Recall@10 | Recall@20 | Recall@30 | NDCG@10 | NDCG@20 | NDCG@30 |
|---|---|---|---|---|---|---|
| SSGCL-M | **0.7143** | **0.7910** | **0.8296** | **0.5546** | **0.5755** | **0.5846** |
| SSGCL-L | 0.5772 | 0.7690 | 0.8143 | 0.5050 | 0.5298 | 0.5505 |
| SSGCL-N | 0.4133 | 0.5140 | 0.5748 | 0.2808 | 0.3072 | 0.3212 |
| SSGCL-O | 0.3706 | 0.4708 | 0.5454 | 0.2455 | 0.2732 | 0.2884 |

*4.6. Hyperparameter Analysis (RQ3)*

In this subsection, we present the results of the experiments that were conducted to explore the sensitivity of several key hyperparameters in our model. Analyzing the parameter sensitivity helped us to better understand the behavior and performance of the model. Through experimenting with and evaluating different parameter values, we can understand how the model's performance changed under different settings, thereby determining the optimal parameter combination.

**The contrastive learning coefficient $\lambda_1$**: We conducted experiments on the contrastive learning coefficient $\lambda_1$, and the results are shown in Figure 4. The model performance peaked on the Last.fm and Douban-book data sets when the contrastive learning coefficient reached $1 \times 10^{-5}$. For the Yelp data set, when the contrastive learning coefficient reached $1 \times 10^{-4}$, the model performance peaked. This shows that adjusting the parameters on different data sets can optimize model performance, as different data sets exhibit varying sensitivities to parameters.

**The regularization coefficient** $\lambda_2$: We conducted experiments on the regularization coefficient $\lambda_2$. The main purpose of the regularization parameter $\lambda_2$ is to control the complexity of the model, thereby helping to prevent overfitting. When the model becomes overly complex, it may perform well on the training data but poorly on unseen data, indicating a lack of generalization to new samples. By introducing the regularization parameter, a penalty term was added to the loss function, penalizing the size of the model parameters, which made the model simpler and improved its generalization capability. The results are shown in Figure 5. We observed that when the regularization parameter was set to $1 \times 10^{-2}$, our model achieved the best performance on all data sets, which was different from the case of the contrastive learning coefficient. Additionally, we found that when we set the parameter between $1 \times 10^{-4}$ and $1 \times 10^{-8}$, the experimental results on the Douban-book and Last.fm data sets remained stable, with the graph lines leveling off. This trend was more rapid on the Yelp data set. When the parameter was set in the range of $[1 \times 10^{-2}, 1 \times 10^{-8}]$, the experimental results stabilized, and the decrease in model performance was minimal. These findings provide guidance for selecting and adjusting regularization parameters, emphasizing the importance of finding optimal parameters within a certain range to achieve stable and excellent model performance.

**The temperature coefficient of InfoNCE** $\tau$: The temperature coefficient $\tau$ plays a crucial role in adjusting the scale of the contrastive size. The main function of temperature coefficient $\tau$ is to control the proportion of positive and negative sample pairs. From a mathematical perspective, the temperature coefficient $\tau$ in Equation (8) is positioned in the denominator. Figure 6 clearly shows that, when the model parameter was set to 0.15, the best performance was achieved on all three data sets. On the Douban-book and Last.fm data sets, the model performance showed an upward trend as the value of parameter $\tau$ increased within the range [0.1, 0.15]. However, when the parameter was set to [0.15, 1], the model performance started to decline. On the Yelp data set, the model performance remained relatively stable within the range [0.1, 0.15], but exhibited a declining trend within the range of [0.15, 1]. Overall, the optimal performance was achieved when the model parameter was set to 0.15.

**Number of GNN layers**: Due to the excessive smoothing issue of GNNs, we conducted experiments to explore the best number of GNN layers for our model. The experimental results are shown in Figure 7. For the Last.fm and Yelp data sets, as the number of GNN layers increased, the model's performance improved, reaching its peak when the number of GNN layers was set to three. However, on the Douban-book data set, the model performance peaked when the GNN layers reached two. This indicates that different data sets exhibited varying sensitivities to the number of GNN layers. The Douban-book data set, being larger and more intricate in its interrelations compared with the other two data sets, further underscored the issue of excessive smoothing in graph neural networks (GNNs). When data sets exhibit denser and more diverse interaction patterns, increasing the number of GNN layers may lead to over-smoothing of the features, resulting in a loss of detail and discriminative power in the learned features.

**Noise radius** $\varepsilon$: We abandoned traditional graph augmentation methods, such as random node deletion or random edge deletion, opting instead to introduce uniform noise into the samples to construct sample pairs and simultaneously enhance the model's robustness. However, the introduction of noise must be constrained, as excessive noise can severely impact the model. Therefore, we imposed a radius constraint on the noise introduced to ensure the effectiveness and stability of the model. We conducted experiments with the noise radius parameter $\varepsilon$ set to 0.01, 0.05, 0.1, 0.2, 0.3, and 0.4. We found that the model achieved optimal performance across all three data sets when the noise radius r was set to 0.1. Moreover, as the noise radius $\varepsilon$ increased, the decreasing trend in performance tended to stabilize. This indicates that our model has a certain level of robustness. The experimental results are shown in Figure 8.

Through the parameter sensitivity experiments, we found that the data distribution varied across each data set, leading to the requirement of different parameter configurations for the model to achieve optimal performance. Therefore, we had to adjust the parameters to obtain the best performance. This also implies that in recommendation systems, we can enhance the generalization performance by adjusting the parameters. In other words, parameter adjustment can improve both the applicability and performance of the recommendation system.

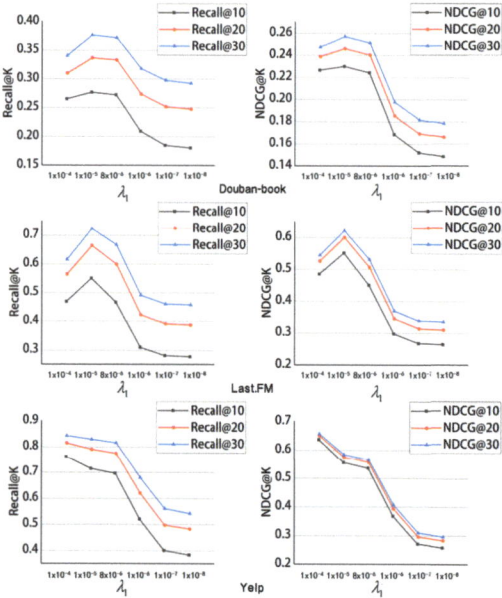

**Figure 4.** Sensitivity analysis of $\lambda_1$.

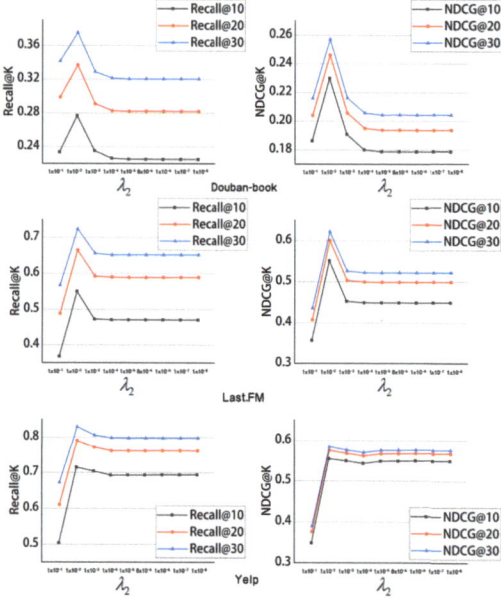

**Figure 5.** Sensitivity analysis of $\lambda_2$.

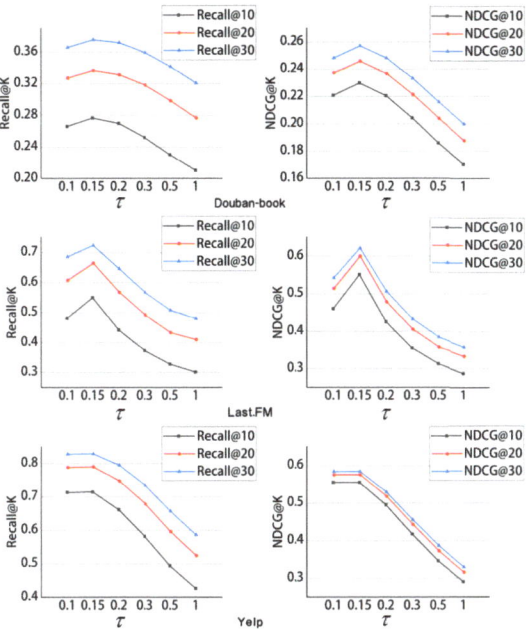

**Figure 6.** Sensitivity analysis of $\tau$.

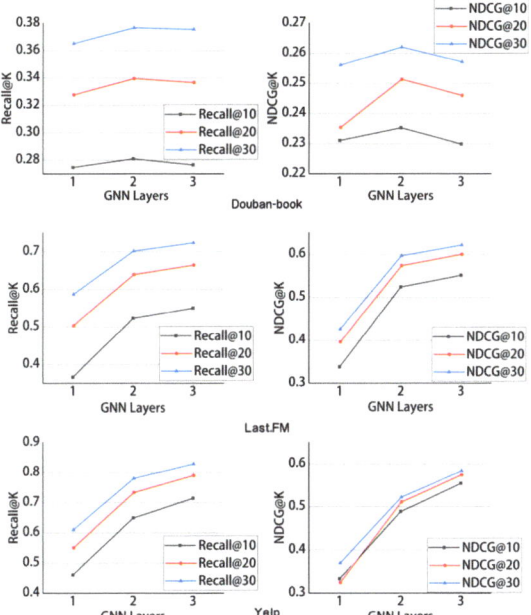

**Figure 7.** Sensitivity analysis of GNN layers.

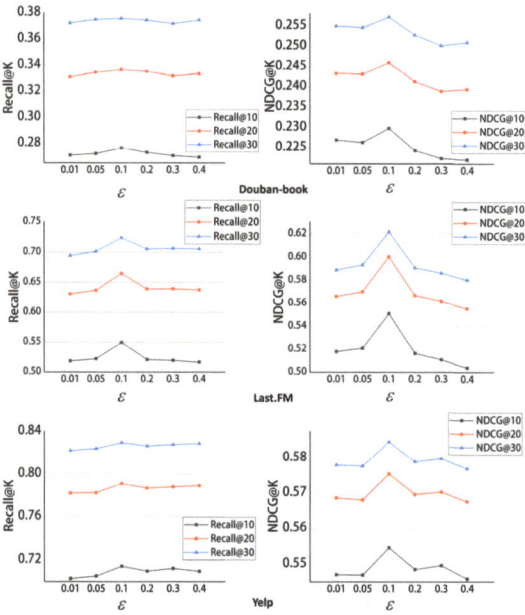

**Figure 8.** Sensitivity analysis of ε.

## 5. Conclusions and Future Work

This paper proposes a simpler and more effective social recommendation system called SSGCL. Specifically, we explore simpler aggregation methods and design a GNN-based influence diffusion module that learns informative user and item representations from both the interest network and the social network. A special contrastive learning module is then employed, which generates positive and negative samples by simply adding noises to the original node embedding to manipulate the learned representations for a better distribution. The experiments demonstrate that some of the strategies in previous social recommendation models are over-designed, while our model is effective and simple. We achieve state-of-the-art results on three public data sets in terms of two evaluation metrics.

While our recommendation model has made significant progress in terms of performance, there are other issues and limitations inherent in recommendation systems that should be recognized. For instance, most existing recommendation systems face the risk of data leakage because they utilize users' private data and do not consider privacy protection, making these data vulnerable to malicious attacks. Some companies choose to completely safeguard data or withhold labels during training to prevent data leakage. However, while this approach ensures data security, it sacrifices data interactivity, leading to sub-optimal model performance during training. Similar issues are addressed in other scenarios but not well explored for recommendation systems yet. Furthermore, social influence and algorithmic bias are also common issues in recommendation systems. Recommendation systems may excessively filter user information, causing users to only encounter information related to their interests, neglecting other important information and leading to societal fragmentation. Ensuring more diverse recommendations while improving recommendation system performance remains a challenge and a focal point for future efforts.

Although these issues are outside the scope of this paper's consideration, we intend to address them in our future work. In our future research, we aim to broaden our focus to explore the robustness of recommendation systems and their security and privacy concerns to better align with real-world applications and offer numerous intriguing avenues for future exploration. Additionally, we would also like to introduce more information, whereas this study focused solely on social recommendation systems, primarily incorporating social information. For example, there has been a surge of interest in knowledge graphs [44] within the field of recommendation systems. In this way, we can potentially uncover more latent relationships and achieve superior performance.

Regarding future work, as mentioned, there has been a surge of interest in knowledge graphs [44] within the field of recommendation systems. Knowledge graphs offer the capability to integrate various types of data, whereas this study focused solely on social recommendation systems, primarily incorporating social information. Introducing knowledge graphs into recommendation systems could potentially enrich the system with a broader range of information, thereby uncovering more latent relationships and achieving superior performance. On the other hand, incorporating additional information into recommendation systems may pose challenges, such as compromising model robustness and introducing excessive noise [19]. In our future research endeavors, we aim to broaden our focus beyond solely self-supervised learning of graphs. Instead, we intend to explore a wider array of topics, including the semi-supervised learning of graphs [45], the security of graph data [46], and privacy concerns in graph recommendation systems [47]. This expansion will enable our recommendation systems to better align with real-world applications and offer numerous intriguing avenues for future exploration.

**Author Contributions:** Methodology, W.Z.; Writing – original draft, Z.D.; Writing—review & editing, C.W. All authors have read and agreed to the published version of the manuscript.

**Funding:** This research received no external funding.

**Data Availability Statement:** The data sets used in our experiments are all publicly available. We have made the code publicly available on github and implemented it using PyTorch. https://github.com/0Nagatuki0/SSGCL.git.

**Conflicts of Interest:** The authors declare no conflicts of interest.

# References

1. Gong, X.; Feng, Q.; Zhang, Y.; Qin, J.; Ding, W.; Li, B.; Jiang, P.; Gai, K. Real-time Short Video Recommendation on Mobile Devices. In Proceedings of the 31st ACM International Conference on Information & Knowledge Management, Atlanta, GA, USA, 17–21 October 2022; pp. 3103–3112.
2. Fan, W.; Ma, Y.; Li, Q.; He, Y.; Zhao, E.; Tang, J.; Yin, D. Graph neural networks for social recommendation. In Proceedings of the World Wide Web Conference, San Francisco, CA, USA, 13–17 May 2019; pp. 417–426.
3. Volokhin, S.; Collins, M.D.; Rokhlenko, O.; Agichtein, E. Augmenting Graph Convolutional Networks with Textual Data for Recommendations. In Proceedings of the European Conference on Information Retrieval, Dublin, Ireland, 2 April 2023; Springer: Berlin/Heidelberg, Germany, 2023; pp. 664–675.
4. Shi, Y.; Larson, M.; Hanjalic, A. List-wise learning to rank with matrix factorization for collaborative filtering. In Proceedings of the Fourth ACM Conference on Recommender Systems, Barcelona, Spain, 26–30 September 2010; pp. 269–272.
5. Koren, Y.; Bell, R.; Volinsky, C. Matrix factorization techniques for recommender systems. *Computer* **2009**, *42*, 30–37. [CrossRef]
6. Abdollahi, B.; Nasraoui, O. Explainable matrix factorization for collaborative filtering. In Proceedings of the 25th International Conference Companion on World Wide Web, Montreal, QC, Canada, 11–15 April 2016; pp. 5–6.
7. Liu, X.; Aggarwal, C.; Li, Y.F.; Kong, X.; Sun, X.; Sathe, S. Kernelized matrix factorization for collaborative filtering. In Proceedings of the 2016 SIAM International Conference on Data Mining, Miami, FL, USA, 5–7 May 2016; pp. 378–386.
8. Baltrunas, L.; Ludwig, B.; Ricci, F. Matrix factorization techniques for context aware recommendation. In Proceedings of the Fifth ACM Conference on Recommender Systems, Chicago, IL, USA, 23–27 October 2011; pp. 301–304.
9. Nguyen, J.; Zhu, M. Content-boosted matrix factorization techniques for recommender systems. *Stat. Anal. Data Min. ASA Data Sci. J.* **2013**, *6*, 286–301. [CrossRef]
10. Yu, H.F.; Hsieh, C.J.; Si, S.; Dhillon, I.S. Parallel matrix factorization for recommender systems. *Knowl. Inf. Syst.* **2014**, *41*, 793–819. [CrossRef]
11. Kumar, R.; Verma, B.; Rastogi, S.S. Social popularity based SVD++ recommender system. *Int. J. Comput. Appl.* **2014**, *87*, 33–37. [CrossRef]
12. Wu, S.; Sun, F.; Zhang, W.; Xie, X.; Cui, B. Graph neural networks in recommender systems: A survey. *ACM Comput. Surv.* **2022**, *55*, 1–37. [CrossRef]
13. Scarselli, F.; Gori, M.; Tsoi, A.C.; Hagenbuchner, M.; Monfardini, G. The graph neural network model. *IEEE Trans. Neural Netw.* **2008**, *20*, 61–80. [CrossRef]
14. Zhou, J.; Cui, G.; Hu, S.; Zhang, Z.; Yang, C.; Liu, Z.; Wang, L.; Li, C.; Sun, M. Graph neural networks: A review of methods and applications. *AI Open* **2020**, *1*, 57–81. [CrossRef]

15. Yin, R.; Li, K.; Zhang, G.; Lu, J. A deeper graph neural network for recommender systems. *Knowl.-Based Syst.* **2019**, *185*, 105020. [CrossRef]
16. Huang, T.; Dong, Y.; Ding, M.; Yang, Z.; Feng, W.; Wang, X.; Tang, J. MixGCF: An improved training method for graph neural network-based recommender systems. In Proceedings of the 27th ACM SIGKDD Conference on Knowledge Discovery & Data Mining, Online, 14–18 August 2021; pp. 665–674.
17. Xia, L.; Huang, C.; Xu, Y.; Dai, P.; Bo, L. Multi-behavior graph neural networks for recommender system. *IEEE Trans. Neural Netw. Learn. Syst.* **2022**, *35*, 5473–5487. [CrossRef]
18. Wang, C.; Pan, S.; Hu, R.; Long, G.; Jiang, J.; Zhang, C. Attributed graph clustering: A deep attentional embedding approach. *arXiv* **2019**, arXiv:1906.06532.
19. Berahmand, K.; Daneshfar, F.; Salehi, E.S.; Li, Y.; Xu, Y. Autoencoders and their applications in machine learning: A survey. *Artif. Intell. Rev.* **2024**, *57*, 28. [CrossRef]
20. Daneshfar, F.; Soleymanbaigi, S.; Nafisi, A.; Yamini, P. Elastic deep autoencoder for text embedding clustering by an improved graph regularization. *Expert Syst. Appl.* **2024**, *238*, 121780. [CrossRef]
21. Chen, T.; Kornblith, S.; Norouzi, M.; Hinton, G. A simple framework for contrastive learning of visual representations. In Proceedings of the International Conference on Machine Learning, PMLR, Online, 13–18 July 2020; pp. 1597–1607.
22. He, K.; Fan, H.; Wu, Y.; Xie, S.; Girshick, R. Momentum contrast for unsupervised visual representation learning. In Proceedings of the IEEE/CVF Conference on Computer Vision and Pattern Recognition, Seattle, WA, USA, 13–19 June 2020; pp. 9729–9738.
23. Wu, J.; Wang, X.; Feng, F.; He, X.; Chen, L.; Lian, J.; Xie, X. Self-supervised graph learning for recommendation. In Proceedings of the 44th International ACM SIGIR Conference on Research and Development in Information Retrieval, Online, 11–15 July 2021; pp. 726–735.
24. Wang, H.; Zhang, J.; Zhu, Q.; Huang, W. Augmentation-free graph contrastive learning with performance guarantee. *arXiv* **2022**, arXiv:2204.04874.
25. Kipf, T.N.; Welling, M. Semi-supervised classification with graph convolutional networks. *arXiv* **2016**, arXiv:1609.02907.
26. Jamali, M.; Ester, M. A matrix factorization technique with trust propagation for recommendation in social networks. In Proceedings of the Fourth ACM Conference on Recommender Systems, Barcelona, Spain, 26–30 September 2010; pp. 135–142.
27. Yang, B.; Lei, Y.; Liu, J.; Li, W. Social collaborative filtering by trust. *IEEE Trans. Pattern Anal. Mach. Intell.* **2016**, *39*, 1633–1647. [CrossRef] [PubMed]
28. Rendle, S.; Freudenthaler, C.; Gantner, Z.; Schmidt-Thieme, L. BPR: Bayesian personalized ranking from implicit feedback. *arXiv* **2012**, arXiv:1205.2618.
29. Yang, L.; Cao, X.; He, D.; Wang, C.; Wang, X.; Zhang, W. Modularity based community detection with deep learning. In Proceedings of the IJCAI, New York, NY, USA, 9–15 July 2016; Volume 16, pp. 2252–2258.
30. Wang, X.; He, X.; Wang, M.; Feng, F.; Chua, T.S. Neural graph collaborative filtering. In Proceedings of the 42nd International ACM SIGIR Conference on Research and Development in Information Retrieval, Paris, France, 21–25 July 2019; pp. 165–174.
31. Wu, L.; Li, J.; Sun, P.; Hong, R.; Ge, Y.; Wang, M. Diffnet++: A neural influence and interest diffusion network for social recommendation. *IEEE Trans. Knowl. Data Eng.* **2020**, *34*, 4753–4766. [CrossRef]
32. Yang, L.; Liu, Z.; Dou, Y.; Ma, J.; Yu, P.S. ConsisRec: Enhancing GNN for social recommendation via consistent neighbor aggregation. In Proceedings of the 44th International ACM SIGIR Conference on Research and Development in Information Retrieval, Online, 11–15 July 2021; pp. 2141–2145.
33. He, X.; Deng, K.; Wang, X.; Li, Y.; Zhang, Y.; Wang, M. LightGCN: Simplifying and powering graph convolution network for recommendation. In Proceedings of the 43rd International ACM SIGIR Conference on Research and Development in Information Retrieval, Online, 25–30 July 2020; pp. 639–648.
34. Xia, J.; Wu, L.; Chen, J.; Hu, B.; Li, S.Z. SimGRACE: A simple framework for graph contrastive learning without data augmentation. In Proceedings of the ACM Web Conference 2022, Online, 25–29 April 2022; pp. 1070–1079.
35. Cai, X.; Huang, C.; Xia, L.; Ren, X. LightGCL: Simple Yet Effective Graph Contrastive Learning for Recommendation. *arXiv* **2023**, arXiv:2302.08191.
36. Yu, J.; Yin, H.; Xia, X.; Chen, T.; Cui, L.; Nguyen, Q.V.H. Are graph augmentations necessary? Simple graph contrastive learning for recommendation. In Proceedings of the 45th International ACM SIGIR Conference on Research and Development in Information Retrieval, Madrid, Spain, 11–15 July 2022; pp. 1294–1303.
37. Chai, T.; Draxler, R.R. Root mean square error (RMSE) or mean absolute error (MAE)?–Arguments against avoiding RMSE in the literature. *Geosci. Model Dev.* **2014**, *7*, 1247–1250. [CrossRef]
38. Oord, A.v.d.; Li, Y.; Vinyals, O. Representation learning with contrastive predictive coding. *arXiv* **2018**, arXiv:1807.03748.
39. Karakayali, N.; Kostem, B.; Galip, I. Recommendation systems as technologies of the self: Algorithmic control and the formation of music taste. *Theory, Cult. Soc.* **2018**, *35*, 3–24. [CrossRef]
40. Zhao, W.X.; Mu, S.; Hou, Y.; Lin, Z.; Chen, Y.; Pan, X.; Li, K.; Lu, Y.; Wang, H.; Tian, C.; et al. RecBole: Towards a unified, comprehensive and efficient framework for recommendation algorithms. In Proceedings of the 30th ACM International Conference on Information & Knowledge Management, Online, 1–5 November 2021; pp. 4653–4664.
41. Yu, J.; Yin, H.; Gao, M.; Xia, X.; Zhang, X.; Viet Hung, N.Q. Socially-aware self-supervised tri-training for recommendation. In Proceedings of the 27th ACM SIGKDD Conference on Knowledge Discovery & Data Mining, Online, 14–18 August 2021; pp. 2084–2092.

42. Yu, J.; Yin, H.; Li, J.; Wang, Q.; Hung, N.Q.V.; Zhang, X. Self-supervised multi-channel hypergraph convolutional network for social recommendation. In Proceedings of the Web Conference 2021, Ljubljana, Slovenia, 19–23 April 2021; pp. 413–424.
43. Gao, Y.; Du, Y.; Hu, Y.; Chen, L.; Zhu, X.; Fang, Z.; Zheng, B. Self-guided learning to denoise for robust recommendation. In Proceedings of the 45th International ACM SIGIR Conference on Research and Development in Information Retrieval, Madrid, Spain, 11–15 July 2022; pp. 1412–1422.
44. Yang, Y.; Huang, C.; Xia, L.; Li, C. Knowledge graph contrastive learning for recommendation. In Proceedings of the 45th International ACM SIGIR Conference on Research and Development in Information Retrieval, Madrid, Spain, 11–15 July 2022; pp. 1434–1443.
45. Daneshfar, F.; Soleymanbaigi, S.; Yamini, P.; Amini, M.S. A survey on semi-supervised graph clustering. *Eng. Appl. Artif. Intell.* **2024**, *133*, 108215. [CrossRef]
46. Sun, L.; Dou, Y.; Yang, C.; Zhang, K.; Wang, J.; Philip, S.Y.; He, L.; Li, B. Adversarial attack and defense on graph data: A survey. *IEEE Trans. Knowl. Data Eng.* **2022**, *35*, 7693–7711. [CrossRef]
47. Zhang, S.; Yin, H.; Chen, T.; Huang, Z.; Cui, L.; Zhang, X. Graph embedding for recommendation against attribute inference attacks. In Proceedings of the Web Conference 2021, Ljubljana, Slovenia, 19–23 April 2021; pp. 3002–3014.

**Disclaimer/Publisher's Note:** The statements, opinions and data contained in all publications are solely those of the individual author(s) and contributor(s) and not of MDPI and/or the editor(s). MDPI and/or the editor(s) disclaim responsibility for any injury to people or property resulting from any ideas, methods, instructions or products referred to in the content.

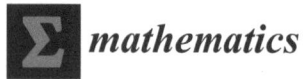

*Article*

# ARS-Chain: A Blockchain-Based Anonymous Reputation-Sharing Framework for E-Commerce Platforms

Yungui Chen [1,2], Li Feng [3,*], Qinglin Zhao [3], Liwei Tian [1,2] and Lei Yang [1,2]

1 School of Computer Science, Guangdong University of Science and Technology, Dongguan 523000, China; chenyungui@gdust.edu.cn (Y.C.); tianliwei@gdust.edu.cn (L.T.); yanglei@gdust.edu.cn (L.Y.)
2 Faculty of Digital Science and Technology, Macau Millennium College, Macao SAR 999078, China
3 School of Computer Science and Engineering, Faculty of Innovation Engineering, Macau University of Science and Technology, Macao SAR 999078, China; qlzhao@must.edu.mo
* Correspondence: lfeng@must.edu.mo

**Abstract:** E-commerce platforms incorporate reputation systems that allow buyers to rate sellers after transactions. However, existing reputation systems face challenges such as privacy leakage, linkability, and multiple rating attacks. The feedback data can inadvertently expose user information privacy because they reveal the buyers' identities and preferences, which deters a significant number of users from providing their ratings. Moreover, malicious actors can exploit data analysis and machine learning techniques to mine user privacy from the rating data, posing serious threats to user security and trust. This study introduces ARS-Chain, a pioneering and secure blockchain-driven anonymous reputation-sharing framework tailored for e-commerce platforms. The core of ARS-Chain is a dynamic ring addition mechanism with linkable ring signatures (LRS), where the number of LRS rings is dynamically added in alignment with the evolving purchase list, and LRS link tags are constructed with the LRS rings and item identifiers. Further, a consortium blockchain is introduced to store these anonymous ratings on e-commerce platforms. As a result, ARS-Chain ensures full anonymity while achieving cross-platform reputation sharing, making rating records unlinkable, and effectively countering multiple rating attacks. The experimental results confirm that ARS-Chain significantly enhances user information privacy protection while maintaining system performance, having an important impact on the construction of trust mechanisms for e-commerce platforms.

**Keywords:** user information privacy; data security; decentralized reputation system; blockchain; linkable ring signatures

**MSC:** 68Uxx

**Citation:** Chen, Y.; Feng, L.; Zhao, Q.; Tian, L.; Yang, L. ARS-Chain: A Blockchain-Based Anonymous Reputation-Sharing Framework for E-Commerce Platforms. *Mathematics* **2024**, *12*, 1480. https://doi.org/10.3390/math12101480

Academic Editor: Antanas Cenys

Received: 6 April 2024
Revised: 26 April 2024
Accepted: 6 May 2024
Published: 10 May 2024

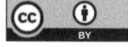

**Copyright:** © 2024 by the authors. Licensee MDPI, Basel, Switzerland. This article is an open access article distributed under the terms and conditions of the Creative Commons Attribution (CC BY) license (https://creativecommons.org/licenses/by/4.0/).

## 1. Introduction

E-commerce is a prevalent feature of modern society, notably in countries like the United States and China, where it constitutes a significant portion of daily consumer purchases [1]. Mainstream e-commerce platforms incorporate reputation systems, which play a crucial role in guiding consumers' decision-making [2]. By enabling users to appraise and critique sellers upon their encounters, these systems provide invaluable perspectives on the quality of products and services. This nurtures trust and mitigates the ambiguities associated with virtual transactions. These assessments serve as instrumental aids for prospective purchasers. However, a notable challenge emerges. Sellers and buyers frequently maintain profiles on several platforms, and the absence of a holistic reputation system that amalgamates feedback from diverse sources hinders a comprehensive grasp of a seller's reliability. This cross-platform reputation synchronization deficit could compromise a consumer's capacity to make astute buying judgments [3]. Therefore, there is a need for a reputation-sharing system based on multiple platforms in the e-commerce industry.

In addition, existing reputation systems face challenges such as privacy breaches, linkability, and multiple rating attacks. Feedback data may unintentionally expose user information privacy as they reveal the buyer's identity and preferences, which can prevent a large number of users from providing their rating. Specifically, malicious actors can use data analysis and machine learning techniques to mine user's private information from rating data [4,5], posing a serious threat to user security and trust. For example, data analysts or hackers can use machine learning techniques to analyze rating data and purchase history, identify specific users' identities, and infer their purchasing preferences and consumption habits. Therefore, it is imperative to design a reputation system that achieves cross-platform reputation sharing while protecting user privacy.

A conventional approach in multi-platform reputation systems involves the deployment of a trusted third-party institution for managing users' reputation data, giving rise to numerous centralization-related issues. Centralized systems, prone to single-point-of-failure problems, are vulnerable to attacks and operational failures [6]. Furthermore, centralized systems' data and authority amalgamation may precipitate power misuse, censorship, and data leakage risks [7]. Simultaneously, the central node's processing capabilities limit the scalability and performance of centralized systems, thereby stunting system advancement [8]. In contrast, decentralized systems provide higher resilience, security, and transparency through distributed architecture [9].

Blockchain technology, specifically consortium blockchain, promises potential solutions to these issues with its inherent advantages in reputation sharing and privacy protection [10]. However, blockchain's anonymity does not guard against linkability and multiple rating attacks. The term "Linkability" refers to the possibility of malicious users linking two pieces of information based on historical rating data. "Multiple rating attacks" occur when a single purchase record is rated in an e-commerce system more than once [11].

*1.1. Motivation*

In mainstream e-commerce frameworks, enterprises' confidentiality is often compromised, necessitating the revelation of specifics like their business identity and location. With such transparency, consumers can make informed decisions and establish trust with merchants. However, ensuring consumers' privacy is paramount in online transactions. There is growing concern among consumers about the safety of their privacy data. This concern indicates that confidence in online shopping platforms could erode if adequate measures are not in place to protect their privacy. Such concerns are particularly pronounced within reputation mechanisms. Here, potential buyers rely on insights and feedback from previous customers to judge a seller's trustworthiness. If privacy is not maintained, consumers might hesitate to engage with these reputation systems or even refrain from transacting on the platform.

Unlinkability is a higher requirement for privacy protection. In Figure 1, Alice provides ratings after purchasing medications on platforms A and B. These ratings entered the e-commerce reputation system, assessing the seller's service and product quality. However, sellers and malicious actors may mine the potential associations of these ratings through manual or data analysis and machine learning methods. Consequently, consumers might worry about personal information security; people might choose silence and discontinue publishing their evaluations, weakening the e-commerce reputation system.

Given the above, our research aims to devise a solution addressing the following challenges:

Multi-platform Reputation Sharing: Our core objective is enabling reputation sharing across multiple e-commerce platforms. In today's segmented digital marketplace, consumers navigate various independent systems, each with unique reputation mechanisms. The absence of a standard reputation system makes it harder for sellers to build trust and complicates the buying process for consumers. We envisage a unified, comprehensive reputation management approach for multi-platform reputation sharing.

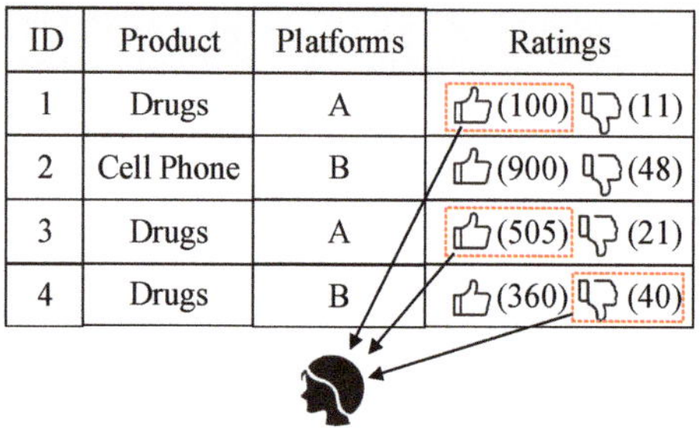

| ID | Product | Platforms | Ratings |
|---|---|---|---|
| 1 | Drugs | A | 👍(100) 👎(11) |
| 2 | Cell Phone | B | 👍(900) 👎(48) |
| 3 | Drugs | A | 👍(505) 👎(21) |
| 4 | Drugs | B | 👍(360) 👎(40) |

**Figure 1.** Malicious users can mine the potential associations of ratings through manual or data analysis and machine learning methods.

Full Anonymity and Rating Validity Verification: Full anonymity in the reputation system implies that the user's personal information remains anonymous to unrelated users, platform administrators, and sellers. Ensuring full anonymity presents a challenge to the validity of ratings: how can one ascertain the legitimacy of anonymous users?

Unlinkability: Unlinkability serves as a safeguard to protect users from potential exploitation. We aim to create a system that effectively prevents malicious entities from linking two different pieces of information (rating records) together using historical data, thus safeguarding users from potential targeted attacks.

Prevention of multiple rating attacks: Our system will prevent users from rating repeatedly upon the same purchase record, thereby avoiding the possibility of distorting reputation scores.

It is crucial to note that our architectural framework does not guarantee sellers' privacy. Buyers need access to sufficient information to assess the seller's reputation, mirroring real-world situations.

*1.2. Contributions*

We propose ARS-Chain, a multi-platform reputation-sharing system based on a consortium blockchain, to address the outlined challenges. E-commerce platforms act as blockchain nodes in ARS-Chain to maintain a distributed ledger through consensus mechanisms. Buyers remain anonymous to sellers, platform administrators, and other users during the evaluation process, utilizing a one-time pseudonym for each evaluation. The system provides unlinkability of evaluation records through one-time pseudonyms, allowing users to participate in evaluations with peace of mind. Furthermore, the system prevents users from repeating their evaluation behavior.

Our research contributes to the body of knowledge in the following ways:

(1) This research proposes ARS-Chain, a novel blockchain-based anonymous reputationsharing system for e-commerce platforms. It is designed to foster reputation sharing among multiple platforms, providing buyers with global reputation data regarding sellers.
(2) This research outlines the design of a new dynamic ring addition mechanism in the linkable ring signatures scheme where the quantity of rings dynamically increases over time. The dynamic ring addition mechanism reduces the LRS group size to a small scale. In addition, the link tags are meticulously constructed using rings and item identifiers. These combined enhancements enable ARS-Chain to achieve full anonymity, unlinkability of rating records, and to resist multiple rating attacks.
(3) This research also involved conducting validity and performance experiments to evaluate the system. The validity experiments demonstrate that ARS-Chain achieves its design goals of anonymity, unlinkability, and prevention of multiple rating attacks. The performance experiments show that the system performs well in terms of runtime, memory consumption, and network overhead under our dynamic ring addition mechanism.

## 2. Related Work

Early research on reputation systems centered on single-platform or centralized models. Blömer [12] leveraged group signatures in designing a reputation management system specific to a single platform. Bethencourt et al. [13] introduced a unique cryptographic primitive termed 'reputation signature'. The reputation signature allows for the efficient proof and verification of reputation without disclosing the user's identity. Zhai et al. [14] introduced 'AnonRep', a system that integrates cryptographic primitives like verifiable shuffle, linkable ring signatures, and homomorphic encryption to streamline reputation calculation, updating, and verification.

Many researchers introduce decentralized technology or blockchain technology to reputation management. PrivBox [15], a decentralized reputation system, harnesses homomorphic encryption and zero-knowledge proofs to safeguard user privacy during online transactions. It eliminates the need for trusted intermediaries or user groups in processing feedback scores.

Attempts have been made to design reputation-sharing systems suitable for specific scenarios. Grinshpoun et al. [16] unveiled models allowing users to migrate their reputation scores between virtual communities based on trust and similarity metrics. Shen et al. [17] constructed a training model for privacy-preserving support vector machines, allowing reputation score sharing without compromising user identity. Wang et al. [18] utilized blockchain for cross-domain reputation sharing, introducing personalized tags as quality indicators. In our previous work, RS-chain [19] used a trusted execution environment (TEE) to ensure reputation integrity during reputation-sharing processes. Despite these strides, existing solutions often neglect challenges like anonymity, unlinkability, and the threat of multiple rating attacks. RepChain [11] and this paper are the closest in addressing the issues mentioned above while focusing on reputation sharing across multiple platforms.

Researchers have looked into how blockchain-based applications can preserve user privacy. Comparing blockchain-based privacy protection reputation systems with traditional reputation systems, Hasan et al. [20] emphasized the benefits of the blockchain-based privacy-preserving reputation system, including its immutability, transparency, and trustlessness. X. Li et al. [21] presented a blockchain privacy protection system based on ring signatures. Utilizing ring signatures on elliptic curves, the author created a private data storage system that guarantees user identification and data security in blockchain applications. The BPP [22] combined blockchain and public key encryption techniques to achieve secure data sharing, data retrieval, and data access while ensuring the interests of users and the correctness of query results. Han et al. [23] introduced a privacy protection scheme for personal credit score calculation based on zero-knowledge proof, which considered the authenticity verification of multi-dimensional user data and proposed a universal verification platform based on blockchain. Wu et al. [24] proposed an efficient and privacy-preserving traceable attribute-based encryption scheme, which used blockchain technology to ensure the integrity and non-repudiation of data. Casino and Patsakis [25] used a decentralized locality-sensitive hashing classification and a series of recommendation methods to improve the efficiency and accuracy of the reputation system. These studies provided us with inspiration for designing a blockchain-based reputation-sharing framework in terms of privacy protection. However, these works did not address the issue of reputation sharing in multi-platform e-commerce scenarios, which is the main focus of our work.

Our work aims to design a reputation-sharing framework across multiple platforms, providing support for decentralization, anonymity, unlinkability of ratings, and prevention of multiple rating attacks. As shown in Table 1, most existing works only focus on a subset of the design goals. RepChain [11] is the closest to our work, but RepChain uses a combination of techniques such as blind signatures, zero-knowledge range proofs, secure multi-party computation, and consensus hashing, which is far more complex than our work.

Table 1. Brief comparison of repchain and existing work.

| Property | Existing Work |
| --- | --- |
| Decentralization | [11,15,18–25] |
| Anonymity | [11–15,17,20,21,23,24] |
| Unlinkability of Ratings | [11,14] |
| Prevention of Multiple Rating Attacks | [11,14] |
| Multi-platform Support | [11,16–19,22] |

## 3. Preliminaries

This section briefly revisits two pivotal technologies: consortium blockchain and linkable ring signatures.

### 3.1. Consortium Blockchain

A consortium blockchain [26] is a semi-decentralized blockchain architecture maintained by a selected group of nodes, typically organizational or corporate entities, regulated through strict permission controls. Compared to public blockchains, consortium blockchains are suitable for scenarios requiring high trust and permission management, such as supply chain management, financial services, and cross-organizational data exchange. Consortium blockchain F can be defined as an ordered triplet $F = (N, T, P)$, where:

$N$ encapsulates the ensemble of nodes within the network.

$T$ represents the aggregation of transactions.

$P$ denotes a set that spells out permissions or governing rules.

Given its semi-decentralized essence, consortium chains are particularly apt for applications like supply chain management, financial services, and cross-organizational data exchange, aligning seamlessly with the objectives of this research. Within the realm of consortium blockchains, Byzantine Fault Tolerance (BFT) or its pragmatic variant, Practical Byzantine Fault Tolerance (PBFT), often emerge as the consensus algorithms of choice [27].

### 3.2. Linkable Ring Signatures

Linkable ring signatures (LRS) [28,29] are a fascinating cryptographic scheme that enables users to sign anonymously yet traceably. This system endows a user with the capability to append an anonymous signature amidst a set of users (i.e., a "ring"), all the while ensuring that a singular user does not produce multiple distinct signatures. Unlike classical ring signatures [30], linkable variants possess a salient attribute: should a user sign the same information multiple times, these signatures can be intricately linked. In this work, buyers use LRS to sign ratings when evaluating sellers or products, and the verifiers (sellers or other users) cannot identify the signer from the signature, thus protecting the signer's privacy. Additionally, if the signer makes two ratings based on the same purchase, the second rating will be recognized by the verifier and discarded by the system. LRS primarily includes the following four algorithms:

1. Key Pair Generation Algorithm: A key pair, delineated as $(SK, PK)$, is composed of a private key, $SK$, intertwined with its public counterpart, $PK$.

$$(SP, PK) \leftarrow KeyGen() \qquad (1)$$

where $KeyGen()$ is the cryptographic key-generating function.

2. Signature Generation Algorithm: As a ring member, a signer orchestrates the signing operation.

$$\sigma \leftarrow Sign(SK, R, m, T) \qquad (2)$$

wherein:

$\sigma$ stands as the signature.

$SK$ is the signer's private key.

$R$ is the ring, characterized by $n$ public keys $\{PK_1, PK_2, \ldots, PK_n\}$.
$m$ is the message awaiting its signature.
$T$ is the link tag.
*Sign()* functions as the signing procedure.

3. Signature Verification Algorithm: The outcome of the signature verification function can either be 1, signifying the legitimacy of the signature and the signer's membership in the ring, or 0, denoting its rejection.

$$0 \mid 1 \leftarrow Verify(\sigma, R, m, T) \quad (3)$$

4. Linkability Verification Algorithm: The *Link()* function, assessing linkability, ingests two signatures, $\sigma_1$ and $\sigma_2$, and exudes a Boolean output, indicating whether these signatures come from the same signer and are based on the same link tag.

$$0 \mid 1 \leftarrow Link(\sigma_1, \sigma_2) \quad (4)$$

## 4. ARS-Chain Overview

This section presents the system architecture, threat model, and security assumptions.

### 4.1. System Architecture

ARS-Chain is a reputation-sharing framework designed for multiple e-commerce platforms, consisting of two parts: e-commerce platforms and blockchain, as shown in Figure 2.

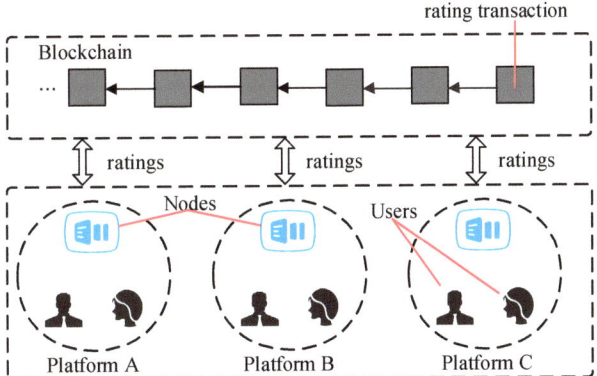

**Figure 2.** System architecture of ARS-Chain.

The platforms are e-commerce websites that join the ARS-Chain framework, such as Amazon. They provide online services for consumers and merchants. In order to provide more comprehensive reputation queries for users, the e-commerce platforms apply to join the ARS-Chain reputation system from a certificate authority (CA). The CA is an e-commerce business association jointly created by all platforms. The CA generates system parameters and encryption keys for users and platforms.

Users: In ARS-Chain, users are categorized into two main groups: buyers and sellers. Acting as the raters, the buyers enjoy the cloak of privacy conferred by the system. Conversely, the sellers, acting as the ratees, have openly disclosed information. In the ARS-Chain ecosystem, both buyers and sellers have the latitude to navigate freely among multiple platforms. Buyers furnish the system with evaluative feedback concerning the sellers.

Rating: Upon receipt of the merchandise, the buyer finalizes his seller rating. The rating should be a real number between a range [low, high], for the sake of conciseness in this study, dichotomized into two distinct values: "+1" or "−1". After formulating this assessment, the buyer employs the linkable ring signatures methodology to sign the ratings. These signed messages are then dispatched to the proximate node in the system.

Blockchain Network Configuration: The blockchain in ARS-Chain is a consortium chain, similar to Hyperledger Fabric [31], maintained by several e-commerce platforms. Each block stores rating transactions in the system.

Nodes: Constituted by servers from various platforms, nodes are vested with the responsibility of aggregating ratings uploaded by buyers, and they also participate in the blockchain consensus mechanism. During the consensus-building phase, each node has the potential to become a consensus node. Consensus nodes are tasked with the duty of block packaging. It should be noted that, in order to ensure the security of the consortium blockchain, it is usually required that at least a sufficient number of consensus nodes participate in the consensus process. Considering this, an e-commerce platform needs to provide multiple servers as blockchain nodes.

Consensus protocol: In alignment with industry consensus, as cited in [27], ARS-Chain adopts the Practical Byzantine Fault Tolerance Algorithm (PBFT) as its consensus protocol.

Rating transactions: The nodes use the signature verification algorithm and the linkability verification algorithm of the linkable ring signature to verify the ratings. The ratings that pass the verifications are valid, called rating transactions, which will be packaged into the blockchain.

### 4.2. Threat Model and Assumptions

The adversaries in the system encompass troublemakers, malicious sellers, malicious buyers, and platform administrators.

(1) Troublemakers: These entities possess an inherent desire to trace sensitive data from other users, such as purchase records of buyers and evaluative feedback given to sellers, and subsequently link these bits of information together.

(2) Malicious Sellers: Upon receipt of negative reviews, these sellers become increasingly inquisitive about the source, prompting them to transform into system adversaries in their quest for identification.

(3) Malicious Buyers: Motivated by excessive admiration or significant disapproval, such buyers might submit redundant ratings.

(4) Platform Administrators: There exists a potential for platform stewards to compromise sensitive platform data for monetary gains [32,33]. While platform investors find such actions deeply concerning, regrettably, these occurrences are not uncommon in reality.

ARS-Chain stands as a system that fosters reputation sharing across multiple platforms. In this ecosystem, the accounts of ratees (sellers) across varying platforms should possess linkability. We postulate that sellers must employ uniform metadata for the registration process when they register on diverse platforms. For corporate sellers, their official registration certificate is deemed viable. ARS-Chain commits to protecting buyer-centric information, sidelining seller privacy—a stance harmonious with prevailing e-commerce platform conventions. We assume that cryptographic tools such as hash functions, key distribution, and signature schemes are secure, and the protection of these tools is beyond the scope of this study. Further, we believe that users are adept at safeguarding their private keys while their public counterparts can be freely disclosed.

## 5. ARS-Chain System Design

In this section, we elucidate the intricacies of the ARS-Chain system design, encompassing the dynamic ring addition LRS Scheme, link tag construction, and the system's operational workflow.

### 5.1. Dynamic Ring Addition Mechanism

We propose a dynamic ring addition mechanism for the LRS scheme in the ARS-Chain. The scheme entails dynamically constructed rings to provide buyers anonymity while forestalling duplicate ratings and ensuring execution efficiency. Under this scheme, buyers are orchestrated into a ring of size *n*, predicated on their purchasing sequence. As illustrated in Figure 3, each signature ring should comprise *j* consensus nodes, one buyer, and *k* sellers. When a buyer acts as a signer to rate a review, the other members in the ring become verifiers of the signature. The ring *R* can be articulated as follows:

$$R_i^{item\_id} = \{PK_{i1},\ PK_{i2},\ldots,PK_{ik}, PK_{item\_id}\} \cup CN \quad (5)$$

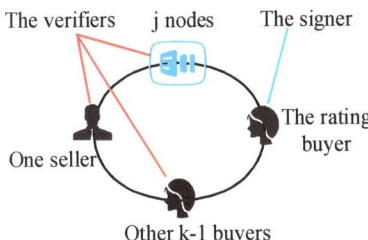

**Figure 3.** Composition of signature rings in ARS-Chain.

Herein, *item_id* denotes the item number, *i* represents the *i*th signature ring under the item number *item_id*, $PK_{item\_id}$ is the public key of the seller of the item numbered *item_id*, and the set $\{PK_{i1}, PK_{i2},\ldots,PK_{ik}\}$ encompasses the public keys of the *k* buyers of the item numbered *item_id*. *CN* represents a collection of the consensus nodes' public keys, defined as follows:

$$CN = \{PK_{N1},\ PK_{N2},\ldots,PK_{Nj}\} \quad (6)$$

The consensus nodes are *j* nodes $\{N1, N1,\ldots, Nj\}$.

The dynamic ring addition LRS scheme, as illustrated in Figure 4, shows that with $n = 100$ and $j = 10$, the number of buyers within the ring, denoted as *k*, is evaluated as $k = n - j - 1 = 89$. In this model, the purchasers of the item numbered *item_id* are allocated into distinct signature rings based on the purchase order: buyers 1 to 89 formulate ring 1, buyers 90 to 178 formulate ring 2, and so on. The benefit of the dynamic ring addition LRS scheme is that it divides large-scale e-commerce transactions into smaller signature rings, thereby reducing the computational overhead within the ring.

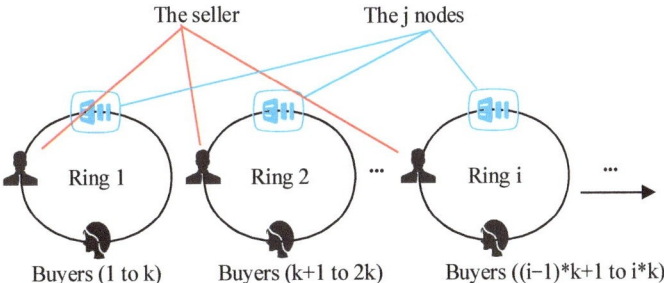

**Figure 4.** Dynamic ring addition LRS scheme.

*5.2. Link Tag Construction*

Link tag [29,34] in LRS addresses issues within ring signatures, such as double-spending or repeated signing. The system can identify whether the same entity has signed multiple times by employing link tags, thereby thwarting malicious activities. The computation formula for the link tag is delineated as follows:

$$Link\ tag = hash\left(R_i^{item\_id}\Big|item\_id\right) \quad (7)$$

where $R_i^{item\_id}$ is a collection of public keys from n members as defined in Section 5.1, and *item_id* denotes the item identifier. The *item_id* is constituted of the platform name and an internal number. For instance, the *item_id* for a product with ASIN code "*B08L8KC1J7*" on Amazon can be represented as "*Amazon-B08L8KC1J7*". The ASIN code is a unique identifier generated for each product by Amazon, autonomously created by the Amazon system without the need for seller input. The uniqueness of $R_i^{item\_id}$ and *item_id* culminates in the uniqueness of the link tag, wherein the system will detect multiple signatures under the same *item_id* by the same entity.

Regarding cases of repurchase, as long as the time interval between two purchases is sufficiently long, the buyer will appear in two distinct rings for the same item. Due to the difference in link tag, both ratings will still be regarded as valid by the LRS system. An extreme scenario is when a buyer purchases the same item twice within a short time and can only provide one rating.

### 5.3. Workflows

As illustrated in Figure 5, the ARS-Chain system's workflows encompass a collection of sub-processes involving multiple stakeholders, including buyers, sellers, and consensus nodes.

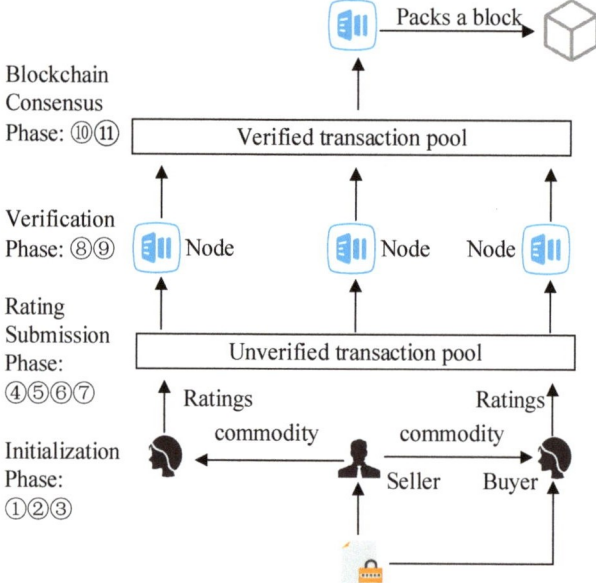

**Figure 5.** The ARS-Chain's workflows.

Initialization Phase:

① Key Generation: Each buyer x generates a pair of private and public keys ($SK_x$, $PK_x$) based on the the *KeyGen()* algorithm.

② Dynamic Ring Formation: The system constructs a ring $R_i^{item\_id}$ for the product identified by *item_id*, where *i* is the ring identifier. According to the definition in Section 5.1, the ring $R_i^{item\_id}$ consists of *k* buyers, *j* consensus nodes, and a seller.

③ Generation of One-time Pseudonyms: One-time pseudonyms are meaningless to the members within the ring and do not serve as inputs for the *Verify()* and *Link()* functions. The one-time pseudonym acts as a part of the rating information *m* to identify the rater, denoted as "*from*". Its calculation method is as follows:

$$from = hash(PK_x | timestamp) \qquad (8)$$

Rating Submission Phase:

④ Rating Creation: Upon receipt of the product, the buyer generates the rating m.

⑤ Link Tag Construction: The buyer utilizes $R_i^{item\_id}$ and $item\_id$ to generate the link tag ($T$).

$$T = hash\left(R_i^{item\_id} \big| item\_id\right) \quad (9)$$

⑥ Signing: Buyer $x$ employs private key $SK_x$, $R_i^{item\_id}$, and $T$ to sign the rating $m$. $T$ will be used as part of the signature data structure for future verification.

$$\sigma \leftarrow Sign\left(SK_x, R_i^{item\_id}, m, T\right) \quad (10)$$

⑦ Transaction Upload: The buyer uploads the transaction $TX$ to the attached blockchain nodes. At this time, the transactions have not been verified by the nodes, and are placed into the local unverified transaction pool by the nodes. $TX$ is the data format after m has been signed, represented as:

$$TX = (item\_id, i, m, \sigma) \quad (11)$$

Verification Phase:

⑧Transaction Legitimacy Verification: The consensus nodes verify the legitimacy of the collected transaction $TX$. A return of 1 from $Verify()$ indicates the signature's legitimacy, passing the verification.

$$0|1 \leftarrow Verify\left(TX.\sigma, TX.m, R_i^{item\_id}, item\_id\right) \quad (12)$$

⑨Transaction Linkability Check: According to $TX.item\_id$ and $TX.i$, the consensus nodes scan all rating transactions generated based on the same $R_i^{item\_id}$, executing $Link()$ to check the linkability of $TX$ with other transactions.

$$0|1 \leftarrow Link(TX\_now.\sigma, TX\_others.\sigma) \quad (13)$$

Here, $TX\_now$ represents the transaction to be checked, while $TX\_others$ represents other rating transactions generated based on the ring $R_i^{item\_id}$. A consistent return of 0 from all calls to $Link()$ indicates no repeated ratings by the same user under the same link tag, passing the check.

Blockchain Consensus Phase:

⑩Transaction Broadcast: Transactions that pass $Verify()$ and $Link()$ are regarded as legitimate transactions, placed into the transaction pool, and then broadcasted to other peers.

⑪ Block Generation and Linkage: Consensus nodes, adhering to the PBFT consensus protocol, reach a consensus to package the rating transactions into a new block and append the new block to the end of the blockchain. At this juncture, the seller's reputation score is updated, and the buyers view the reputation score based on multi-platform global data.

## 6. Validity Analysis

This section analyzes whether the ARS-Chain system meets the design goals we proposed in Section 1.1.

Multi-platform Reputation Sharing: ARS-Chain achieves this goal by storing reputation data in a consortium blockchain maintained by multiple platforms.

Full Anonymity and Evaluation Validity Verification: ARS-Chain uses linkable ring signature technology to achieve the signer's anonymity to the seller, platform administrators, and other members within the ring. In addition, as shown in Section 5.3, the system generates a one-time pseudonym for the user during the initialization phase. This helps to achieve the signer's anonymity to outsiders. We conducted validity experiments in Section 7.2 to test this design goal.

Unlinkable Rating Records: ARS-Chain ensures that the identity presented by the user in each rating is different by introducing one-time pseudonyms, thus ensuring that rating records are unlinkable. It should be noted that the linkability in LRS and the unlinkability in our design goals are not contradictory. The unlinkability in the design goals refers to the unlinkability between two different purchase records, while the linkability in LRS refers to the linkability between two ratings of the same purchase record.

Preventing Multiple Rating Attacks: ARS-Chain achieves this goal through our novel dynamic ring addition LRS scheme and link tag construction method. As shown in Table 2, two legitimate ratings are based on different link tags. Conversely, two ratings based on the same link tag will be considered as multiple rating attacks. When the system detects repeated ratings, the second rating will be discarded. In addition, the experiments (Section 7.2) shows that ARS-Chain effectively prevents multiple rating attacks.

**Table 2.** The value of the link tag($T$) based on different rating situations.

| Situation | $R_i^{item\_id}$ and $item\_id$ | Link Tag ($T$) |
|---|---|---|
| two ratings based on different products | different $R_i^{item\_id}$ / different $item\_id$ | different T |
| two ratings based on repurchase records | different $R_i^{item\_id}$ / same $item\_id$ | different T |
| two ratings based on a purchase record | same $R_i^{item\_id}$ / same $item\_id$ | same T |

Preventing Multiple Rating Attacks: ARS-Chain achieves this goal through our novel dynamic ring addition LRS scheme and link tag construction method. As shown in Table 1, two legitimate ratings are based on different link tags. Conversely, two ratings based on the same link tag will be considered as multiple rating attacks. When the system detects repeated ratings, the second rating will be discarded. In addition, the experiments (Section 7.2) shows that ARS-Chain effectively prevents multiple rating attacks.

Sybil attacks: In ARS-Chain, the blockchain stores reputation information and does not compete for control over user accounts with e-commerce platforms. We assume that e-commerce platforms can resist Sybil attacks through measures such as real-name authentication, and ARS-Chain is responsible for anonymizing real-name accounts during the process of reputation data being put on the blockchain.

## 7. Experiments and Evaluation

The primary algorithms encompassed within the framework of LRS consist of three pivotal components: signature generation, signature verification, and linkability verification. To assess the performance metrics of these algorithms, we conducted empirical evaluations in three areas: runtime, memory consumption, and signature size. Both runtime and memory consumption are indicative parameters for gauging the computational burden imposed on user hardware. The signature constitutes a seminal factor contributing to blockchain network communication overhead. Recognizing that the performance of LRS is intricately correlated with the LRS group size, our experimental framework was judiciously executed under both large-scale (100–5000 members) and small-scale (<100 members) LRS group sizes. It should be pointed out that the dynamic ring addition LRS scheme described in Section 5.1 transforms the large-scale group size LRS, corresponding to large-scale e-commerce transactions, into small-scale group size LRS, corresponding to small-scale e-commerce transactions. In actuality, the LRS within ARS-Chain operates under the small-scale group size condition.

### 7.1. Experimental Setup

Parameters Configuration. Unsigned blockchain transactions (the rating from buyer to seller) are delineated as follows:

*const m = {*

*timestamp: "May-19-2023 08:17:35 AM +UTC",*

*from*: "0x1114c78d5de672996d812dc2e1a05b5f33eacdfb",
*to*: "0x000000d40b595b94918a28b27d1e2c66f43a51d3",
*value*: "+1"
};

In this structure, the "timestamp" signifies the initiation time of the blockchain transaction, which concurrently serves as the moment at which the buyer rates the seller. The "from" field represents the rater's one-time pseudonym. Adopting this one-time pseudonym obfuscates the evaluator's identity, impeding malicious actors from tracking evaluations. Furthermore, the 'to' field distinctly identifies the seller, while the 'value' parameter denotes the appraisal score. Given the structural confines of our model, this score is rigorously limited to the binary choices of "+1" or "−1".

The item identifier is configured as a string similar to "*Amazon-B08L8KC1J7*", representing a product from Amazon.

Hardware Specifications. For the empirical analysis, we conducted our experiments on a machine equipped with an Intel® Core™ i5-7300HQ CPU @ 2.50 GHz, 8.0 GB of memory, running Windows 10.

Experimental Framework. Our experimental framework is implemented in two programming languages, PureScript and JavaScript, each catering to distinct aspects of the LRS algorithm. More specifically, the framework is partitioned into the following modules: (1) PureScript Component: This segment takes on the onus of actualizing the core logic of the LRS algorithm, encompassing key pair generation, message signing, signature verification, and linkability verification. The code for this module is encapsulated in approximately 300 lines of PureScript statements and further augmented by a plethora of PureScript library references. (2) JavaScript Component: This section serves as interface calls and benchmarking. The JavaScript component consists of about 400 lines of code.

*7.2. Validity Experiments*

As described in Section 1.1, the design goal of ARS-Chain is to achieve anonymity, unlinkability and prevent multiple rating attacks while sharing reputation across multiple platforms. We introduce the validity experiments in this section.

In LRS, *Verify()* returns "*true*" to indicate that the signature is valid, i.e., the signer belongs to the signature ring, and *Link()* returns "*true*" to indicate that the two signatures are signed by the same signer under the same link tag, i.e., the system detects that the user rated multiple times. As shown in Table 3, ARS-Chain correctly judged the legitimacy of the users and successfully detected the multiple ratings. When the system detects multiple ratings, the second rating will be discarded, thus avoiding the multiple rating attack. The experiments show that ARS-Chain effectively achieves legitimacy verification and prevents multiple rating attacks.

**Table 3.** Results of *Verify()* and *Link()* based on different rating situations.

| Situation | Results of *Verify()* | Results of *Link()* |
|---|---|---|
| Legal and illegal users rate the same product | First signature: true<br>Second signature: false | Linkability of two signatures: false |
| A legal user rates the same product twice | First signature: true<br>Second signature: true | Linkability of two signatures: true |
| A legal user rates two different products | First signature: true<br>Second signature: true | Linkability of two signatures: false |
| Different legal users rate the same product | First signature: true<br>Second signature: true | Linkability of two signatures: false |

*7.3. Performance Evaluation under Large-Scale LRS Group Size*

The numbers of participants ($n$) in experiments under the large-scale LRS group size are 100, 200, 400, 800, 1200, 1600, 2400, 3200, and 5000, respectively.

The runtimes of signature generation, signature verification, and linkability verification algorithms increase with the number of participants, exhibiting an approximately linear relationship, as shown in Figure 6. The runtimes of signature generation and verification are very close to each other and much larger than the runtimes of linkability. This indicates that signature generation and verification processes involve more computation, while the linkability verification algorithm is relatively simple.

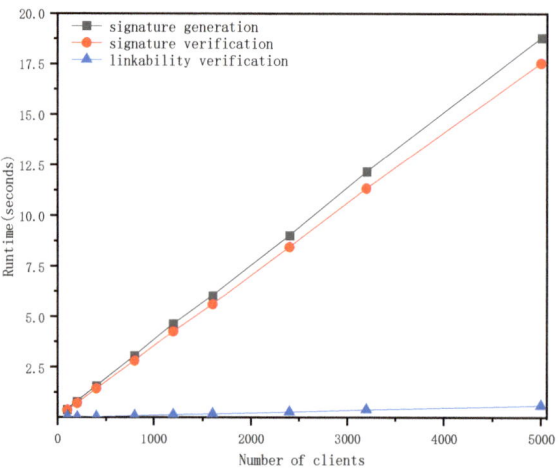

**Figure 6.** Algorithm runtime with different numbers of participants.

As can be discerned from Figure 7, several noteworthy patterns emerge in memory consumption across the three algorithms. In the signature generation algorithm, memory usage escalates as the number of participants increases; however, the trajectory of this increase does not strictly adhere to a linear pattern. In stark contrast, the memory utilization for the signature verification algorithm demonstrates considerable fluctuation across varying participant counts, defying any conspicuous systematic trend. For the linkability verification algorithm, it is apparent that the memory overhead is markedly lower compared to the other two algorithms, an attribute that may be due to its relative algorithmic simplicity.

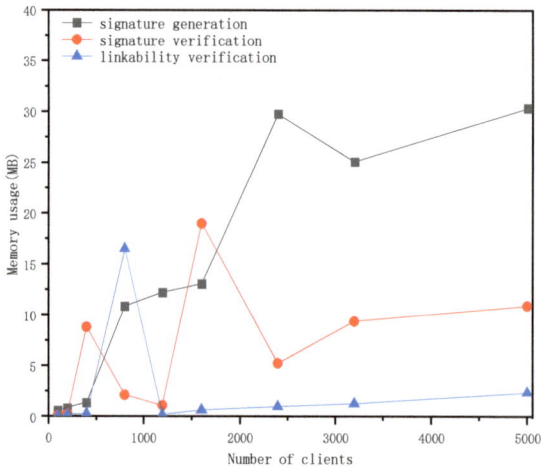

**Figure 7.** Algorithm memory consumption with different numbers of participants.

Viewed holistically, the hierarchy of memory consumption from highest to lowest aligns well with the algorithms' inherent code complexities. It is sequenced as follows: signature generation, signature verification, and linkability verification. Additionally, each algorithm manifests episodic spikes in memory usage, which are subsequently followed by a decrement. This oscillatory behavior could potentially be correlated with the garbage collection and optimization mechanisms intrinsic to the node.js runtime environment.

The signature constitutes a seminal factor contributing to blockchain network communication overhead. Figure 8. shows a linear correlation between the signature size ($y$) and the number of participants ($n$). Mathematically, the best-fit function for the signature size ($y$) and the number of participants ($n$) can be expressed as follows:

$$y = 0.1884 * n + 0.3808 \tag{14}$$

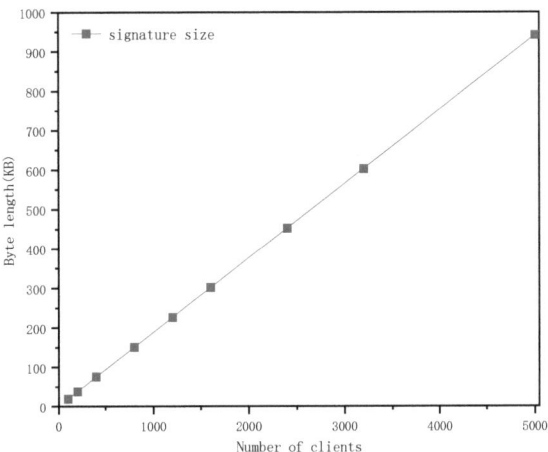

**Figure 8.** Signature size with different numbers of participants.

Given these findings, managing the number of ring participants is necessary to ensure operational efficiency.

*7.4. Performance Evaluation under Small-Scale LRS Group Size*

In light of the observations presented in Section 7.3, it becomes evident that large-scale LRS group size not only elongates the algorithm's runtime but also inflates the communication overhead within the blockchain network. As a direct countermeasure, we introduce the dynamic ring addition mechanism described in Section 5.1. The dynamic ring addition mechanism reduces the LRS group size to a small scale. In this section, we test the system performance when the LRS group size is small (less than 100).

Table 4 unequivocally elucidates that when the group size is curtailed to under 100, the signature size and the algorithmic runtime exhibit an incremental ascent in correlation with increasing group size. Although memory consumption generally trends upwards, it demonstrates a degree of irregularity, potentially attributable to the idiosyncrasies of the runtime environment's memory garbage collection mechanisms. With a group size restricted to fewer than 100, all 3 performance metrics remain within the bounds of reduced overhead. Considering the ubiquitous flood-fill propagation characteristic inherent in blockchain systems, it is necessary to limit the byte size of transactions to be sufficiently small. We surmise that fixing the group size to less than 50 is optimal.

Table 4. Performance metrics correlation with group size under 100.

| Group Size | Signature Size (KB) | The Runtime of Sign() (s) | The Runtime of Verify() (s) | The Runtime of Link() (s) | Memory Usage of Sign() (MB) | Memory Usage of Verify() (MB) | Memory Usage of Link() (MB) |
|---|---|---|---|---|---|---|---|
| 10 | 2.25 | 0.0783 | 0.0521 | 0.0017 | 0.6633 | 0.4267 | 0 |
| 20 | 4.14 | 0.1172 | 0.0827 | 0.0029 | 0.32 | 0.0833 | 0 |
| 30 | 6.03 | 0.1503 | 0.1186 | 0.0041 | 0.2067 | 0.09 | 0 |
| 40 | 7.91 | 0.1909 | 0.1535 | 0.0054 | 0.33 | 0.1367 | 0.0267 |
| 50 | 9.79 | 0.2273 | 0.1859 | 0.0067 | 0.3967 | 0.13 | 0.0167 |
| 60 | 11.68 | 0.2687 | 0.2215 | 0.0082 | 0.3533 | 0.0867 | 0.02 |
| 70 | 13.56 | 0.3113 | 0.257 | 0.009 | 0.52 | 0.0967 | 0.02 |
| 80 | 15.44 | 0.3443 | 0.291 | 0.0101 | 0.5267 | 0.0967 | 0.03 |
| 90 | 17.32 | 0.3841 | 0.3308 | 0.0115 | 0.5967 | 0.1233 | 0.0367 |
| 100 | 19.2 | 0.4217 | 0.3627 | 0.013 | 0.6067 | 0.12 | 0.0467 |

## 8. Discussion

### 8.1. Waiting Time for LRS Ring Generation

As discussed in Section 5.1, the generation of a signature ring is based on the buyer list of a particular commodity, which includes one seller, j consensus nodes, and k buyers. The ring generation time will correspondingly increase when the commodity is less prevalent.

We denote $h_i(t)$ as the popularity of the ith commodity at time t, where the popularity of a commodity is generally an indicator of its appeal or sales velocity. $T(h_i)$ represents the time required for this commodity to form a LRS ring independently. We can infer that there exists a functional relationship between $T(h_i)$ and $h_i(t)$, as follows:

$$T(h_i) = \frac{a}{h_i(t) + b} \tag{15}$$

In situations where the popularity of a single commodity is insufficient to form a LRS ring within a reasonable time frame, we consider combining the buyers of N commodities to form a LRS ring. Assuming H(t) represents the total popularity of these N commodities at time t, then:

$$T(H(t)) = \frac{a}{\sum_{i=1}^{n} h_i(t) + b} \tag{16}$$

This approach will significantly reduce the waiting time for forming a LRS ring.

### 8.2. Performance Optimization

In Section 7, performance experiments were conducted regarding the LRS group size under large-scale and small-scale scenarios. The experimental results show that the algorithms' runtime and signature size exhibit a linear relationship with the group size. Thanks to the dynamic ring addition mechanism (described in Section 5.1), ARS-Chain achieves the optimal state of runtime and memory consumption by increasing the number of rings, but the signature size is still the bottleneck of the system. We propose the following methods to address the issue of excessive signature size:

1. SBFT Consensus Protocol: SBFT [35] protocol adopts threshold signature technology and collector technology, modifying P2P broadcasting across the network to message collection through a collector. Once the collector collects a certain number of signatures, aggregation is performed, followed by the dissemination of the aggregated signature by the collector, thereby reducing the message complexity to a polynomial level. The SBFT protocol effectively addresses the issue of oversized signatures, significantly reducing network communication overhead.

2. Optimized Signature Size LRS: Beullens et al. [36] proposed a logarithmic-size LRS, while Subhra Mazumdar et al. [37] introduced a constant signature size LRS. These variants provide technical support for LRS with a large number of members.

*8.3. Technical and Economic Barriers That May Be Encountered during Integration*

In the process of integrating ARS-Chain with existing e-commerce platforms, we are facing several technical challenges and economic barriers. Firstly, the scalability issue of blockchain is a key factor. Currently, the transaction processing speed of ARS-Chain may not meet the demands of large-scale e-commerce platforms, and sharding technology [38] could be a solution. Sharding divides the blockchain network into multiple smaller segments, each handling a portion of transactions, thereby improving the overall processing speed. Additionally, when integrating ARS-Chain, we must also consider economic barriers. This includes the initial technological investment, operational costs, and potential market resistance. To overcome these barriers, we propose the following: (1) Establishing partnerships with e-commerce platforms to jointly develop and maintain ARS-Chain, sharing the costs. (2) Reducing operational costs by enhancing the efficiency of ARS-Chain and minimizing resource consumption. (3) Through flexible design, enabling ARS-Chain to adapt to e-commerce platforms of different scales and needs, enhancing market competitiveness.

## 9. Conclusions and Future Work

This paper proposes ARS-Chain, a blockchain-based anonymous reputation-sharing system for e-commerce platforms. ARS-Chain utilizes a novel dynamic ring addition mechanism in the LRS scheme where the number of LRS rings increases over time based on the purchase list. In addition, we propose a practical method for constructing link tags with the LRS rings and item identifiers.

ARS-Chain addresses the critical challenges of enabling reputation sharing across platforms while protecting buyers' privacy through anonymity and unlinkability of ratings. It prevents multiple rating attacks through the link tag mechanism. The experimental results confirm that ARS-Chain achieves its design goals, and the dynamic ring addition mechanism ensures the system's performance.

The anonymous reputation systems have profound impacts on both social and ethical levels. Socially, they can promote more honest and transparent communication, but may also lead to a lack of accountability and misuse. Ethically, such systems could affect individual privacy rights and fairness. Therefore, future research should focus on how to balance anonymity with a sense of responsibility, ensuring that the design and implementation of these systems protect users' rights while promoting the overall well-being of society.

For future work, we plan to extend our framework to support more complex and diverse reputation models, such as multi-dimensional, multi-faceted, and multi-level reputation. We also intend to explore the possibility of applying our framework to other domains that require anonymous and secure data sharing, such as healthcare, social networks, and IoT. Furthermore, we aim to conduct more comprehensive experiments and evaluations to demonstrate the effectiveness and efficiency of our framework in real-world scenarios.

**Author Contributions:** Conceptualization, Y.C., L.F. and Q.Z.; methodology, Y.C. and L.F.; software, Y.C. and L.F.; validation, Y.C., L.T. and L.Y.; formal analysis, Y.C. and Q.Z.; investigation, Y.C., Q.Z. and L.F.; resources, Y.C. and L.F.; writing—original draft preparation, Y.C. and Q.Z.; writing—review and editing, L.F., L.T. and L.Y.; supervision, L.F. All authors have read and agreed to the published version of the manuscript.

**Funding:** This work is supported by the National Key Research and Development Program of China (2023YFB2703800) and the Science and Technology Development Fund, Macau SAR (0093/2022/A2, 0076/2022/A2, and 0008/2022/AGJ), Department of Education of Guangdong Province (2021ZDZX1075, 2022ZDJS146), Guangdong University of Science and Technology (GKY-2022KYZDK-12, GKY-2022CQTD-4).

**Data Availability Statement:** The original contributions presented in the study are included in the article, further inquiries can be directed to the corresponding author.

**Conflicts of Interest:** The authors declare no conflicts of interest.

## References

1. Statista-Research-Department. E-Commerce in the United States—Statistics & Facts. 2023. Available online: https://www.statista.com/topics/2443/us-ecommerce/ (accessed on 15 March 2024).
2. Huang, N.; Sun, T.; Chen, P.-Y.; Golden, J. Social Media Integration and E-Commerce Platform Performance: A Randomized Field Experiment. 2017. Available online: https://ssrn.com/abstract=2969670 (accessed on 15 March 2024).
3. He, Y.; Zhang, C.; Wu, B.; Yang, Y.; Xiao, K.; Li, H. A cross-chain trusted reputation scheme for a shared charging platform based on blockchain. *IEEE Internet Things J.* **2021**, *9*, 7989–8000. [CrossRef]
4. Nassar, A.; Kamal, M. Machine Learning and Big Data analytics for Cybersecurity Threat Detection: A Holistic review of techniques and case studies. *J. Artif. Intell. Mach. Learn. Manag.* **2021**, *5*, 51–63.
5. Sabir, B.; Ullah, F.; Babar, M.A.; Gaire, R. Machine learning for detecting data exfiltration: A review. *ACM Comput. Surv. (CSUR)* **2021**, *54*, 1–47. [CrossRef]
6. Huang, J.; Kong, L.; Dai, H.-N.; Ding, W.; Cheng, L. Blockchain-based mobile crowd sensing in industrial systems. *IEEE Trans. Ind. Inform.* **2020**, *16*, 6553–6563. [CrossRef]
7. Allen, S.; Čapkun, S.; Eyal, I.; Fanti, G.; Ford, B.A.; Grimmelmann, J.; Juels, A.; Kostiainen, K.; Meiklejohn, S.; Miller, A. *Design Choices for Central Bank Digital Currency: Policy and Technical Considerations*; National Bureau of Economic Research: Cambridge, MA, USA, 2020.
8. Nasir, M.H.; Arshad, J.; Khan, M.M.; Fatima, M.; Salah, K.; Jayaraman, R. Scalable blockchains—A systematic review. *Future Gener. Comput. Syst.* **2022**, *126*, 136–162. [CrossRef]
9. Asante, M.; Epiphaniou, G.; Maple, C.; Al-Khateeb, H.; Bottarelli, M.; Ghafoor, K.Z. Distributed ledger technologies in supply chain security management: A comprehensive survey. *IEEE Trans. Eng. Manag.* **2021**, *70*, 713–739. [CrossRef]
10. Xu, M.; Chen, X.; Kou, G. A systematic review of blockchain. *Financ. Innov.* **2019**, *5*, 27. [CrossRef]
11. Li, M.; Zhu, L.; Zhang, Z.; Lal, C.; Conti, M.; Alazab, M. Anonymous and verifiable reputation system for E-commerce platforms based on blockchain. *IEEE Trans. Netw. Serv. Manag.* **2021**, *18*, 4434–4449. [CrossRef]
12. Blömer, J.; Juhnke, J.; Kolb, C. Anonymous and publicly linkable reputation systems. In Proceedings of the Financial Cryptography and Data Security: 19th International Conference, FC 2015, San Juan, Puerto Rico, 26–30 January 2015; Revised Selected Papers; pp. 478–488.
13. Bethencourt, J.; Shi, E.; Song, D. Signatures of reputation. In Proceedings of the Financial Cryptography and Data Security: 14th International Conference, FC 2010, Tenerife, Spain, 25–28 January 2010; Revised Selected Papers 14; pp. 400–407.
14. Zhai, E.; Wolinsky, D.I.; Chen, R.; Syta, E.; Teng, C.; Ford, B. Anonrep: Towards tracking-resistant anonymous reputation. In Proceedings of the 13th {USENIX} Symposium on Networked Systems Design and Implementation ({NSDI} 16), Santa Clara, CA, USA, 16–18 March 2016; pp. 583–596.
15. Azad, M.A.; Bag, S.; Hao, F. PrivBox: Verifiable decentralized reputation system for online marketplaces. *Future Gener. Comput. Syst.* **2018**, *89*, 44–57. [CrossRef]
16. Grinshpoun, T.; Gal-Oz, N.; Meisels, A.; Gudes, E. CCR: A model for sharing reputation knowledge across virtual communities. In Proceedings of the 2009 IEEE/WIC/ACM International Joint Conference on Web Intelligence and Intelligent Agent Technology, Milan, Italy, 15–18 September 2009; pp. 34–41.
17. Shen, M.; Tang, X.; Zhu, L.; Du, X.; Guizani, M. Privacy-preserving support vector machine training over blockchain-based encrypted IoT data in smart cities. *IEEE Internet Things J.* **2019**, *6*, 7702–7712. [CrossRef]
18. Wang, L.-E.; Ma, S.; Sun, Z. Blockchain-Based Reputation Sharing for High-Quality Participant Selection of MCS. *Secur. Commun. Netw.* **2023**, *2023*, 6120860. [CrossRef]
19. Chen, Y.; Feng, L.; Liang, H.; Yao, S.; Tian, L.; Yuan, X. RS-chain: A decentralized reputation-sharing framework for group-buying industry via hybrid blockchain. *Clust. Comput.* **2022**, *25*, 4617–4632. [CrossRef]
20. Hasan, O.; Brunie, L.; Bertino, E. Privacy-preserving reputation systems based on blockchain and other cryptographic building blocks: A survey. *ACM Comput. Surv. (CSUR)* **2022**, *55*, 1–37. [CrossRef]
21. Li, X.; Mei, Y.; Gong, J.; Xiang, F.; Sun, Z. A blockchain privacy protection scheme based on ring signature. *IEEE Access* **2020**, *8*, 76765–76772. [CrossRef]
22. Zhang, S.; Yao, T.; Arthur Sandor, V.K.; Weng, T.-H.; Liang, W.; Su, J. A novel blockchain-based privacy-preserving framework for online social networks. *Connect. Sci.* **2021**, *33*, 555–575. [CrossRef]
23. Han, Y.; Chen, H.; Qiu, Z.; Luo, L.; Qian, G. A Complete Privacy-Preserving Credit Score System Using Blockchain and Zero Knowledge Proof. In Proceedings of the 2021 IEEE International Conference on Big Data (Big Data), Orlando, FL, USA, 15–18 December 2021; pp. 3629–3636.
24. Wu, A.; Zhang, Y.; Zheng, X.; Guo, R.; Zhao, Q.; Zheng, D. Efficient and privacy-preserving traceable attribute-based encryption in blockchain. *Ann. Telecommun.* **2019**, *74*, 401–411. [CrossRef]
25. Casino, F.; Patsakis, C. An efficient blockchain-based privacy-preserving collaborative filtering architecture. *IEEE Trans. Eng. Manag.* **2019**, *67*, 1501–1513. [CrossRef]
26. Yao, W.; Deek, F.P.; Murimi, R.; Wang, G. SoK: A Taxonomy for Critical Analysis of Consensus Mechanisms in Consortium Blockchain. *IEEE Access* **2023**, *11*, 79572–79587. [CrossRef]
27. Wu, X.; Jiang, W.; Song, M.; Jia, Z.; Qin, J. An efficient sharding consensus algorithm for consortium chains. *Sci. Rep.* **2023**, *13*, 20. [CrossRef]

28. Liu, J.K.; Wei, V.K.; Wong, D.S. Linkable spontaneous anonymous group signature for ad hoc groups. In Proceedings of the Information Security and Privacy: 9th Australasian Conference, ACISP 2004, Sydney, Australia, 13–15 July 2004; Proceedings 9; pp. 325–335.
29. Odoom, J.; Huang, X.; Zhou, Z.; Danso, S.; Zheng, J.; Xiang, Y. Linked or unlinked: A systematic review of linkable ring signature schemes. *J. Syst. Archit.* **2023**, *134*, 102786. [CrossRef]
30. Rivest, R.L.; Shamir, A.; Tauman, Y. How to leak a secret. In Proceedings of the Advances in Cryptology—ASIACRYPT 2001: 7th International Conference on the Theory and Application of Cryptology and Information Security, Gold Coast, Australia, 9–13 December 2001; Proceedings 7; pp. 552–565.
31. Androulaki, E.; Barger, A.; Bortnikov, V.; Cachin, C. Hyperledger Fabric: A Distributed Operating System for Permissioned Blockchains. In Proceedings of the Eurosys '18: Proceedings of the Thirteenth Eurosys Conference, Porto, Portugal, 23–26 April 2018.
32. Song, H.; Li, J.; Li, H. A cloud secure storage mechanism based on data dispersion and encryption. *IEEE Access* **2021**, *9*, 63745–63751. [CrossRef]
33. Theodouli, A.; Arakliotis, S.; Moschou, K.; Votis, K.; Tzovaras, D. On the design of a blockchain-based system to facilitate healthcare data sharing. In Proceedings of the 2018 17th IEEE International Conference on Trust, Security and Privacy in Computing and Communications/12th IEEE International Conference on Big Data Science and Engineering (TrustCom/BigDataSE), New York, NY, USA, 1–3 August 2018; pp. 1374–1379.
34. Ren, Y.; Guan, H.; Zhao, Q. An efficient lattice-based linkable ring signature scheme with scalability to multiple layer. *J. Ambient. Intell. Humaniz. Comput.* **2022**, *13*, 1547–1556. [CrossRef]
35. Gueta, G.G.; Abraham, I.; Grossman, S.; Malkhi, D.; Pinkas, B.; Reiter, M.; Seredinschi, D.-A.; Tamir, O.; Tomescu, A. SBFT: A scalable and decentralized trust infrastructure. In Proceedings of the 2019 49th Annual IEEE/IFIP International Conference on Dependable Systems and Networks (DSN), Portland, OR, USA, 24–27 June 2019; pp. 568–580.
36. Beullens, W.; Katsumata, S.; Pintore, F. Calamari and Falafl: Logarithmic (linkable) ring signatures from isogenies and lattices. In Proceedings of the 26th International Conference on the Theory and Application of Cryptology and Information Security, Daejeon, Republic of Korea, 7–11 December 2020; pp. 464–492.
37. Mazumdar, S.; Ruj, S. Design of anonymous endorsement system in hyperledger fabric. *IEEE Trans. Emerg. Top. Comput.* **2019**, *9*, 1780–1791. [CrossRef]
38. Wang, J.; Wang, H. Monoxide: Scale out blockchains with asynchronous consensus zones. In Proceedings of the 16th USENIX Symposium on Networked Systems Design and Implementation (NSDI 19), Boston, MA, USA, 26–28 February 2019; pp. 95–112.

**Disclaimer/Publisher's Note:** The statements, opinions and data contained in all publications are solely those of the individual author(s) and contributor(s) and not of MDPI and/or the editor(s). MDPI and/or the editor(s) disclaim responsibility for any injury to people or property resulting from any ideas, methods, instructions or products referred to in the content.

MDPI AG
Grosspeteranlage 5
4052 Basel
Switzerland
Tel.: +41 61 683 77 34

*Mathematics* Editorial Office
E-mail: mathematics@mdpi.com
www.mdpi.com/journal/mathematics

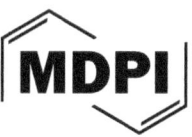

Disclaimer/Publisher's Note: The title and front matter of this reprint are at the discretion of the Guest Editors. The publisher is not responsible for their content or any associated concerns. The statements, opinions and data contained in all individual articles are solely those of the individual Editors and contributors and not of MDPI. MDPI disclaims responsibility for any injury to people or property resulting from any ideas, methods, instructions or products referred to in the content.

www.ingramcontent.com/pod-product-compliance
Lightning Source LLC
LaVergne TN
LVHW072351090526
838202LV00019B/2521